**Cardiovascular
Clinical Trials**

Cardiovascular Clinical Trials

PUTTING THE EVIDENCE INTO PRACTICE

Edited by

Marcus D. Flather, MBBS, FRCP

Professor of Medicine and Clinical Trials
University of East Anglia and Norfolk and Norwich University Hospital
Norwich, UK

Deepak L. Bhatt, MD, MPH, FACC, FAHA, FESC

Chief of Cardiology, VA Boston Healthcare System;
Director, Integrated Interventional Cardiovascular Program, Brigham and Women's
Hospital & VA Boston Healthcare System;
Professor of Medicine, Harvard Medical School;
Senior Investigator, TIMI Study Group
Boston, MA, USA

Tobias Geisler, MD

Associate Professor of Medicine
Consultant, Cardiology
University Hospital Tübingen
Tübingen Medical School
Tübingen, Germany

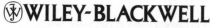
WILEY-BLACKWELL
A John Wiley & Sons, Ltd., Publication

BMJ|Books

BMJ Books is an imprint of BMJ Publishing Group Limited, used under licence by Blackwell Publishing which was acquired by John Wiley & Sons in February 2007. Blackwell's publishing programme has been merged with Wiley's global Scientific, Technical and Medical business to form Wiley-Blackwell.

Registered office: John Wiley & Sons, Ltd, The Atrium, Southern Gate, Chichester, West Sussex, PO19 8SQ, UK

Editorial offices: 9600 Garsington Road, Oxford, OX4 2DQ, UK
The Atrium, Southern Gate, Chichester, West Sussex, PO19 8SQ, UK
111 River Street, Hoboken, NJ 07030-5774, USA

For details of our global editorial offices, for customer services and for information about how to apply for permission to reuse the copyright material in this book please see our website at www.wiley.com/wiley-blackwell

The contents of this work are intended to further general scientific research, understanding, and discussion only and are not intended and should not be relied upon as recommending or promoting a specific method, diagnosis, or treatment by physicians for any particular patient. The publisher and the author make no representations or warranties with respect to the accuracy or completeness of the contents of this work and specifically disclaim all warranties, including without limitation any implied warranties of fitness for a particular purpose. In view of ongoing research, equipment modifications, changes in governmental regulations, and the constant flow of information relating to the use of medicines, equipment, and devices, the reader is urged to review and evaluate the information provided in the package insert or instructions for each medicine, equipment, or device for, among other things, any changes in the instructions or indication of usage and for added warnings and precautions. Readers should consult with a specialist where appropriate. The fact that an organization or Website is referred to in this work as a citation and/or a potential source of further information does not mean that the author or the publisher endorses the information the organization or Website may provide or recommendations it may make. Further, readers should be aware that Internet Websites listed in this work may have changed or disappeared between when this work was written and when it is read. No warranty may be created or extended by any promotional statements for this work. Neither the publisher nor the author shall be liable for any damages arising herefrom.

Library of Congress Cataloging-in-Publication Data

Cardiovascular clinical trials : putting the evidence into practice / edited by Marcus D. Flather, Deepak L. Bhatt, Tobias Geisler.
  p. ; cm.
  Includes bibliographical references and index.
  ISBN 978-1-4051-6215-9 (pbk. : alk. paper)
  I. Flather, M. II. Bhatt, Deepak L. III. Geisler, Tobias.
  [DNLM: 1. Cardiovascular Diseases–prevention & control. 2. Clinical Trials as Topic. WG 120]

  616.100724–dc23

                                        2012009758

A catalogue record for this book is available from the British Library.

Wiley also publishes its books in a variety of electronic formats. Some content that appears in print may not be available in electronic books.

Cover images: iStock © Christian Jasiuk and Anthony A. Bavry et al. Eur Heart J (2008) 29(24): 2989–3001 by permission of Oxford University Press
Cover design by Grounded Design

Set in 9.5 on 12 pt Palatino by Toppan Best-set Premedia Limited
Printed and bound in Malaysia by Vivar Printing Sdn Bhd

1 2013

Contents

List of contributors

Aiden Abidov, MD, PhD, FACC, FAHA
Associated Professor of Medicine and Radiology
The University of Arizona College of Medicine
Tucson, AZ, USA

Thanos Athanasiou, MD, PhD, FETCS,
FRCS
Cardiothoracic Surgeon
Hammersmith Hospital
Imperial College
London, UK

Thomas M. Bashore, MD
Professor of Medicine
Division of Cardiology
Duke University Medical Center
Durham, NC, USA

Daniel S. Berman, MD, FACC, FAHA,
FSCCT
Professor of Medicine
Department of Imaging and Department of
Medicine
Cedars-Sinai Medical Center;
Department of Medicine
David Geffen School of Medicine, UCLA
Los Angeles, CA, USA

Deepak L. Bhatt, MD, MPH, FACC,
FAHA, FESC
Chief of Cardiology, VA Boston Healthcare
System;
Director, Integrated Interventional Cardiovascular
Program, Brigham and Women's Hospital & VA
Boston Healthcare System;
Professor of Medicine
Harvard Medical School;
Senior Investigator, TIMI Study Group
Boston, MA, USA

William E. Boden, MD, FACC, FAHA
Professor of Medicine, Albany Medical College;
Chief of Medicine
Samuel S. Stratton VA Medical Center;
Vice-Chairman, Department of Medicine,
Albany Medical Center
Albany, NY, USA

Ralph B. D'Agostino, Sr
Department of Mathematics
Boston University
Boston, MA, USA

Sabine Ernst, MD, PhD, FESC
National Heart and Lung Institute
Imperial College;
Royal Brompton and Harefield Hospital
London, UK

Marcus D. Flather, MBBS, FRCP
Professor of Medicine and Clinical Trials
University of East Anglia and Norfolk and
Norwich University Hospital
Norwich, UK

Tobias Geisler, MD
Associate Professor of Medicine
Consultant, Cardiology
University Hospital Tübingen
Tübingen Medical School
Tübingen, Germany

J. Kevin Harrison, MD
Professor of Medicine
Division of Cardiology
Duke University Medical Center
Durham, NC, USA

Chee W. Khoo, MRCP
Research Fellow
University of Birmingham Centre for
Cardiovascular Sciences
City Hospital
Birmingham, UK

Dharam J. Kumbhani, MD, SM
Division of Cardiovascular Medicine
Brigham and Women's Hospital
Harvard Medical School
Boston, MA, USA

Gregory Y.H. Lip, MD, FRCP
Professor of Cardiovascular Medicine
University of Birmingham Centre for
Cardiovascular Sciences
City Hospital
Birmingham, UK

Christopher M. O'Connor, MD
Professor of Medicine and Director
Duke Heart Center
Duke University Medical Center
Durham, NC, USA

Alice J. Owen, PhD
Department of Epidemiology & Preventive
Medicine
Monash University
Melbourne, VIC, Australia

John Pepper, MA, MChir, FRCS
Cardiothoracic Surgeon
Royal Brompton Hospital
London, UK

Christopher M. Reid, PhD
Professor of Cardiovascular Epidemiology
Department of Epidemiology & Preventive
Medicine
Monash University
Melbourne, VIC, Australia

Amir Sepehripour, BSc, MBBS, MRCS
Specialist Registrar Cardiothoracic Surgery
Imperial College
London, UK

Wendy Gattis Stough, PharmD
Assistant Consulting Professor
Duke University Medical Center
Durham, NC;
Associate Professor of Clinical Research
Campbell University School of Pharmacy
Buies Creek, NC, USA

Irina Suman-Horduna, MD, MSc
National Heart and Lung Institute
Imperial College;
Royal Brompton and Harefield Hospital
London, UK

Sabu Thomas, MD, FACC, FRCPC
Assistant Professor
Division of Cardiology
University of Rochester School of Medicine
Rochester, NY, USA

Cary Ward, MD
Assistant Professor
Division of Cardiology
Duke University Medical Center
Durham, NC, USA

Preface

Randomized controlled trials (RCTs) represent the highest standard to test whether a therapeutic intervention is safe and effective. RCTs are of pivotal importance for regulatory authorities, healthcare providers, and medical associations for the introduction of new treatments in clinical practice. Cardiovascular medicine is a rapidly growing field with enormous innovation in the last decade. RCTs in cardiovascular medicine are usually performed under enormous time pressure to keep up with the dynamic advances in this field, but they need to comply with standards of quality. This apparent conflict between timely completion and reporting of RCTs, and the growing demands on good clinical research practice, creates a clear challenge to investigators and sponsors of clinical research. Additionally, as healthcare steadily improves, it is more difficult to show superiority of new treatments compared with established therapies; larger patient cohorts are often required to show that a new treatment is superior to its comparator. Despite these barriers, a myriad of landmark RCTs have been conducted in the last few years, leading to a major change in the treatment landscape and contributing to current guidelines in the cardiovascular field.

This book provides a unique overview of quality standards for clinical trials and guides the reader through methodological design, results, and interpretation of RCTs, using examples of recent important trials in major fields of cardiovascular medicine. Each of the major cardiovascular specialties is covered and modern concepts of diagnosis and management are described. This book is intended for clinicians who want an update on current developments in clinical trials in cardiovascular medicine, for those who plan to conduct a clinical trial, and last but not least, to assist in translating the evidence into practice. We would like to thank all the chapter authors for sharing their expert insights in this book. We would also like to thank Helen Whyte of the Royal Brompton Hospital for administrative support, Mary Banks (Wiley-Blackwell) for encouraging us to pursue the book, and Jon Peacock (Wiley-Blackwell) for editorial support in completing the manuscript.

Marcus D. Flather, Deepak L. Bhatt and Tobias Geisler

List of abbreviations

A-HeFT	African American Heart Failure Trial
A4	Atrial fibrillation ablation versus antiarrhythmic drugs study
ABSORB	Clinical Evaluation of the BVS everolimus eluting stent system
ACCOMPLISH	Avoiding Cardiovascular Events through Combination Therapy in Patients Living with Systolic Hypertension
ACCURACY	Assessment by Coronary Computed Tomographic Angiography of Individuals Undergoing Invasive Coronary Angiography
ACME	Angioplasty Compared to Medicine
ACTIVE-A	Clopidogrel plus aspirin vs. aspirin alone in atrial fibrillation
ACTIVE-W	Clopidogrel plus aspirin vs. oral anticoagulants in atrial fibrillation
ACUITY	Bivalirudin vs. heparin and GP IIb/IIIa inhibitors in acute coronary syndromes
ACUITY-timing trial	Routine upfront initiation vs. GP IIb/IIIa inhibitors in acute coronary syndromes
ADHERE registry	Acute Decompensated Heart Failure National Registry
AF-CHF	Rate control vs. rhythm control in atrial fibrillation and congestive heart failure
AFASAK	Atrial Fibrillation, Aspirin, Anticoagulation
AFFIRM	Atrial Fibrillation Follow-Up Investigation of Rhythm Management
AIM-HIGH	Atherothrombosis Intervention in Metabolic syndrome with low HDL/high triglycerides: impact on Global Health outcomes
AIMI	AngioJet Rheolytic Thrombectomy In Patients Undergoing Primary Angioplasty for Acute Myocardial Infarction
ALLHAT	Antihypertensive and Lipid-Lowering Treatment to prevent Heart Attack Trial
AMEthyst	Assessment of the Medtronic AVE Interceptor Saphenous Vein Graft Filter System
AMIGO	Atherectomy before Multi-link Improves lumen Gain and clinical Outcomes

AMRO	Amsterdam-Rotterdam study
APAF	A randomized trial of circumferential pulmonary vein ablation vs. antiarrhythmic drug therapy in paroxysmal atrial fibrillation
APPRAISE-2	Apixaban for Prevention of Acute Ischemic Events 2
ARISTOTLE	Apixaban vs. Warfarin in Patients with Atrial Fibrillation
ARTIST	Angioplasty versus Rotational Atherectomy for Treatment of Diffuse In-stent Restenosis Trial
ARTS	Arterial Revascularization Therapies Study
ASCOT-BPLA	Anglo-Scandinavian Cardiac Outcomes Trial–Blood Pressure Lowering
ASPARAGUS	Comparison of thrombectomy to percutaneous coronary intervention alone for myocardial infarction
ASPREE	Aspirin in Reducing Events in the Elderly
ATLAS-1-TIMI 46	Anti-Xa Therapy to Lower cardiovascular events in Addition to standard therapy in Subjects with Acute Coronary Syndrome–Thrombolysis in Myocardial Infarction 46
ATLAS-TIMI 51	Rivaroxaban in addition to standard care for acute coronary syndromes
AVERROES	Apixaban Versus Acetylsalicylic acid (ASA) to Prevent Strokes
AVERT	Atorvastatin VErsus Revascularization Treatment
AVID	Antiarrhythmic Versus Implantable Defibrillators
AWESOME	Angina With Extremely Serious Operative Mortality/ Evaluation
BAATAF	Boston Area Anticoagulation Trial for Atrial Fibrillation
BAFTA	Birmingham Atrial Fibrillation Treatment of the Aged
BARI	Bypass Angioplasty Revascularization Investigation
BARI-2D	Bypass Angioplasty Revascularization Investigation 2D
BASKET	Basel Stent Kosten Effektivitats Trial
BEAUTIFUL	Morbidity-Mortality Evaluation of the If Inhibitor Ivabradine in Patients With Coronary Artery Disease and Left Ventricular Dysfunction
BENESTENT	BElgian NEtherlands STENT
BREATHE-5	Bosentan Therapy in Patients With Eisenmenger Syndrome
CABANA	Catheter Ablation versus Antiarrhythmic Drug Therapy for Atrial Fibrillation
CABRI	Coronary Artery versus Bypass Revascularization Investigation

CACAF	Catheter ablation treatment in patients with drug refractory atrial fibrillation
CACTUS	Coronary Angiography by Computed Tomography with the use of a Submillimeter resolution
CAFA	Canadian Atrial Fibrillation Anticoagulation trial
CAPPP	Captopril Prevention Project
CAPRIE	Clopidogrel versus Aspirin in Patients at Risk of Ischaemic Events
CAPS	Cardiac Arrhythmia Pilot Study
CARDIoGRAM	Coronary Artery Disease Genome-wide Replication and Metaanalysis
CARE-HF	Cardiac Resynchronisation Heart Failure
CARESS-in-AMI	Combined Abciximab REteplase Stent Study in Acute Myocardial Infarction
CARISA	Combination Assessment of Ranolazine in Stable Angina
CASH	Cardiac Arrest Study Hamburg
CAST	Cardiac Arrhythmia Suppression Trial
CAVEAT I	Coronary Angioplasty vs Excisional Atherectomy trial I
CCAT	Canadian Coronary Atherectomy trial
CHARISMA	Clopidogrel for High Atherothrombotic Risk and Ischemic Stabilization, Management, and Avoidance
CHARM	Candesartan in Heart Failure Assessment of Reduction in Morbidity and Mortality
CIBIS	Cardiac Insufficiency Bisoprolol Study
CIDS	Canadian Implantable Defibrillator Study
COMMIT-CCS-2	ClOpidogrel and Metoprolol in Myocardial Infarction Trial
COMPANION	Comparison of Medical Therapy, Pacing, and Defibrillation in Heart Failure
CONSENSUS	Cooperative North Scandinavian Enalapril Survival Study
CONSORT	Consolidated Standards of Reporting Trials
COPERNICUS	Carvedilol Prospective Randomized Cumulative Survival
COURAGE	Clinical Outcomes Utilizing Revascularization and Aggressive druG Evaluation
CTAF	Canadian Trial of Atrial Fibrillation
CURE	Clopidogrel in Unstable angina to prevent Recurrent Events
CURRENT-OASIS 7	Clopidogrel optimal loading dose Usage to Reduce Recurrent EveNTs/Optimal Antiplatelet Strategy for Intervention
DART	Dilatation vs Ablation Revascularization Trial Targeting Restenosis

DASH	Dietary Approaches to Stop Hypertension
DEAR-MI	Dethrombosis to Enhance Acute Reperfusion in Myocardial Infarction
DECODE	Diabetes Epidemiology: Collaborative Analysis of Diagnostic Criteria in Europe
DEDICATION	Drug Elution and Distal protection In ST-elevation Myocardial Infarction
DESSERT	Sirolimus-eluting stents versus bare-metal stents in patients with diabetes mellitus
DIABETES	Diabetes and sirolimus-eluting stent trial
DINAMIT	Defibrillator in Acute Myocardial Infarction Trial
DIPLOMATE	Comparison of Angioguard vs conventional PCI in patients with acute myocardial infarction
EAFT	European Atrial Fibrillation Trial
EARLY-ACS	Early Glycoprotein IIb/IIIa Inhibition in Non–ST-Segment Elevation Acute Coronary Syndrome
EAST	Emory Angioplasty versus Surgery trial
EHFS	Euro Heart Failure Survey
EMERALD	Enhanced Myocardial Efficacy and Recovery by Aspiration of Liberated Debris
EMPHASIS HF	Eplerenone in patients with systolic heart failure and mild symptoms
ENDEAVOR	Randomized Comparison of Zotarolimus-Eluting and Paclitaxel-Eluting Stents in Patients with Coronary Artery Disease
EPHESUS	Eplerenone Post-Acute Myocardial Infarction Heart Failure Efficacy and Survival Study
ERACI II	Coronary Angioplasty with Stenting versus Coronary Bypass Surgery
ERBAC	Excimer Laser, Rotational Atherectomy, and Balloon Angioplasty Comparison
ESCAPE	Evaluation Study of Congestive Heart Failure and Pulmonary Artery Catheterization Effectiveness
ESPS	European Stroke Prevention Study
EUROASPIRE	European Society of Cardiology survey of secondary prevention of coronary heart disease
EXTRACT-TIMI 25	Enoxaparin and Thrombolysis Reperfusion for Acute Myocardial Infarction Treatment—Thrombolysis in Myocardial Infarction 25
FIBISTEMI	Firebird DES stent versus bare metal stent in ST segment elevation myocardial infarction
FINESSE	Facilitated Intervention with Enhanced Reperfusion Speed to Stop Events
FIRE	FilterWire EX Randomized Evaluation
FUTURA-OASIS-8	Low vs. standard dose unfractionated heparin for percutaneous coronary intervention in acute

coronary syndrome patients treated with
fondaparinux

FUTURE-1	First Use To Underscore Restenosis Reduction with Everolimus-1
GISSI	Gruppo Italiano per to studio delta streptochinasi nell'infarto miocardico
GISSOC II-GISE	Gruppo Italiano di Studio sullo Stent nelle Occlusioni Coronariche
GRACE	Global Registry of Acute Coronary Events
HAAMU-STENT	Helsinki Area Acute Myocardial Infarction Treatment Reevaluation
HERS	Heart and Estrogen/Progestin Replacement Study
HF-ACTION	Heart Failure and A Controlled Trial Investigating Outcomes of Exercise Training
HOPE	Heart Outcomes Prevention Evaluation
HORIZON AMI	Harmonizing Outcomes with Revascularization and Stents in Acute Myocardial Infarction
HORIZON-HF	Hemodynamic, Echocardiographic, and Neurohormonal Effects of Istaroxime, a Novel Intravenous Inotropic and Lusitropic Agent: A Randomized Control Trial in Patients Hospitalized with Heart Failure
HPS-2 THRIVE	Treatment of HDL to Reduce the Incidence of Vascular Events
I-PRESERVE	Irbesartan in Heart Failure with Preserved Ejection Fraction
I-REVIVE	Initial Registry of Endovascular Implantation of Valves in Europe
IMPROVE HF	Registry to Improve the Use of Evidence-Based Heart Failure Therapies in the Outpatient Setting
IMPROVE-IT	Outcomes in Subjects With Acute Coronary Syndrome: Vytorin (Ezetimibe/Simvastatin) vs Simvastatin
INITIATIVE	INternatIonal TrIAl on the Treatment of angina with IVabradinE vs. atenolol
INSIGHT	Intervention as a Goal in Hypertension Treatment
INSPIRE	adenosINe Sestamibi Post-InfaRction Evaluation
INTERHEART	Effect of potentially modifiable risk factors associated with myocardial infarction in 52 countries
INVEST	International Verapamil-Trandolapril Study
ISAR LEFT MAIN	Intracoronary Stenting and Angiographic Results: Drug-Eluting Stents for Unprotected Coronary Left Main Lesions
ISAR-REACT	Intracoronary Stenting and Antithrombotic-Regimen Rapid Early Action for Coronary Treatment
ISIS-1	International Study of Infarct Survival 1

JAST	Japan Atrial Fibrillation Stroke Trial
JETSTENT	Comparison of AngioJET Rheolytic Thrombectomy Before Direct Infarct Artery STENTing in Patients with Acute Myocardial Infarction
JUPITER	Justification for the Use of Statins in Primary Prevention: an Intervention Trial Evaluating Rosuvastatin
LANCELOT-ACS	Lessons from Antagonizing the Cellular Effect of Thrombin—Acute Coronary Syndrome
LASAF	Low-dose Aspirin, Stroke, Atrial Fibrillation
LAVA	Laser Angioplasty Versus Angioplasty
LEADERS	Limus Eluted from A Durable versus ERodable Stent coating
LIFE	Losartan Intervention For Endpoint reduction in hypertension study
LIFE-ISH	Losartan Intervention for Endpoint Reduction sub-study
LOCAL TAX	Local intracoronary delivery of paclitaxel after stent implantation for prevention of restenosis in comparison with implantation of a bare metal stent alone or with implantation of a paclitaxel-coated stent
MADIT	Multicenter Automatic Defibrillator Implantation Trial
MASS II study	Medicine Angioplasty or Surgery Study
MERIT-HF	Metoprolol Randomized Intervention Trial in Congestive Heart Failure
MERLIN	Metabolic Efficiency with Ranolazine for Less Ischemia in Non–ST-elevation acute coronary syndromes
MIAMI	Metoprolol In Acute Myocardial Infarction
MICADO	Multicenter investigation of coronary artery protection with a distal occlusion device in acute myocardial infarction
MISSION	Sirolimus-eluting stents versus baremetal stents in patients with ST-segment elevation myocardial infarction
MIST	Migraine Intervention With STARFlex Technology
MONICA	Multinational MONItoring of trends and determinants in CArdiovascular disease
MRFIT	Multiple Risk Factor Intervention Trial
MUSTT	Multicenter Unsustained Tachycardia Trial
NONSTOP	Comparison of rescue vs conventional PCI in patients with acute myocardial infarction
NORDIL	Nordic Diltiazem study

OASIS	Organization to Assess Strategies in Acute Ischemic Syndromes
OAT	Occluded Artery Trial
ON-TIME 2	Ongoing Tirofiban in Myocardial Infarction Evaluation
ONTARGET	Ongoing Telmisartan Alone and in Combination with Ramipril Global Endpoint Trial
OPTIME-CHF	Outcomes of a Prospective Trial of Intravenous Milrinone for Exacerbations of Chronic Heart Failure
OPTIMIZE-HF	Organized Program to Initiate Lifesaving Treatment in Hospitalized Patients with Heart Failure
PACCOCATH ISR	Treatment of In-Stent Restenosis by Paclitaxel-Coated Balloon Catheters
PARTNER EU	Placement of Aortic Transcatheter Valve
PASSION	Paclitaxel-Eluting Stent versus Conventional Stent in Myocardial Infarction with ST-Segment Elevation
PCI-CURE	Clopidogrel in Unstable angina to prevent Recurrent Events substudy
PEACE	Prevention of Events with ACE inhibition
PEPCAD II	Paclitaxel-Eluting PTCA Balloon Catheter in Coronary Artery Disease II
PIAF	Pharmacological Intervention in Atrial Fibrillation
PICCS	PFO in Cryptogenic Stroke Study
PLATO	Platelet Inhibition and Patient Outcomes
PREMIA	Protection of Distal Embolization in High-Risk Patients with Acute ST-Segment Elevation Myocardial Infarction
PRISON II	Prospective Randomized Trial of Sirolimus-Eluting and Bare Metal Stents in Patients With Chronic Total Occlusions II
PROBE endpoint	Prospective, randomized, open-label, blinded endpoint
PROMISE	PROspective Imaging Study for Evaluation of Chest Pain
RAAFT	Radiofrequency ablation versus antiarrhythmic drugs as first line treatment of symptomatic atrial fibrillation: A randomised trial
RACE	Rate Control vs Electrical cardioversion
RALES	Randomized Aldactone Evaluation Study
RAVEL	Randomized Study with the Sirolimus-Coated Bx Velocity Balloon-Expandable Stent in the Treatment of Patients with de Novo Native Coronary Artery Lesions
REACH	Reduction of atherothrombosis for continued health
RECAST	Registry of Endovascular Critical Aortic Stenosis Treatment

REDUCE III	Restenosis Reduction by Cutting Balloon Evaluation – III
RELY	Randomized Evaluation of Long-Term Anticoagulant Therapy
REMATCH	Randomized Evaluation of Mechanical Assistance for the Treatment of Congestive Heart Failure
REMEDIA	Randomized evaluation of the effect of mechanical reduction of distal embolization by thrombus-aspiration in primary and rescue angioplasty
REST	Bare metal stent vs. percutaneous coronary intervention
REVIVAL-II	Transcatheter Endovascular Implantation of Valves II
REVIVE-II	Registry of Endovascular Implantation of Valves in Europe II
RITA-2	Randomised Intervention Treatment of Angina-2
RIVAL	Radial versus femoral access for coronary angiography and intervention in patients with acute coronary syndromes
ROCKET-AF	Rivaroxaban versus warfarin in nonvalvular atrial fibrillation
ROMICAT	Rule Out Myocardial Infarction using Computer Assisted Tomography
ROSTER	Rotational Atherectomy versus Balloon Angioplasty for Diffuse In-Stent Restenosis
4S	Scandinavian Simvastatin Survival Study
SAFE	Screening for Atrial Fibrillation in the Elderly
SAFER	Saphenous Vein Graft Angioplasty Free of Emboli Randomized
SAVED	Bare metal stent vs. percutaneous coronary intervention
SCANDSTENT	Stenting Coronary Arteries in Non-stress/benestent Disease
SCD-HeFT	Sudden Cardiac Death in Heart Failure Trial
SCORE	Systematic Coronary Risk Estimation
SCORPIUS	effectiveness of sirolimus-eluting stents in diabetic patients
SELECTION	Single-center randomized evaluation of paclitaxel-eluting versus conventional stent in acute myocardial infarction
SENIORS	Study of the Effects of Nebivolol Intervention on Outcomes and Rehospitalization in Seniors with Heart Failure
SES-SMART	Sirolimus-eluting vs uncoated stents for prevention of restenosis in small coronary arteries
SESAMI	Sirolimus-Eluting Stent Versus Bare-Metal Stent in Acute Myocardial Infarction

SIRIUS	Sirolimus-Eluting Stent in De-Novo Native Coronary Lesions (C-SIRIUS = Canadian arm, E-SIRIUS = European arm)
SOLVD-T	Studies of Left Ventricular Dysfunction Treatment
SORT OUT III	Efficacy and Safety of Zotarolimus-Eluting and Sirolimus-Eluting Coronary Stents in Routine Clinical Care III
SoS	Stent or Surgery
SOURCE	European Registry of Transcatheter Aortic Valve Implantation Using the Edwards SAPIEN Valve
SPAF-1	Stroke Prevention in Atrial Fibrillation
SPINAF	Stroke Prevention in Non-rheumatic Atrial Fibrillation
SPIRIT	Clinical Evaluation of the Xience V Everolimus Eluting Coronary Stent System in the Treatment of Patients With de Novo Native Coronary Artery Lesions
STAF	Strategies of Treatment of Atrial Fibrillation
STICH	Surgical Treatment for Ischaemic Heart Failure
STRATEGY	Tirofiban with a sirolimus-eluting stent in percutaneous coronary intervention
STRATUS	Study to Determine Rotablator and Transluminal Angioplasty Strategy
STRESS	Stent Restenosis Study
SURVIVE	Survival of Patients With Acute Heart Failure in Need of Intravenous Inotropic Support
SWISS II	Swiss Interventional Study on Silent Ischemia Type II
SYNTAX	Synergy Between Percutaneous Coronary Intervention with TAXUS and Cardiac Surgery
TAPAS	Thrombus Aspiration during Percutaneous Coronary Intervention in Acute Myocardial Infarction Study
TAXUS	Treatment of De Novo Coronary Disease Using a Single Paclitaxel-Eluting Stent
TIMI	Thrombolysis in Myocardial Infarction
TOSCA	Total Occlusion Study of Canada
TRACER	Thrombin Receptor Antagonist for Clinical Event Reduction in Acute Coronary Syndrome
TRANSFER-AMI	Transfer for urgent percutaneous coronary intervention early after thrombolysis for ST-elevation myocardial infarction
TREND	Trial on Reversing Endothelial Dysfunction
TRITON-TIMI-38	Trial to Assess Improvement in Therapeutic Outcomes by Optimizing Platelet Inhibition with Prasugrel—Thrombolysis in Myocardial Infarction

TYPHOON | Trial to Assess the Use of the CYPHer Sirolimus-Eluting Coronary Stent in Acute Myocardial Infarction Treated With BallOON Angioplasty

UK-TIA | United Kingdom Transient Ischaemic Attack

UKPDS | United Kingdom Prospective Diabetes Study

UNLOAD | Ultrafiltration versus Intravenous Diuretics for Patients Hospitalized for Acute Decompensated Heart Failure

UpFlow MI | Comparison of thrombectomy with PCI alone for primary percutaneous coronary intervention

URGENT | Ularitide Global Evaluation in Acute Decompensated Heart Failure

Val-HeFT | Valsartan benefits left ventricular structure and function in heart failure

VALIANT | Valsartan in Acute Myocardial Infarction

VAMPIRE | VAcuuM asPIration thrombus REmoval

VANQWISH | Veterans Affairs Non–Q-Wave Infarction Strategies In Hospital

VMAC | Vasodilation in the Management of Acute CHF

WARRS | Warfarin-Aspirin Recurrent Stroke Study

X AMINE ST | X-sizer in AMI for negligible embolization and optimal ST resolution

CHAPTER 1

Introduction to randomized clinical trials in cardiovascular disease

Tobias Geisler,[1] Marcus D. Flather,[2] Deepak L. Bhatt,[3] and Ralph B. D'Agostino, Sr[4]
[1]University Hospital Tübingen, Tübingen Medical School, Tübingen, Germany
[2]University of East Anglia and Norfolk and Norwich University Hospital, Norwich, UK
[3]VA Boston Healthcare System; Brigham and Women's Hospital and Harvard Medical School, Boston, MA, USA
[4]Boston University, Boston, MA, USA

What is a randomized clinical trial?

The question "does it work" is common when a treatment is being considered for a patient. How do we know whether treatments "work" and what is the best way to demonstrate the efficacy and safety of new treatments? The main rationale behind a clinical trial is to perform a prospective evaluation of a new treatment in a rigorous and unbiased manner to provide reliable evidence of safety and efficacy. This is done by comparing the new treatment to a comparator or control treatment. Defining the term "clinical trial" is not as straightforward as it seems. In its simplest form, a clinical trial is any comparative evaluation of treatments involving human beings. Randomized clinical trials (RCTs) are the optimal means we use to achieve this demonstration. In this chapter we explore the relevance of RCTs to modern medicine and review strengths and weaknesses of this methodology (Table 1.1). As we will discuss below, RCTs represent the highest form of a clinical trial. Since the results of RCTs inform clinical practice guidelines, it is increasingly important for clinicians to understand their methodology, including their strengths and weaknesses. In this chapter we provide an overview of the main methodological aspects of well-designed RCTs.

Cardiovascular Clinical Trials: Putting the Evidence into Practice, First Edition.
Edited by Marcus D. Flather, Deepak L. Bhatt, and Tobias Geisler.
© 2013 Blackwell Publishing Ltd. Published 2013 by Blackwell Publishing Ltd.

Table 1.1 Issues for design/conduct and analysis of randomized clinical trials.

• Study objective	• Unit of analysis
• Study populations	• Missing data
• Efficacy variables	• Analysis methods
• Control groups	• Sample size/power
• Study design (bias)	• Safety
• Study design (samples)	• Subsets and more
• Comparisons	• Number of studies
• Trial monitoring	• Clinical significance
• Data analysis sets	

Concept of randomization

The RCT is the most powerful design to prove whether or not there is a valid effect of a therapeutic intervention compared to a control. Randomization is a process of allocating treatments to groups of subjects using the play of chance. It is the mechanism that controls for factors except for the treatments, and allows comparison of the treatment under investigation with the control in an unbiased manner. It is important that information on the process of randomization is included in the trial protocol. The number of subjects allocated to each group, those who actually received the assigned treatment and reasons for non-compliance need to be recorded. In a representative analysis of trials listed in the free MEDLINE reference and abstract database at the United States National Library of Medicine (PubMed) in 2000, an adequate approach to random sequence generation was reported in only 21% of the trials [1]. This increased to 34% for a comparable cohort of PubMed-indexed trials in 2006 [2].

The procedure to assign interventions to trial participants is a critical aspect of clinical trial design. Randomization balances for known and unknown prognostic factors (covariates) allows the use of probability theory to express the likelihood that any difference in outcome between intervention groups merely reflects chance [3]. It facilitates blinding the identity of treatments to the investigators, participants, and evaluators, possibly by use of a placebo, which reduces bias after assignment of treatments [4]. Successful randomization is dependent on two related elements—generation of an unpredictable allocation sequence and concealment of that sequence until assignment takes place [5].

There are many procedures for randomization in the setting of a clinical trial and these will be discussed in detail below [see Study design (bias)]. For now we call attention to its importance in allowing the unbiased comparison of the investigational treatment and a control in a clinical trial.

Clinical trial phases

Preclinical studies

Preclinical studies of potentially useful treatments are usually carried out to understand mechanisms of action, effect of different doses, and possible unwanted effects. There are two main types of preclinical studies—those using whole animal models and those using components of living tissue, usually cells or organs. Preclinical studies help to build up hypotheses about how and why treatments may work. Most of these experiments are not randomized and there may be substantial reporting bias (i.e., only interesting results are reported), but they are an essential step in the development of new treatments.

Phase 1 clinical trials

The first step to evaluate the safety of a new drug or biological substance after successful experiments in animals is to evaluate how well it can be tolerated in a small number of individuals. This phase is intended to test the safety, tolerability, pharmacokinetics (PK), and pharmacodynamics (PD) of a drug. Although it does not strictly meet the definition criteria of a clinical trial, this phase is often termed a phase 1 clinical trial. Usually, if the drug has a tolerable toxicological profile, a small number of healthy volunteers are recruited. If the drug has an increased toxicological profile, often critically ill patients are included in whom standard, guideline-based therapy fails. The design of phase 1 clinical trial is usually simple. In general, drugs are tested at different doses to determine the maximum tolerated dose (MTD) before signs of toxicity occur. The most difficult challenge in the planning of phase 1 trials is finding ways to adequately translate the animal experimental data into a dosing scheme and not to exceed the maximum tolerated dose in humans. Phase 1 clinical trials are dose-ranging studies to identify a tolerable dose range that can be evaluated further for safety in phase 2 trials. There are different ways to adjust doses in a phase 1 clinical trial, e.g., single ascending and multiple ascending dosing schemes. Studies in apparently healthy human volunteers usually involve short exposure to new treatments to understand the effects of different doses on human physiology. Starting at low or sub-therapeutic doses, especially with novel immunogenic agents, is essential to ensure that unexpected serious side effects are reduced.

Phase 2 clinical trials

Phase 2 clinical trials refer to the results of phase 1 trials. Once the maximum tolerated dose has been defined and an effective and tolerable dose range has been determined, phase 2 trials are designed to investigate how well a drug works in a larger set of patients (usually 100–600 subjects and sometimes up to 4000 patients, depending on the number of groups to be investigated) and to continue measurements of PK and PD in a more global population. Some phase 2 trials are designed as case series where selected patients all receive the drug or as randomized trials where candidate doses of a drug are tested against placebo. Usually, different doses of a pharmacological treatment will be compared against placebo in a randomized study design with outcomes based on the mechanistic action of the treatment being evaluated. For example, phase 2 trials of anticoagulants will usually document laboratory measures of anticoagulant effect, incidence of major and minor bleeding, and effects on relevant clinical outcomes. Minimizing risk to patients is essential as most treatments evaluated in phase 2 trials will never be approved for human use. Strategy-based treatments such as new methods for percutaneous coronary intervention (PCI) or surgical procedures also have their equivalent "phase 2" trials in which the new techniques are systematically tested in smaller number of patients to ensure safety and feasibility before being tested in larger trials. For obvious reasons these trials cannot be "placebo controlled," but should compare the new strategy with an established one. Sometimes "phase 2" trials of treatment strategies are not randomized, which often makes it difficult to draw conclusions about safety and feasibility, and to plan further larger trials.

As an example, in the phase 2 trial Anti-Xa Therapy to Lower cardiovascular events in Addition to standard therapy in Subjects with Acute Coronary Syndrome–Thrombolysis in Myocardial Infarction 46 (ATLAS-1-TIMI 46 trial), the oral factor Xa inhibitor rivaroxaban was tested in several doses (5 mg, 10 mg, or 20 mg total daily dose, given either once or twice daily) in a total of 3491 patients with acute coronary syndromes (ACS) being treated with aspirin or aspirin and clopidogrel and compared with placebo. There was a dose-related increase in bleeding and a trend toward a reduction in ischemic events with the addition of rivaroxaban to antiplatelet therapy in patients with recent ACS. The researchers found that patients assigned to 2.5 mg and 5.0 mg twice-daily rivaroxaban in both the aspirin alone and aspirin plus clopidogrel groups had the most efficacious results versus placebo [6]. These results led to a selection of these dosing groups for transition into a large phase 3 trial that enrolled 15 526 patients (ATLAS-2-TIMI-51) [7].

Phase 3 clinical trials

Phase 3 trials are usually RCTs, often multicenter, and including up to several thousand patients (the sample size depending upon the disease and medical condition being investigated). Due to the study size and duration, phase 3 trials are the most expensive, time-consuming, and complex trials to design and run, especially in therapies for chronic medical conditions, and are usually the "pivotal" trials for registration and marketing approval. Other possible motives for conducting phase 3 trials include plans to extend the label by the sponsor (i.e., to demonstrate the drug is effective for subgroups of patients/disease conditions beyond the use for which the drug was originally approved); to collect additional safety data; or to secure marketing claims for the drug. Trials at this stage are sometimes classified as "phase 3B trials" in contrast to "phase 3A trials," denoting RCTs performed before marketing approval [8]. Once a drug has proved acceptable in phase 3 trials, the trial results are usually combined into a large comprehensive document describing the methods and results of animal (preclinical) and human (clinical studies), manufacturing processes, product characteristics (e.g., formulation, shelf-life). This document serves as a "regulatory submission" to be reviewed by the appropriate regulatory authorities in different countries before providing approval to market the drug.

Phase 4 clinical trials

In phase 4 trials, post-marketing studies delineate additional information, including the drug's risks, benefits, and optimal use. They also aim to see if a treatment or medication can be used in other circumstances beyond the originally approval indications. Phase 4 clinical trials are done after a treatment has gone through all the other phases and is already approved by the regulatory health authorities. Phase 4 clinical trials may not necessarily be RCTs. A large body of phase 4 trials is made up of registries and observational studies.

The following discussion about the methodology will mainly focus on phase 3 confirmatory RCTs.

Study objective

The search for new treatments is an evolutionary process, starting with a series of questions and eventually providing answers through a complex route that involves epidemiology (pattern and impact of disease in the population), basic science (cellular, mechanical, and genetic nature of the disease), and clinical trials to understand the response of patients to the new treatment. Trials that show clear benefits of treatments are usually followed by an assessment of cost and "affordability" to understand if the new treatment can actually be used in clinical practice. Some of these pathways are illustrated in Figure 1.1.

The quest to find effective and safe treatments arises from the needs of patients who present with illness and suffering. Thus, most clinical research is responsive in nature; we are not trying to improve on the healthy human but rather to treat and prevent illness and disease. However, in order to find an effective treatment, it is essential to understand the cause and pathology of the disease. Once specific causes are identified, whether they are protein deficiencies, transport errors, metabolic problems or genetic defects, it becomes possible to identify potential treatments that can then be tested in clinical trials. The challenge is that clinical trials take time and are costly to run, which means that they should be reserved for clinically important questions. Most clinical trials are set up and run by industry for commercial gain—often as industry/academic partnerships—but it should be emphasized that important health issues should be supported by the major healthcare providers, including governments and insurance agencies as part of their programs to

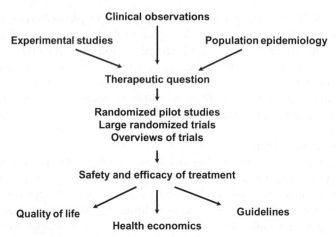

Figure 1.1 Generating evidence for new treatments.

improve health [1]. At present, most independent, non-commercial medical research is funded by competitive grants from governments or charities. While the competitive process helps to maintain high standards, it is an unpredictable method of funding and can lead to delays in carrying out important clinical trials. Lastly, well-intentioned but bureaucratic regulations applied to medical research are actually leading to substantial delays in important and effective treatments reaching patients in a timely manner. Thus, randomized trials are needed as the final pathway to test the hypothesis "Does it work?". To answer this question reliably, large trials involving many patients from many centers are needed, which means that trial procedures including data collection and analysis need to be as simple and streamlined as possible [9,10].

Given all the above, when a specific phase 3 clinical trial is being designed, the first question is "What is the specific objective?". For example, with the ATLAS-2 trial mentioned above, the objective was to establish the safety and effectiveness of rivaroxaban with both aspirin alone and aspirin and clopidogrel in reducing ischemic events in patients with ACS. The study objective must be explicitly stated in the study protocol (see below) and drives the study design, implementation, and analysis.

Study populations

The characteristics and features of the subjects to be enrolled in the clinical trial becomes the next issue and should be defined beforehand, using unequivocal inclusion (eligibility) criteria. A complete report of the eligibility criteria used to enrol the trial participants is required to assist readers in the interpretation of the study. In particular, a clear knowledge of these criteria is needed to evaluate to whom the results of a trial apply, i.e., the trial's generalizability (applicability) and importance for clinical or public health practice [11,12]. Since eligibility criteria are applied before randomization, they do not have an impact on the internal validity of a trial, but they are central to its external validity. It is important to differentiate between sample population and target population with regard to generalizability of results. The *sample population* is the population from which study subjects will be enrolled. The *target population* is the population to which the clinical trial results will be generalized. These are not necessarily the same. The eligibility criteria create a sample population that might significantly deviate from the target population. Thus, eligibility criteria should be kept as general and as realistic as possible. Ideally, study subjects should correspond to those to whom the product will be marketed. Demographic factors (age, gender, and race) and, when appropriate, socioeconomic status should be representatively covered. In addition, there is a sentiment that the study conditions should be realistic. For example, for over-the-counter drugs, regulatory authorities often require, before a drug is approved, the performance of clinical trials in settings similar to those in which the drug will actually be taken. These studies are called "actual use" studies.

Typical selection criteria include the nature and stage of the disease being studied, the exclusion of persons who may be harmed by the study treatment, and issues required to ensure that the study satisfies legal and ethical norms. Informed consent by study participants, for example, is a mandatory inclusion criterion in all clinical trials. The information about the number of patients being screened and meeting the eligibility criteria should be provided in flow diagrams (an example according to the CONSORT statement is shown in Figure 1.2).

Efficacy variables

Clinical trials can have numerous efficacy variables. However, it is essential that the primary efficacy variables should be kept to a minimum. The study objectives and efficacy variables should relate clearly and sharply to each other. Since large amounts of data can be collected and stored electronically, weighting their importance and relevance to the study objectives is crucial, and excess data collection is an important cause of poor trial performance. The primary efficacy variable should be the variable capable of providing the most clinically relevant and convincing evidence directly related to the primary objective of the trial. Ideally, there should only be one or a small number of primary variables. Multiple primary efficacy variables, however, are sometimes used in clinical trials with the hope of increasing the statistical power while keeping the sample size low. These can be counterproductive and increase the chance of producing inconclusive results. Careful consideration of how to deal with "multiple testing" or "alpha spending" is recommended [13,14]. The latter term describes how to distribute the type I or alpha error associated with testing the primary efficacy variables. Other efficacy

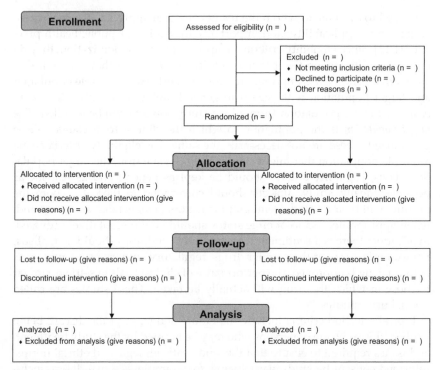

Figure 1.2 Flow diagram showing the progress through different stages of a parallel randomized trial of two groups (i.e., enrolment, intervention allocation, follow-up, and data analysis). (According to http://www.consort-statement.org/consort-statement and Moher *et al.* [106].)

variables are classified as secondary and usually summarize variables that further support the primary variables and/or provide more information on the study objectives. Quality of life scales are an example of standard secondary efficacy variables in many clinical trials.

Remarkable effort has been made to solve the multiple testing problems associated with the primary variables. Exclusive testing of individual variables is one approach. The development of composite variables has been shown to be very helpful. These range from the combinations of endpoints, such as combining ischemic stroke, fatal and non-fatal coronary events ,and hospitalizations in cardiovascular studies, to scoring scales developed by sophisticated psychometric techniques. Global assessment variables are also used to measure an overall composite.

Another issue of focus concerns the allocation of the alpha error to secondary variables, especially when the effects on the primary variables are not statistically significant [15–17]. For example, in a cardiovascular disease trial, how should the results be interpreted when the primary outcome variable (e.g., exercise testing or improvement of NYHA classification) is not significant at the 0.05 level, but the significance level for a secondary variable related to overall mortality is highly significant at 0.001? [18]. It is hard to ignore such a finding when it refers to a hard clinical endpoint such as mortality. A prior allocation of alpha may need to be applied to major secondary endpoints. Future clinical trials in the same field should have the latter variables as the primary variables.

Surrogate variables

A surrogate endpoint is an intermediate endpoint that serves as a surrogate for a true endpoint if it can be used *in lieu* of the true endpoint to assess treatment benefit (i.e., reliable predictor of the clinical benefit). A surrogate variable should also be able to capture adverse effects. More specifically, it is a laboratory parameter or a physical sign used as a substitute for a clinically meaningful endpoint (e.g., measures of brain natriuretic peptide or 6-minute walking distance as surrogate for worsening heart failure; blood pressure or cholesterols levels as surrogates for coronary events; cardiac necrosis marker levels, Holter-detected ischemia, or microvascular obstruction detected on MRI as surrogates for severity of ischemic heart disease). As a surrogate variable usually represents an intermediate endpoint, it is obtained much sooner than the clinical endpoint of interest. It is usually much cheaper to obtain and has a more frequent incidence than the original endpoint. Surrogate variables have received increasing attention [19,20]. The challenge is to choose a surrogate variable that correlates strongly with the desired clinical endpoint. As an example, a commonly proposed intermediate surrogate variable for stroke is common carotid artery intima–media thickness (IMD) progression as measured by carotid ultrasound [21]. The progression of IMD occurs much earlier than stroke. The question is how well this relates to later development of the event. The value of measuring surrogate variables has been questioned, e.g., regulatory agencies claim that if the surrogate parameter has an effect on a "hard" clinical outcome (e.g., death or myocardial infarction), then the surrogate outcome should be a direct measurement of these. Additionally, history tells us that surrogate outcomes are not always related to the desired clinical outcome [25]. In the classic examples of the Cardiac Arrhythmia Pilot Study (CAPS) and the Cardiac Arrhythmia Suppression Trial (CAST), a combination of encainide/flecainide showed a reduction of the surrogate endpoint of ventricular extrasystoles and arrhythmias, but total mortality and arrhythmic deaths were significantly increased in the treatment arm [22,23]. More recently, in the Heart and Estrogen/Progestin Replacement Study (HERS), estrogen use in post-menopausal women with coronary disease was associated with a modest reduction in cholesterol, but this was not associated with any reduction in cardiovascular deaths or myocardial infarction [24]. Finally, in the Antihypertensive and Lipid-Lowering Treatment to prevent Heart Attack Trial (ALLHAT), of a total of 44 000 patients, 9067 were randomized to doxazosin and 15 268 to chlorthalidone. Blood pressure was lowered by both treatments. However, treatment with doxazosin was significantly associated with a higher incidence of congestive heart failure, whereas chlorthalidone had beneficial effects on heart failure incidence [25]. Analysis of the data suggests that chlorthalidone may have some beneficial effect beyond the blood pressure effect. If blood pressure reduction, a surrogate endpoint, had been the primary endpoint variable, this conclusion would not have been reached.

Control groups

In principle, there are two ways to show that a therapy is effective. One can demonstrate that a new therapy is better or roughly equivalent to a known effective treatment, or better than a placebo. In many RCTs, one group of patients is given an experimental drug or treatment, while the control group receives either a standard treatment for the illness or a placebo. Control groups in clinical trials can be defined using two different classifications: the type of treatment allocated and the method of determining who will be in the control group. The type of treatment can be categorized as followed: placebo or vehicle; no treatment; different dose or regimen from the study treatment, or different active treatment. The principal methods of creating a control group are by randomized allocation of a prospective control group or by selection of a control population separate from the investigated population (external or historical control) [26].

Placebo-controlled trials

A placebo-controlled trial is a way of testing a therapy against a separate control group receiving a sham "placebo" treatment, which is specifically designed to have no real pharmacological effect, and is a key strategy to reduce bias by avoiding knowledge of treatment allocation. Placebo treatment is usually a characteristic of blinded trials, where subjects and/or investigators do not know whether they are receiving a real or placebo treatment. The main purpose of the placebo group is to take account of the "placebo" effect, which consists of symptoms or signs that occur through the taking of a placebo treatment.

Active-control trials

In an active-control (also called positive-control) trial, subjects are randomly assigned to the test treatment or to an active-control drug. Such trials are usually double blind, but this is not always possible due to different treatment regimens, routes of administration, monitoring of drug effects, or obvious side effects. Active-control trials can have different objectives with respect to demonstrating efficacy.

The ability to conduct a placebo-controlled trial ethically in a given situation does not necessarily mean that placebo-controlled trials should be conducted when effective therapy exists. Patients and treating physicians might still favor a trial in which every participant receives an active treatment. Still, placebo-controlled trials are frequently needed to demonstrate the effectiveness of new treatments and often cannot be replaced by active-control trials that show that a new drug is equivalent or non-inferior to an established agent. The limitations of active-control equivalence trials that are intended to show the effectiveness of a new drug have long been recognized [27–29], but are perhaps not as widely appreciated as they should be.

Study design (bias)

Bias can be loosely defined as "any influence that causes the results of a trial to deviate from the truth." This broad definition implies that any element of study design or conduct (including analysis of results) could contribute to bias. In practice, we are particularly concerned about the method of randomization, compliance with treatment, systematic differences in concomitant treatments after randomization (especially in unblinded trials), completeness of follow-up, quality of data, and reporting of outcome measures . Systematic bias occurs when there is a difference in the treatment groups that does not occur by chance, and therefore the measurement of treatment effect may be unduly influenced. Systematic biases are mainly observed in non-randomized comparisons of treatment effects, such as those carried out in observational studies. Randomization, if performed correctly, can balance group differences and minimize systematic bias, to enable the quantification of the true effects of the interventions. Random allocation does not, however, protect RCTs against other types of bias.

Methods of randomization

Several methods exist to generate allocation sequences. Besides true random allocation, the sequence may be generated by the process of minimization, a non-random but generally acceptable method (see Table 1.2).

Simple (unrestricted) randomization

This method is the most basic of allocation approaches. Analogous to repeated fair coin-tossing, this method is associated with complete unpredictability of each intervention assignment. No other allocation generation approach, irrespective of its complexity and sophistication, surpasses the unpredictability and bias prevention of simple randomization.

Restricted randomization

Restricted randomization procedures control the probability of obtaining an allocation sequence with an undesirable sample size imbalance in the intervention groups. In other words, if researchers want treatment groups of equal sizes, they should use restricted randomization.

Table 1.2 Methods of sequence generation [30].

- Simple (unrestricted) randomization
- Restricted randomization
- Stratified randomization
- Minimization

Stratified randomization

Randomization can create chance imbalances on baseline characteristics of treatment groups. Investigators sometimes avert imbalances by using prerandomization stratification on important prognostic factors, such as age or disease severity. In such instances, researchers should specify the method of restriction (usually blocking). To reap the benefits of stratification, investigators must use a form of restricted randomization to generate separate randomization schedules for stratified subsets of participants defined by the potentially important prognostic factors.

Minimization

Minimization is a dynamic randomization algorithm designed to reduce disparity between treatments by taking stratification factors into account. Important prognostic factors are identified before the trial starts and the assignment of a new subject to a treatment group is determined in order to minimize the differences between the groups regarding these stratification factors. In contrast to stratified randomization, minimization intends to minimize the total imbalance for all factors together, instead of considering only predefined subgroups [31].Concerns over the use of minimization have focused on the fact that treatment assignments may be anticipated in some situations and on the impact on the analysis methods being used [32].

The practicality of randomization in a clinical trial can be complicated [33]. The conventional method is for a random number list to be generated by computer and a then treatment allocation list drawn up using the last digit (even or odd) to determine the treatment group. Patients entering the trial are then allocated according to the preprepared randomization list. It is essential that investigators do not have access to this list as they will of course then know the next allocation which can lead to a range of biases. Most trials use a method of central randomization using a telephone- or internet-based system for investigators to randomize patients. This method ensures that all patients are registered in the trial database and that prior knowledge of treatment allocation is not possible. Trials of double-blind pharmacological treatments (i.e., those in which the "active" and "placebo" treatments appear identical) have additional practical issues as the randomization list is used in the production and labeling process. Drug supplies must be provided to centers in "blocks" usually consisting of even amounts of active and placebo in identical packages, except for unique study identification numbers that can be used in emergencies to link the drug pack to the original randomization list for unblinding purposes.

The term "random" is often misused in the literature to describe trials in which non-random, deterministic allocation methods were applied, such as alternation or assignment based on date of birth, case record number, or date of presentation. These allocation techniques are sometimes referred to as "quasi-random." A central weakness with all systematic methods is that concealing the allocation is usually impossible, which allows anticipation of intervention and biased assignments. The application of non-random methods in clinical trials likely yields biased results [4,34,35].

Readers cannot judge adequacy from terms such as "random allocation," "randomization," or "random" without further elaboration. Thus, investigators should clarify the method of sequence generation, such as a random-number table or a computerized random number generator.

In some trials, participants are intentionally allocated in unequal numbers to each intervention and control: e.g., to gain more experience with a new procedure or to limit the size and costs of the trial. In such cases, the randomization ratio (e.g., 2:1 or two treatment participants per each control participant) is reported.

Random and systematic error

When the clinical trial results are produced, the differences observed between treatments may represent true outcome differences. However, it is essential that the investigator (and the reader) consider the chance that the observed effects are due to either random error or systematic error. *Random error* is the result of either biological or measurement variation, whereas *systematic error* is the result of a variety of biases that can affect the results of a trial (Table 1.3). The process of analyzing the outcomes of a study for random error includes both estimation and statistical testing. Estimates describing the distribution of measured parameters may include point estimates (such as means or proportions) and measures of precision (such as confidence intervals).

Study design issues to overcome systematic bias

As stated above, the most important design techniques to overcome bias in clinical trials are blinding and randomization. Most trials follow a double-blind approach in which treatments are prepacked in accordance with a suitable randomization schedule, and supplied to the trial center(s) labeled only with the subject number and the treatment period: no one involved in the

Table 1.3 Potential sources of systematic bias at different stages in the course of a trial.

Planning phase
- Choice of research question
- Type of research study

Recruitment phase
- Allocation of participants to study groups
- Selection bias (eligible individuals are excluded, because the investigator knows the allocation to treatment group)
- Delivery of interventions
- Measurement of outcomes

Post-recruitment phase
- Loss to follow-up
- Analysis
- Dissemination of results
- Interpretation of the results by the study group or external persons (e.g., reviewer)

conduct of the trial is aware of the specific treatment allocated to any particular subject, not even as a code letter. Bias can also be reduced at the design stage by specifying procedures in the protocol aimed at minimizing any anticipated irregularities in trial conduct that might impair a satisfactory analysis, including various types of protocol violations, withdrawals, and missing values. The study design should consider ways both to minimize the frequency of such problems, and also to handle the problems that do occur in the analysis of data.

Blinding

Blinding or masking is used in clinical trials to curtail the occurrence of conscious and unconscious bias in the conduct and interpretation of a clinical trial, caused by the impact that the insight into treatment may have on the enrolment and allocation of subjects, their subsequent care, the compliance of subjects with the treatments, the evaluation of endpoints, the handling of drop-outs, the analysis of data, etc.

A double-blind trial is a trial in which neither the investigator nor the study participant or sponsor who is involved in the treatment or investigation of the subjects is aware of the treatment received. This includes anyone who evaluates eligibility criteria or analyses endpoints, or assesses protocol. The principle of blinding is maintained throughout the whole course of the trial, and only when the data are cleaned to an appropriate level, can particular personnel can be unblinded. If unblinding to the allocation code to any staff who are not involved in the treatment or clinical evaluation of the subjects is required (e.g., bioanalytical scientists, auditors, those involved in serious adverse event reporting), adequate standard operating procedures should exist to guard against inappropriate publication of treatment codes. In a single-blind trial, the investigator and/or his/her staff are conscious of the treatment but the subject is not, or *vice versa*. In an open-label trial, the identity of treatment is known to all participants/study personal. Double-blind trials are the optimal approach, but are associated with greater complexity in providing placebo and the process of drug supply and packaging.

Difficulties in pursuing a double-blind design can be caused by: the different nature of treatments, e.g., surgery compared to drug therapy, or comparison of different drug formulations (e.g., an oral drug compared to an intravenous one). Additionally, the daily pattern of administration of two treatments and the method used to monitor pharmacological effects may differ. A possible way of achieving double-blind conditions despite these circumstances is to apply a "double-dummy" technique. This technique may sometimes imply an administration scheme that is unusual and thus adversely influences the motivation and compliance of the subjects. Ethical difficulties may also arise, e.g., if dummy operative procedures are performed. Nevertheless, it is recommended to make extensive efforts to implement methods to maximize blinding. The double-blind nature of some clinical trials may be jeopardized by obvious treatment-induced effects. In these cases, blinding may be improved by blinding investigators and relevant sponsor staff to particular test results (e.g., selected clinical laboratory measures). If a double-blind trial is not possible, then the single-blind option should be considered. In some cases, only an open-label trial is practically or ethically possible, or cost constraints preclude producing and packaging a placebo. Consideration should be given to the use of a centralized randomization method, such as telephone- or internet-based randomization, to administer the assignment of randomized treatment and to ensure that all patients are registered in the trials. Furthermore, clinical assessments should be made by medical staff who are not involved in the treatment of the subjects and who remain blinded to treatment. In single-blind or open-label trials, every effort should be undertaken to minimize the various known sources of bias and primary variables should be as objective as possible. The reasons for the degree of blinding should be explained in the protocol, together with actions taken to reduce bias by other means. The PROBE (prospective, randomized, open-label, blinded endpoint) was developed to adopt a more "real-world" principal. By using open-label therapy, the drug intervention and its comparator can be clinically titrated, as would occur in every day clinical practice. Blinding is maintained for the outcome assessment. In a meta-analysis of PROBE trials and double-blind trials in hypertension [36], changes in mean ambulatory blood pressure from double-blind controlled studies and PROBE trials were statistically equivalent; however, the impact of the PROBE design on clinical trial design is still being evaluated.

Unblinding of a single subject should be considered only when knowledge of the treatment assignment is necessary to provide information to the subject's physician for further therapeutic actions. Any unintended breaking of the blinding should be reported and explained at the end of the trial, irrespective of the reason for its occurrence. The procedure for and timing of unmasking the treatment allocations should be documented.

Study design (samples)

Major study designs in RCTs are:
- *Parallel group design*: each study subject is randomly assigned to a treatment or an intervention
- *Crossover design*: within a certain period of time each study subject receives all study treatments in a random sequence (possibly separated by a washout period in case of delayed offset of the study drug action)
- *Factorial*: each study subject is randomly assigned to a fixed combination of treatment (e.g., 2 x 2 factorial design: study drug A + study drug B, study drug A + placebo B, placebo A + study drug B, placebo A + placebo B).

The parallel group design is the preferred design in RCTs with two treatment arms. In a representative analysis of published RCTs, the parallel group design was the most frequently chosen design—more than two-thirds of trials [37]. In case of more than one treatment arm, the parallel group design requires a larger sample size and does not allow for investigation of effects and interactions of study drug combinations of interest; a factorial design might be a good choice of study design to answer this question. A crossover design may be considered as it may yield more efficient comparison of treatments, e.g., fewer patients required for the same statistical power since every patient serves as his/her own control. However, there are problems with crossover designs in clinical outcome trials because the effects of treatment B are dependent on treatment A, meaning that if treatment A heals the patients or prevents cardiovascular events then treatment B might not have the opportunity to show its effectiveness or the prognostic effects may not be specifically attributable to treatment B. Crossover designs are mainly used for assessing responses to treatment, e.g., blood pressure, blood values or exercise capacity.

Besides the adequate choice of study design to avoid bias, careful selection of sample composition, types of control, and sequence of different treatments (or exposures) for samples are essential to ensure the quality of a clinical trial. In detail, this includes:

- Recruitment, patient population studied, and number of patients to be included
- Eligibility (inclusion and exclusion)
- Measurements of treatment compliance
- Prophylaxis at baseline
- Administration of treatment(s) (specific drugs, doses, and procedures)
- Level and method of blinding/masking (e.g., open, double-blind, single-blind, blinded evaluators, and unblinded patients and/or investigators)
- Type of control(s) (e.g., placebo, no treatment, active drug, dose–response, historical) and study configuration (parallel, crossover, factorial design)
- Method of assignment to treatment (randomization, stratification)
- Sequence and duration of all study periods, including prerandomization and post-treatment periods, baseline periods, therapy withdrawal/washout periods, and single and double-blind treatment periods. When patients were randomized should be specified. It is usually helpful to display the design graphically with a flow chart that includes timing of assessments
- Any safety, data monitoring, or special steering or evaluation committees
- Any interim analyses.

In the past, many clinical trials were restricted to two treatments only, and the choice between parallel samples or a crossover study design was the major decision. In most cases, a parallel-group design was chosen in most RCTs. Nowadays, there is an increasing trend toward using factorial approaches that may allow more than one major question to be answered. For example, when comparing the effects of two antihypertensive treatments in those who also have cholesterol problems, a comparison of the effect of lipid-lowering drugs could also be performed. Accurate use of a factorial design allows for independent assessment of both of these comparisons. Additionally, clinical trials are increasingly designed as large multicenter and often multinational studies to ensure generalizability, and also, for regulatory issues, to justify the need for only one study for approval.

Comparisons

Trials to show superiority

Scientifically, efficacy is established by demonstrating superiority to placebo in a placebo-controlled trial, by demonstrating superiority to an active-control treatment or by proving a dose–response relationship. This type of trial is referred to as a "superiority" trial. When a therapeutic treatment that has been shown to be efficacious in superiority trial(s) exists for treatment of serious illnesses, a placebo-controlled trial may be considered unethical. In that case, the scientifically sound use of an active treatment as a control should be considered. The appropriateness of placebo control versus active control should be considered on a trial-by-trial basis.

Trials to show equivalence or non-inferiority

This type of trial design might be the preferred strategy of the sponsor when there is the suspicion that an experimental treatment is not superior in terms of efficacy but may offer safety or compliance advantages compared to the active control [38]. According to its objective, two major types of trial are described: "equivalence" trials and "non-inferiority" trials. Bioequivalence trials belong to the first category. Sometimes, clinical equivalence trials are also undertaken for the purpose of other regulatory issues, such as proving the clinical equivalence of a generic product to the marketed product. In a non-inferiority trial, putative placebo comparisons are essential:

• (Historical) Effect of control drug versus placebo is of a specified size and there is a belief that this would be maintained in the present study if the placebo were included as a treatment.

• The trial has the ability to recognize when the test drug is inferior to the control drug.

• There is sufficient belief that the test drug would be superior to a placebo by a specified amount.

Many active-control trials are designed to show that the efficacy of an investigational product is not worse than that of the active comparator. Another possibility is a trial in which various doses of the investigational drug are compared with the recommended dose. Active-control equivalence or non-inferiority trials may also incorporate a placebo treatment arm, thus pursuing multiple goals in one trial; e.g., they may establish superiority to placebo and hence simultaneously validate the trial design and evaluate the degree of similarity of efficacy and safety to the active comparator. There are well-known difficulties connected with the use of an active-control equivalence (or non-inferiority) trial that does not include a placebo or does not incorporate multiple doses of the new drug. These relate to the inherent lack of any measure of internal validity (in contrast to superiority trials), thus making external validation necessary. A particularly important issue is establishing a credible non-inferiority "margin" to decide the usefulness of the new treatment and estimate the sample size, which should be discussed with a statistician. Equivalence (or non-inferiority) trials are not robust in nature, making them particularly susceptible to flaws in the design of a trial or its conduct, thus leading to biased results and the conclusion of equivalence. For these reasons, the design aspects of non-inferiority trials deserve particular recognition and their conduct needs special attention. For example, it is especially important to minimize the incidence of violations of the entry criteria, non-compliance, withdrawals, losses to follow-up, missing data, and other deviations from the protocol, and also to reduce their impact on subsequent analyses. Active comparators should be carefully chosen. A suitable active comparator would be a widely applied therapy whose efficacy for the same indication has been clearly established and measured in well-designed and well-reported superiority trial(s), and which can be reliably anticipated to exhibit similar efficacy in the planned active-control trial. As a consequence, the new trial should have the same important features (primary variables, dose of the active comparator, eligibility criteria, etc.) as the previously conducted superiority trials in which the active comparator clearly demonstrated clinically relevant efficacy, taking into consideration relevant advances in medical or statistical practice.

It is crucial that the protocol of an equivalence or non-inferiority trial contains an explicit statement about its intention. An equivalence (non-inferiority) margin should be specified in the protocol; this margin is the largest difference between the test treatment and active control that can be judged as being clinically tolerable, and it should be smaller than differences observed in superiority trials between the active comparator and the placebo. For the active-control equivalence trial, both the upper and lower equivalence margins are needed, while only the lower margin is needed for the active-control non-inferiority trial. The choice of equivalence margins should be justified clinically. For equivalence trials, two-sided confidence intervals should be used. Equivalence can be concluded when the entire confidence interval lies within the equivalence margins. There are also special issues regarding the choice of analysis sets. Subjects who withdraw consent or drop out of any treatment or comparator group will be predisposed to have a lower treatment response, and hence the results of using the full analysis set may be biased toward showing equivalence. This is discussed further below.

Trials to show a dose–response relationship

Dose–response trials may serve several objectives, most importantly: confirmation of efficacy; investigation of the shape and location of the dose–response curve; evaluation of an optimal starting dose; definition of strategies for individual dose adjustments; and determination of a maximal dose beyond which surplus benefit would be unlikely to occur. For these purposes the use of procedures to estimate the relationship between dose and response, including the calculation of confidence intervals and the use of graphical methods, is as important as the use of statistical tests. The hypothesis tests that are used may need to be tailored to the natural ordering of doses or to particular questions regarding the shape of the dose–response curve (e.g., monotonicity).

The details of the applied statistical methods should be provided in the protocol.

Study protocol

In the above we have discussed a number of features and considerations necessary to mount a clinical trial. The study protocol pulls it all together.

The protocol is the "recipe" for a clinical trial, describing in detail the scientific rationale, patient eligibility, trial treatments, study investigations, outcome measures, sample size, statistical analysis, and management of safety issues [39]. The protocol should be understandable to investigators and research staff taking part in clinical trials, so brevity and simplicity are key objectives when preparing the protocol. As stated above (see Study populations) one of the most important sections is eligibility (inclusion and exclusion criteria), since this governs how many patients can be entered and is the main driver for enrolment (or lack of it). Inclusion criteria should provide a simple guide to the population that should be screened for eligibility, and exclusion criteria should explain which patients should not be enrolled for safety reasons. Exclusion criteria "rule out patients" and generally make trials less applicable to clinical practice [40]. The usual justification for an extensive list of exclusion criteria is that a "homogeneous" population is needed to test the hypothesis. Since this is not the situation in clinical practice (i.e., patients with a particular disease are often heterogeneous in terms of age, gender, and co-morbidities), there seems little logic in supporting this practice. We propose a simple "rule" that no trial should have more than 10 exclusion criteria; this should allow better enrolment and greater generalizability of results. All of the features and issues listed in Table 1.1 also have importance and must be considered and dealt with seriously in the protocol.

Trial monitoring

In the past, the monitoring of a trial's progress was essentially the function of the study sponsor. Today, this is less and less common. Monitoring the quality of the study is still the responsibility of the sponsor; however, this function is often shared with another institution, the Independent Data Monitoring Committee (IDMC), also called the Data and Safety Monitoring Board (DSMB). This committee usually consists of at least three people, and includes no less than two clinicians and one biostatistician [41,42]. Other persons, including epidemiologists, ethicists, and patient advocates, might also belong to the DSMS, depending on the type of clinical trial.

In contrast to monitoring for quality, monitoring for safety and efficacy has shifted from the sponsor towards the IDMC. If unblinded interim analyses are performed for evaluation of efficacy or safety, they are done solely for the IDMC. These interim analyses affect alpha spending [43], and the IDMC has to take into account this issue. Also, usually, the IDMC alone can view unblinded data and its reports may form the basis of the safety information provided to regulatory authorities. Interim analyses for efficacy and safety have become standard features of clinical trials, and the role of the IDMC has steadily increased. Other activities, such as decisions whether to adjust sample size or study length, may be recommended by the IDMC.

Data monitoring

The process of evaluating and analyzing data accruing from a clinical trial can be prone to systematic bias and/or type I error. Therefore, all interim analyses, formal or informal, preplanned or unplanned, by any study partici-pant, sponsor staff member, or data monitoring group need to be explained in full, even if the treatment groups were not identified. The requirements for statistical adjustments due to such additional analyses should be adequately mentioned. Any operating instructions or procedures used for such analyses should be described in detail. Data monitoring without code breaking should also be described, even if this type of monitoring is considered to cause no increase in type I error.

Data analysis sets

Ultimately, the data from the clinical trial will be analyzed. Ideally all rand-omized subjects will be analyzed. The data set that includes all subjects as randomized is called the intention-to-treat (ITT) data set or analysis set. This data set retains all the optimal features of the randomization and permits valid statistical analysis. In practice, the complete ITT analysis data set is not achieved due to premature termination, safety concerns, drop-outs, lack of adherence, etc. Below and in the section Analysis methods, we elaborate more on the implication of the lack of the ideal ITT data set.

Intention-to-treat analysis and data set

The particular strength of RCTs is the avoidance of various sources of bias. In order to safeguard the full protective effect of randomization against bias, inclusion of all randomized patients regardless of further study adherence is the preferred strategy [44]. Thus, analysis of the ITT data set or, equivalently, the ITT analysis refers to the analysis performed exactly according to initial randomization on all those randomized. Some trialists prefer to exclude patients in the analysis for whom outcome data are missing. This is not a rare problem since in half of RCTs more than 10% of outcome data are missing [45]. Sometimes this approach is reasonable, but strictly speaking, this kind of analysis does not represent an ITT analysis and, instead, should be claimed as a "complete case" (or "available case") analysis. Alternatively, it is possible to impute missing outcome data and perform the analysis on available cases plus the imputed data. The validity of this analysis depends upon the extent of the missing data and the reasons for missing data (see section on Missing data below). The modified ITT (mITT) analysis data set is a subset of the ITT data set and allows for the post-randomization exclusion of some subjects in a justified manner, e.g. those who never receive the treatment drugs. Analysis of this data set is at times reasonable, but can contain biases and has been recently reported to be associated with industry funding and authors' conflicts of interest [46].

Per protocol analysis and on-treatment analysis data sets

The per-protocol (PP) data set is restricted only to those "ideal" study subjects who fulfil the protocol in terms of the eligibility criteria, study interventions, and outcome measures. On-treatment analysis refers to an approach stratified according to the real allocated treatment regardless of randomization. Though a per-protocol and on-treatment analysis may be reasonable in some settings, it should be emphasized that this analysis approach represents a non-randomized, observational comparison.

Subgroup analysis data sets

Whether the main results of a clinical trial do or do not support the null hypothesis, it is inevitable that the sample will be analyzed based on clinical subgroups of interest to determine the response to treatment [33,34]. Typical subgroups include gender (binary), age (continuous but may be divided into categories), and diabetes (categorical). Subgroups of interest may be specified prior to the study being analyzed (prospectively defined or *a priori* subgroups) or after the main results have been analyzed (*post hoc* or retrospective). Subgroups can be exploratory in post-hoc analysis of clinical trials and then usually do not have sufficient power to provide reliable estimates of treatment effect, but can be hypothesis generating. Important subgroups of interest (like diabetic or ST-elevation myocardial infarction subgroups in cardiovascular trials) are often predefined per protocol in large phase 3 RCTs, and sample size and power calculations can be performed considering these predefined subgroup analyses. Subgroups that have more than 500 events may have greater reliability, e.g. in large trials with extremely favorable p-values (<0.001) or subgroups in a meta-analysis of large trials. However, the unreliability of even large subgroups has been demonstrated in the ISIS-2 trial, which showed that aspirin was highly effective in reducing mortality after myocardial infarction in the group overall, but when data for patients with the star signs Libra and Gemini were analyzed, there was no apparent benefit of aspirin in contrast to the other star signs [47]. Using such a non-medical subgroup emphasizes the unreliability of subgroup analysis, so in general subgroups should be considered hypothesis generating, not hypothesis testing.

Unit of analysis

It should be precisely stated which patients are to be included in each efficacy analysis. For example, as discussed above, depending on the analysis set the included patients can be those with any efficacy observation or with a minimum number of observations; all patients receiving any test drugs/investigational products; only patients completing the trial; all patients with an observation during a particular time window; or only patients with a specified degree of compliance.

In all of the above cases, the subject (patient) is the unit of analysis. Recognition of this is important in applying statistical analyses procedures to the data. Often there is a single outcome associated with the patient (e.g., does or does not develop a myocardial infarction). The analysis considers this outcome as coming from a single subject. In contrast, there are situations where an outcome is measured repeatedly in a subject (e.g., blood pressure on monthly visits). A proper statistical analysis must consider these multiple, repeated measurements on a single subject. The unit of analysis is still the patient, but now there are correlated measures on him/her. Confusion has accrued over how to deal with multiple measurements collected either at a single time point or at several time points during the course of a trial. Methods such as generalized estimating equations and random-effects models can effectively deal with the problem of correlation within subjects and across time [48–50].

Missing data

As mentioned above, numerous factors may influence drop-out rates: study duration, efficacy and toxicity of the study drug, disease nature, and other individual factors. Ignoring those patients who "dropped out" (i.e., who did not complete the study for whatever reason) and only analyzing patients who completed the study can be misleading. A large number of drop-outs, however, even if included in the analysis, may cause bias, particularly if there are differences in the timing of drop-outs between the treatment groups or the reasons for dropping out are related to outcome. Although the effects of early drop-outs can be difficult to evaluate, any possible impact should be investigated as fully as possible. In case the drop-out rate is high, it might be helpful to concentrate on analyses at time points when most of the patients were still under observation and when the full effect of the drug could be expected. It may also be helpful to consider modeling approaches that have been developed for analysis of such incomplete data sets. The results of a clinical trial should be analyzed not only for the subgroup of subjects who completed the study, but also for the entire patient population as randomized (*intention-to-treat*) or at least for all those with any on-study measurements (*on-treatment*). Several factors should be taken into account and compared for the treatment groups in analyzing the effects of drop-outs. These include the reasons for the drop-outs, the time to drop-out, and the proportion of drop-outs among treatment groups at various time points. Procedures for dealing with missing data, e.g., use of estimated or derived data, should be described. Detailed explanation should be given as to how such estimations or derivations were performed and what underlying assumptions were made.

Sensitivity analysis
Sensitivity analyses refer to broad-spectrum of computational analyses in which certain inputs are modified to see how this will affect the outcome.

They address the following questions: How confident are the results? How great will be the impact on the results if the basic data are slightly wrong? Will this give a completely different outcome? Unused categories like missing data, conflicting data derived from various sources (e.g. different results reported by the general practitioner and the investigator), or uncertain cases (no disease versus disease) might have a major impact on the general results if included in the analysis. Advanced statistical imputation methods can be applied to check the impact of these unused categories by substituting uncertain cases and missing values, e.g., on the basis of best guess estimates.

Analysis methods

For data analysis, the patients included in each efficacy analysis should be precisely described, e.g., all patients receiving any test drugs/investigational products; all patients with any efficacy observation or with a certain minimum number of observations; only patients completing the trial; all patients with an observation during a particular time window; or only patients with a specified degree of compliance. It should be clear, if not defined in the study protocol, when (relative to study unblinding) and how inclusion/exclusion criteria for the data sets analyzed were developed. Even if it was proposed that primary analysis would be based on a reduced subset of the patients with complete follow-up data, there should also be, for any trial aimed at establishing efficacy, an additional analysis using all randomized (or otherwise entered) patients with any on-treatment data. Ideally, there should be a figure or table listing all patients, visits, and observations excluded from the efficacy analysis. The reasons for exclusion should also be analyzed for the whole treatment group over time. The Consort diagram (with extensions as needed) in Figure 1.2 is a useful device for this.

Demographic and other baseline characteristics

Group data for the relevant demographic and baseline characteristics of the patients, as well as other factors identified during the study that could affect response, should be presented, and the comparability of the treatment groups for all relevant characteristics should be displayed using graphs or tables. Analysis of the ITT data set is the only analysis justified by the randomization and should be the primary analysis. This may be followed by data on other groups used in principal analyses, such as the "per-protocol" analysis, "complete case," or other analyses, e.g., groups defined by compliance, concomitant disease/therapy, or demographic/baseline characteristics. When such groups are analyzed, data for the complementary excluded cohort should also be provided. In a multicenter study, where appropriate, comparability between centers should be assessed. A diagram showing the relationship between the entire sample and any other analysis groups should be provided. The critical variables will usually depend on the specific nature of the disease and on the protocol, but should usually cover:

- *Demographic variables:*
  - Age
  - Sex
  - Race.
- *Disease factors:*
  - Specific entry criteria (if not uniform), duration, stage, and severity of disease, and other clinical factors and subgroups of known prognostic significance
  - Baseline values for critical clinical measurements performed during the course of a study or identified as important indicators of prognosis or response to therapy
  - Concomitant illness at trial initiation, such as renal disease, diabetes, heart failure
  - Relevant previous illness
  - Relevant previous treatment for the illness treated in the study
  - Concomitant treatment maintained, even if the dose was changed during the study, including oral contraceptive and hormone replacement therapy; treatments stopped at entry into the study period (or changed at study initiation)
  - Other factors that might affect response to therapy (e.g., weight, renal and hepatic status, antibody levels, metabolic status)
  - Other possibly relevant variables (e.g., smoking, alcohol intake, special diets) if pertinent to the study.

Measurements of treatment compliance

Any measurements of compliance of individual patients with the treatment regimen under study and drug concentrations in body fluids should be summarized, and analyzed by treatment group and time interval.

Analysis of efficacy

Treatment groups should be compared for all relevant measures of efficacy (primary and secondary endpoints; any pharmacodynamic endpoints studied), as well as benefit/risk assessment(s) in all patients where these are utilized. In general, the results of all analyses implemented in the protocol and an analysis including all patients with on-study data should be performed in studies aimed at establishing efficacy. The analysis should provide results to estimate the size (point estimate) of the difference between the study treatments, the associated confidence interval, and the results of the predefined hypothesis testing. Analyses based on continuous variables (e.g., mean blood pressure, levels of cardiac necrosis markers at time point X, etc.) and categorical factors (e.g., worsening of heart failure, hospital admission, or occurrence of event) can be equally valid. For a multicenter study, where appropriate, data display and analysis of larger individual sites or more sites per geographic region should be included for critical variables to give a clear picture of trends between the recruitment sites and to evaluate possible differences in study conduct.

It is important for clinicians to avoid an obsession with a "P value less than 0.05" and develop an understanding of how statistical methods can be applied in a valid way to clinical trials. Experienced statisticians will emphasize that many of the assumptions in the design and interpretation of a clinical trial are actually *clinical* rather than *statistical*, and it is surprising how often clinical assumptions are carried out in a sloppy manner. For example, the key driver for sample size estimation is the expected difference between the two groups and this is determined by careful scrutiny of the literature. Similarly, subgroup analysis and interpretation can be heavily influenced by seeing analyses from a completed trial. Analyses that are triggered by seeing "interesting results" are often called "data derived" and experience tells us that data-derived analyses often lead to biased conclusions, in contrast to analyses that are prespecified prior to seeing the results.

An understanding of basic statistical issues applied to clinical trials is essential for clinicians. We provide a short introduction to these issues below.

Distribution of data

Understanding how to classify measurements in a clinical trial according to accepted statistical methods is an important starting point. Results obtained in a clinical trial can be expressed in two main ways: "continuous" or "categorical." Measurement of blood pressure, weight, height, plasma cholesterol, serum creatinine, and left ventricular ejection fraction are examples of "continuous" variables. Continuous variables can be expressed at different levels of precision depending on the scale of the measurement methods (e.g., centimeters or millimeters). Common biological data such as height, weight, and cholesterol have a "normal" or Gaussian distribution. For example, in a sample population where height is measured there will be a clustering of measurements around the average ("mean") and fewer measurements further away from the mean. The shape of the normal distribution curve can be described mathematically and the key variables are the mean, variance, and standard deviation (discussed below). Data that are not normally distributed are commonly found in clinical trials of biomarkers, especially those that are found at low levels in individuals without disease, such as C-reactive protein and troponin. Analysis of these data requires statistical tests suitable for nonparametric analysis.

Measurements of death, hospital admission, stroke, and myocardial infarction are examples of categorical variables. When there are only two possibilities, categorical variables are called "dichotomous" or "binary." Thus in a trial evaluating the effects of a new treatment on mortality, patients can be classified as having one of two outcomes: dead or alive. Most measurements in clinical trials can be classified as continuous or dichotomous. Other ways of expressing measurements include assigning grades or "ranks." For example, when asked "Do you feel depressed?," a patient may be asked to select the most appropriate answer from the following: "never, sometimes, often, always." The patient's response has four possible categories that can be ranked from mild to severe. The New York Heart Association classification of heart failure also has four possible categories. When managing patients, it is helpful to know whether a treatment is indicated or not, even when there is uncertainty about the benefits and risks of treatment, which may require dichotomizing continuous variables, e.g., a persistent systolic blood pressure above 140 mmHg may be an indication for pharmacological treatment for hypertension, implying that pressures below 140 mmHg do not require treatment. The reality is more complex, but it is common practice to convert a continuous variable into a dichotomous variable, although this often leads to loss of statistical power.

The importance of understanding the classification of measurements is that different statistical assumptions and tests are used for continuous data and categorical data. When data from a clinical trial have been collected, it is important to present them in a logical and clear manner, which requires the use of tables and figures. Data showing key variables (or "covariates"), which describe the population sample enrolled into a clinical trial (including age, gender, medical history, disease severity, etc.), are called "descriptive" or "summary" statistics.

Statistical analysis of clinical trials (elementary concepts)

Figure 1.3 shows a simplified, but helpful, decision tree for statistical comparisons depending on the type of variable measured in a RCT.

The comparison of categorical variables from a two-group clinical trial (parallel sample design with treatment versus control) using the Chi-square test is relatively simple and can be performed on a hand calculator. The first step is to populate the "2 x 2" table, which has the number of subjects with the outcome of interest (yes or no) in the columns, and treatment and control in the rows. The "observed minus expected" is a common method for estimating the Chi-square value in which the average values of the events rates are calculated for each of the four cells (estimated or E). These are then subtracted from the actual value (observed or O), squared, and divided by the expected value for that cell. The four values are added and this provides the Chi-square statistic. Reference to standard tables will provide the associated p-value. This Chi-square test is equivalent to the test of differences in proportions of outcomes for the two treatments, where the proportion of events in the test treatment is compared to the proportion of events in the control.

When treatment effects on changes of a categorical variable are evaluated (i.e., comparing before and after treatment effects), the McNemar test is useful. It is applied to 2 x 2 contingency tables with a dichotomous distribution and matched pairs, and tests the hypothesis whether or not the row and column marginal frequencies are equal (also called marginal homogeneity) [51].

For normally distributed data the key measurements for comparison are means and their associated standard deviations. Standard deviation describes the "spread" of the data, which includes the difference between highest and lowest values, and the variability around the mean. Data which are clustered

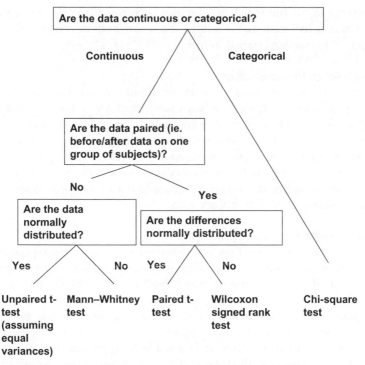

Figure 1.3 Decision tree for analysis of comparative data from a clinical trial.

around the mean will have smaller standard deviations. Standard deviation is the square root of the variance, which is the sum of all the differences between the mean and actual value divided by the number of observations minus one. The appropriate tests are indicated in Figure 1.3 and are called t-tests.

For non-normally distributed data there are equivalent tests called non-parametric test; they are the Wilcoxon Rank Sum and Mann–Whitney tests.

The above discussion may give the impression that for categorical and continuous data, rigid selection of Chi-square test, t-tests, Mann–Whitney or Wilcoxon tests is imperative. This is not the case and there is a substantial literature showing that, for example, the t-test is valid (robust) when used on simple five-point scale data. Here the five points may measure, for example, pain ranging from no pain (score 1) to maximum pain (score 5) [52–57]. The above discussion was given to indicate the need to select an appropriate statistical test that is valid for the data.

More advanced statistical concepts applied to trials include: when to stop a trial early ("stopping rules"), exploring the strength of association between variables (logistic regression), comparison of events over time (survival analysis), and introducing new treatments which may be safer and more convenient to use but which are not more effective than existing treatments ("non-inferiority" testing). For a fuller discussion of these concepts the reader is referred to standard statistical texts.

Adjustments for covariates

Selection of, and adjustments for, demographic or baseline characteristics, concomitant medical therapy, or any other covariates or prognostically relevant factors should be explained in the analysis report, and methods of adjustment, results of analyses, and supportive information (e.g., ANCOVA, linear regression models) should be addressed in the detailed description of statistical methods. Although not a mandatory part of the trial report, comparisons of covariate adjustments and prognostic factors can have informative value in the summary of clinical efficacy data.

Time to event ("survival") analysis

In many clinical trials the time to the occurrence of an event represents the main outcome measure of interest. This is the case for a binary outcome where the time at which an outcome occurs is built into the analysis. Examples are when the events are adverse, like cardiovascular death, non-fatal myocardial infarction or stent thrombosis, or positive, such as improvement of left ventricular function or heart failure symptoms, or neutral, such as freedom from arrhythmia. In all these cases, it is suitable to apply survival analysis for evaluation of endpoints; the term survival can be misleading as this method could be applied to any event, although originally it was planned for mortality evaluation. Events in survival analysis are defined by a "conversion" from one state (in its simplest form, no event) to another (i.e., occurrence of the event) at an instantaneous time point. Typically, not all the study participants will have experienced the event at the end of the follow-up period. This feature is defined as censoring, meaning that the observation period ended without occurrence of the predefined event, either because the subject has not experienced the event within the follow-up period, has dropped out event-free prior to termination of follow-up, or experiences a different type of event that makes further follow-up impossible (e.g., the patient died from a non-cardiovascular cause and the survival analysis was planned for analysis of cardiovascular death as event). In case of censoring, it is not feasible to know whether and when the subject would have experienced the event. Right censoring means that a subject's follow-up terminates before occurrence of the event; while left censoring refers to when the event has taken place before the subject has entered the study. Classical statistical tests, such as t-test, Mann–Whitney test or Chi-square test, are not suitable to analyze such survival data because they are not designed to take censoring into account. All trial subjects (including those with censored follow-up) can provide important information for event analysis, and should therefore not be excluded from the analysis. However, considering the censoring time as an equivalent survival time might lead to biased estimate of survival time and event probability. Therefore, specific statistical methods to handle survival data need to be applied. In clinical practice, all the subjects are not enrolled at the same time and thus the follow-up period can vary from one subject to another.

To estimate the proportion of subjects surviving the event (i.e., being event free) at a specified time point, and hence to calculate the survival probability to that time in relation to the generic population from which the sample derives, the Kaplan–Meier method [58,59] is commonly used, which permits censored information to be dealt with. In some situations it is not possible to know or to record the precise time when the event occurs; the only available information is that the event occurred in a certain time window. If this is the case, the survival probability cannot be updated every time an event happens, and the derived survival curve and probability are called life table or actuarial estimates. Comparisons of survival distribution between two samples are commonly applied in clinical trials to establish the efficacy of a new treatment compared to a control treatment. These can be analyzed using a non-parametric test method, the Mantel–Cox test or log-rank test. Sophisticated models based on the linear regression analysis (like the Cox regression analysis) are applied to compare survival data from different samples, mostly in non-randomized clinical trials to adjust for differences in group compositions, but these analyses require certain assumptions for data distribution [60].

Sample size and power

For scientific, ethical, and practical reasons, the sample size for a trial needs to be planned carefully, with a balance between statistical, medical, and resource considerations. Ideally, a clinical trial should be large enough to have a high probability (statistical power) of detecting with sufficient significance any clinically relevant difference of a given size. For clinical trials with a categorical outcome measure and two comparison groups, we need to know the expected event rate in the control group, the expected difference between groups, and the assumed values for alpha and beta (see below for definitions of these). Obtaining reliable estimates for the expected treatment difference and event rate is probably the most important and difficult aspect of the sample size calculation. Clinical trials, for illustration say superiority trials, start with the null hypothesis that states there is no difference in event rates between the two groups (this refers to the true state of nature if the null hypothesis is true) and attempt to prove the alternative hypothesis (the research hypothesis) that there will be a difference. The hypothesis test is attempting to decide which is the more plausible hypothesis based on the trial's data. The alpha value, which equates with the p-value and often set at 0.05 or less, is the probability that we will commit a type 1 (alpha) error when the null hypothesis is true. That is, it is the probability of saying the null hypothesis is false, when in fact it is true. In other words, if the null hypothesis is true, we have a 0.05 chance of the data and statistical test telling us to reject the null hypothesis. The alpha error is also known as the "false positive" rate. The type II (beta) error rate is the chance of saying the null hypothesis is true when, in fact, it is not. This error rate t is often set at 0.2 or 20% (i.e., the false negative rate). The "power" of a study is loosely defined as the ability of a study to detect the expected difference in terms of the estimated number of events during the trial and is described by the function 1—beta, which is conventionally 0.8 (or 80%). Formally the power of the statistical test is the probability that the statistical test will tell us to reject the null hypothesis when the null hypothesis is false. Alpha and power values can be modified to be more stringent than 0.05 and 0.8, respectively, and are sometimes set at 0.01 or 0.9, respectively, but the consequence of this additional precision is that sample sizes are much larger. When calculating sample size, the values for alpha and power are converted to function values, which appear as constants in the sample size equation. In addition to calculating the statistical power of a study to detect an expected numeric difference, it is important to determine a "minimal clinically significant difference" or "minimal important difference," defined as the smallest difference that clinicians and patients would care about. This parameter should be considered in the sample size estimation and should be stated in the clinical trial report, so that any statistically significant difference in outcome can be judged for clinical relevance.

Some trialists have postulated that "underpowered" trials may be acceptable as they could be used later in combined analyses in systematic reviews and meta-analyses [61–63]. Of note, this implies important caveats—the trial should be reported adequately, follow principles of minimizing bias, and published irrespective of the results. Underpowered trials with indeterminate results often remain unpublished. Ideally, all trials should individually have sufficient power to address the primary hypothesis. Irrespective of the power, authors need to properly report their intended sample size and expected difference between treatment and control with all their methods and assumptions. That gives transparency to readers and a measure by which to assess whether the trial achieved its planned sample size.

Safety evaluation

Analysis of safety-related data can be performed at three levels:
1. Extent of exposure (dose, duration, number of patients) should be explored to determine the degree to which safety can be assessed from the study.
2. Typical adverse events and laboratory test changes should be identified, compared for treatment groups, and analyzed, as appropriate, for factors that may affect the frequency of adverse reactions/events, such as time dependence, relation to demographic characteristics, and relation to dose or drug concentration.
3. Serious adverse events and other relevant adverse events should be identified, usually by detailed examination of patients who died or who left the study prematurely due to an adverse event, whether or not this was identified as drug related.

The International Conference on Harmonisation (ICH) guideline "Clinical Safety Data Management: Definitions and Standards for Expedited Reporting" defines serious adverse events as follows: "A serious adverse event (experience) or reaction is any untoward medical occurrence that at any dose: results in death, is life-threatening, requires inpatient hospitalization or prolongation of existing hospitalization, results in persistent or significant disability/incapacity, or is a congenital anomaly/birth defect."

Safety data have always been important, but are often not consequently analyzed. Most clinical trials designed to show efficacy of a treatment (difference between treatment and a control) are not large enough, either in terms of sample size or follow-up, to identify serious safety concerns. Recent developments regarding health regulatory issues have led to more rigorous analyses. For instance, data mining techniques have been generated and successfully applied to safety data from previously unrevealed structures [64,65]. Drug approval does not only involve efficacy studies, but also complete analyses of safety studies. Furthermore, because there are so many effective treatments in cardiovascular disease, the choice among them may ultimately rest upon the safety issues.

Subsets and more

Evaluation of any "efficacy subset" of patients should be devoted to the effects of dropping patients with available data from analyses because of their poor compliance, missed visits, ineligibility, or any other reasons. As noted above, an analysis using all available data should be performed for all studies that aim to establish efficacy, even if it is not the primary analysis planned by the investigators. In general, it is of advantage to confirm the robustness of the principal trial results with respect to alternative subsets of patient populations. Any relevant differences deriving from the choice of patient population for analysis should be the subject of explicit discussion. If the size of the study allows, any subgroups based on important demographic or baseline characteristics should be examined for unusually large or small responses and the results presented, e.g., comparison of effects by age, gender, race, disease condition, or cardiovascular risk groups. These analyses are not intended to retrieve an otherwise negative study, but may reveal hypotheses worth examining in other trials or be helpful in refining labeling information, or patient or dose selection. Where there is a preceding hypothesis of a differential effect in a particular subgroup, this hypothesis and its assessment should be part of the planned statistical analysis and considered in the sample size calculation.

Types of significance

Statistical significance

Statistical significance tends to be used in the context of null hypothesis significance testing. The null hypothesis (e.g., for a superiority trial) states that there is no effect (or in other words the effect is zero) in a given population. Rejection of the null hypothesis means that we have a statistically significant reason to believe the null hypothesis is false. If the null hypothesis were true, there is only a 0.05 (the alpha value is set usually at 0.05 and p-value at ≤0.05) chance of reaching this conclusion. Testing of the null hypothesis is often misunderstood in some way: that the p-value is the likelihood that the null hypothesis is wrong; it has to emphasized that null hypothesis testing only yields information about whether results are statistically likely given some assumption about the population (the truth of the null hypothesis). In terms of testing clinical treatments, if a treatment is actually ineffective, statistical significance can only provide an answer to the question, "How likely is it that the statistical test of the treatment would falsely indicate that the treatment is effective?" It does not give any information about practical or clinical significance.

Practical or "clinical" significance

In broader terms, "practical significance" answers the question, "How effective is the intervention or treatment, or how much change does the treatment cause?". In terms of testing clinical treatments, practical significance ideally provides quantified information about the importance of a finding, using metrics such as effect size, number needed to treat (NNT), and preventive fraction.

Calculation of practical significance

Effect size is one type of practical significance. It is a measure between two variables in a statistical population and quantifies the extent to which a trial result deviates from expectations. Effect sizes have their own sources of bias, are subject to change based on population variability of the dependent variable, and tend to focus on group effects, not individual changes. Effect size can provide important information about the results of a study, and are recommended for inclusion in addition to statistical significance [66].

Clinical significance usually refers to two related but different concepts either by (1) being of a magnitude of effect that conveys practical (in this case there is an interchangeability with practical significance) or (2) more technically and restrictively, addressing whether an intervention or treatment may or may not fully correct previous findings. There are a variety of statistical methodologies to calculate clinical significance. For detailed description of these analysis methods the reader is referred to the statistical literature.

How have trials contributed to medical care?

Many trials have influenced practice in cardiovascular disease and we provide some examples. It is important to note that it is unusual for a *single* trial to change practice—usually a series of trials taken together provide clear evidence of benefit of using a new treatment paradigm. In addition, good trials build on a wealth of epidemiology, basic science, and clinical studies, which have elucidated the nature of the disease and provided preliminary evidence of the benefit of a potential new treatment. The modern era of clinical trials started in the late 1970s with investment from the National Institutes of Health to identify and combat major health threats, including cardiovascular disease and cancer. In the 1980s the need for larger studies and cooperation between hospitals was established, leading to many large trials which have provided reliable evidence about benefits and risks of promising treatments.

Clinical trials for treatment of high blood pressure (see also Chapter 12)

Many major trials of antihypertensive drug therapy have been performed in the last 10–15 years: CAPPP (Captopril Prevention Project) [67]; STOP Hypertension 2 and NORDIL [68,69], ALLHAT [70], Intervention as a Goal in Hypertension Treatment (INSIGHT) [71], INVEST [72], LIFE [73], LIFE-ISH [74], Anglo-Scandinavian Cardiac Outcomes Trial (ASCOT) [75], ONTARGET [76], and ACCOMPLISH [77]. All of them belong to the category of active-control RCTs. Among these trials, two different concepts are followed in the comparison with the active control. In the first group of trials, the aim was to show the preservation of a clinically meaningful efficacy and safety margin (equivalence or non-inferiority trials). Examples are CAPPP, INSIGHT, INVEST, LIFE and LIFE-ISH, STOP Hypertension 2 and NORDIL, and ONTARGET. In the second group of studies using an active control, the margin of clinically meaningful effect has been exceeded, as seen in superiority trials. The ACCOMPLISH trial demonstrated superiority of initiating antihypertensive therapy with an angiotensin converting enzyme (ACE) inhibitor combined with a calcium channel blocker (CCB) over initiating therapy with a thiazide-type diuretic, and the ALLHAT trial showed that the diuretic chlorthalidone, as the active control standard treatment, was superior to amlodipine, lisinopril or doxazosin.

All recent trials assessing the efficacy and safety of antihypertensive drugs have been designed and conducted as randomized, blinded trials. Such trials not only minimize experimental bias, but also implement many important aspects of controlled clinical trials. Many large antihypertensive trials, such as INVEST and ALLHAT, were designed to include a prospective, randomized, open, blinded endpoint evaluation (PROBE) in a large number (thousands) of patients in multiple countries. In some studies, there is also a focus on demonstrating reduction of mortality and/or cardiovascular morbidity rather than simply measuring the blood-lowering effects.

Hypertension is associated with a higher stroke risk, and several early trials, including the MRC Blood Pressure trials, showed that beta-blockers and thiazides could effectively lower blood pressure and reduce the risk of stroke [78]. Several subsequent trials in elderly patients showed that these benefits were not confined to "younger" hypertensives, and that the elderly could also be protected from stroke and death with effective antihypertensive treatment [79]. More recently, combinations of ACE inhibitors and calcium antagonists have been shown to be more effective than the more traditional combinations of beta-blockers and thiazides in the ASCOT trial [80]. Thus, larger randomized trials have the ability to reliably evaluate the efficacy and safety of treatments.

Clinical trials of atherosclerosis, lipid lowering, and statins (see also Chapter 12)

Understanding the main components of atherosclerosis, including the biochemistry of cholesterol and, low density lipoprotein (LDL) oxidation, role of monocytes and activated macrophages, and uptake of oxidized LDL into the arterial wall, took four to five decades, with several groups providing important insights into these processes [81]. Epidemiological studies including Keys' "7 countries study" also provided evidence of the link between cholesterol and coronary heart disease [82]. Early studies in the 1970s and 1980s of strategies to lower cholesterol (including diet and fibrates) did not show clear benefit because the amount of cholesterol lowering was modest (in the order of 10–15% proportional reduction) and the studies were too small to detect moderate but important benefits [83]. Synthesis of agents that could reduce cholesterol production in the liver by inhibiting a key enzyme, HMG Co-A reductase, led to the development of statins, which were found to reduce cholesterol by 20% or more [84]. The first trial to show that cholesterol lowering could reduce mortality and major morbidity was the 4S study, which randomized 4444 patients to simvastatin or placebo, and demonstrated a proportional reduction of 25% in death over a mean 4 years of follow-up in patients with prior myocardial infarction and cholesterol above 6.5 mmol/L (260 mg/dL) [85]. This led to the widespread uptake of statin use, with other trials confirming these results in a wider range of patients [86].

Clinical trials of acute myocardial infarction, coronary thrombosis, aspirin, and fibrinolysis (see also Chapter 4)

Acute coronary syndromes (ACS), including myocardial infarction (MI) and unstable angina, are responsible for about 15% of all deaths globally per year, and complications related to ACS cause 20–30% of all hospital admissions globally each year [87]. The main pathophysiological cause of ACS is plaque rupture leading to activation of platelets and intracoronary thrombus formation. Prior to 1985 standard treatments for MI were pain relief, glyceryl trinitrate (GTN), bed rest, monitoring, and usually heparin to prevent deep venous thrombosis. The ISIS-1 (first International Study of Infarct Survival) and MIAMI (Metoprolol In Acute Myocardial Infarction) trials demonstrated the benefits of beta-blockers early in MI [88,89], and were followed by the GISSI (Gruppo Italiano per to studio delta streptochinasi nell'infarto miocardico)-1 and ISIS-2 trials, which showed the benefits of early fibrinolysis; the latter trial confirmed that aspirin given early in MI could reduce all-cause mortality by about one-fifth [90,91]. Subsequent trials have added to knowledge about the benefits of antiplatelet therapy in ACS and the role of primary PCI in acute ST-segment elevation MI. Primary PCI has replaced fibrinolytic therapy in centers that can deliver it in a timely manner on a 24-hour basis [92].

Conducting reliable trials: issues of size and simplicity

The most common design issues in clinical trials have been discussed in the literature [93–95] and there is wide agreement on many key aspects. Practical issues are a major challenge, including cost, regulation (and its associated bureaucracy which can impede progress in trials), and complex project management. By definition, clinical trials involve patients in a clinical setting, so it is essential to keep trial procedures streamlined and simple and data collection to a minimum. It is noteworthy that clinical trials operate in somewhat artificial environments that do not entirely reflect real-world behavior. Most trials are complicated and not run efficiently: excessive and unnecessary tests (increasing patient discomfort and the time needed to administer and report tests) and excess data collection waste time and resources. A simple rule of thumb for data collection is to limit the number of data points to 300 per study subject (excluding repetitions that may occur with multiple follow-up visits). This approach provides a discipline to the length and complexity of case report forms by ensuring there is clear justification for all data points collected. Clinical trials are costly (small trials cost hundreds of thousands of dollars and large phase 3 trials cost millions of dollars) and this is a major limitation to the number of patients that can be enrolled. Several features of clinical trials require similar time and effort irrespective of trial size, including preparing the protocol, programming the database, and statistical analysis. Large multicenter trials will require more time and effort to set up and run than trials involving fewer centers, but much of this can be streamlined by simplifying the protocol and data collection. Trials that are too small to reliably answer the question are usually a waste of time and money, and making trials larger is an essential priority. "Simple" streamlined trials do not need to be complicated and can be cost-effective to carry out. The term "simple" refers to the outcome measure and not to the conduct of the study; thousands of patients from hundreds of centers and different countries may be followed for long periods of time (up to 5 or more years).

Costs, cost-effectiveness, and health economics

If a large clinical trial has shown that a certain treatment has a beneficial action with an acceptable safety profile, "How much does it cost" is usually the next question. Of course "cost" and "price" are different but related issues, where the upfront "cost" of a treatment is hopefully offset by downstream reduced costs of healthcare, improved quality of life, and better productivity. Health economics is a growing specialty that evaluates the costs and healthcare impact of introducing new treatments. It is a key part of modern clinical trials that provides accurate assessments of cost and cost-effectiveness within the trial [96,97]. This information forms the basis of sensible extrapolations beyond the trial in terms of longer lengths of treatments and management of larger populations with the same disease. Health economics attempts to model the costs and benefits of introducing new and effective treatments and is used by many healthcare funders to help make decisions about which treatments should and should not be provided.

Practical issues: managing a trial, funding, and regulation

Trial management, including trial design, securing funds, obtaining approvals, coordinating sites, and data management, is a complex and time-consuming activity. The current view is that all clinical trials should be managed by specialist clinical trial units (CTUs) with the appropriate expertise and capacity. Academic clinical trial units usually specialize in a disease area like cancer or cardiology, but there is a growing trend for larger units to undertake trial management in broader disease areas. Academic CTUs are made up of multidisciplinary teams, including trial managers, administrators, data managers, clinicians, and statisticians. A well-conducted trial will address an important question reliably and, given sufficient resources, most experienced CTUs can carry out trials to a high standard. The main barriers to conducting good trials are insufficient funds, unrealistic timelines, and excess bureaucracy and "red tape." The other issue facing academic CTUs is the cost of preparing grants and funding applications that may take several years, and this activity usually is not funded through grants. Thus, academic CTUs need to be hosted in institutions that have an understanding of the complex and long-term nature of clinical trials, and, of course, the enormous health benefits from the results of well-conducted trials. Most host institutions receive major benefits from CTUs through methodological and statistical expertise, which are often undervalued, and the long-term financial security of most academic CTUs remains uncertain. There has been a longstanding collaboration between industry and academic CTUs in the evaluation of new and promising cardiovascular drugs and devices, and many of these trials are discussed in this book.

In the 1980s most of the methodological expertise for trials was located in academic CTUs. During the 1990s and 2000s, increasing expertise and capacity for running trials was developed in the industry sector. Contract research organizations (CROs) work with companies developing devices and drugs to carry out the practical aspects of clinical trials, but are usually not involved in developing the scientific rationale for trials or publishing results in peer-reviewed journals. The CRO market was estimated to turn over more than 20 billion dollars per annum during 2011, indicating that this is an important and growing commercial activity [98].

The academic research organization (ARO) is an alternative model that often employs university faculty members as clinical trial investigators. Since they must comply with university regulatory requirements, AROs are also likely to ensure that investigators own the right to publication of findings, whereas publication rights for RCTs conducted by CROs usually belong to the drug company by contract. AROs are considered to be more independent, especially with regard to presentation of trial results and communication with health regulatory authorities during drug approval processes [99]. Academic–

industry collaboration in trials has many advantages, including the sharing of expertise to improve the quality of trials, but also raises issues of conflicts of interest if academic groups or individuals stand to gain disproportionate financial rewards in the form of direct payments, intellectual property rights, or stock options [100–102]. There is a growing trend for universities and large hospitals to develop long-term partnerships with industry for financial gain, which is a sensible way forward if these partnerships lead to measurable health improvements and are openly declared. However, the "ground rules" for such collaborations are still in development.

What does the future hold?

Clinical trials are an essential tool of modern healthcare evaluation and the demand for new trials both in the commercial and non-commercial sector is growing year on year. There are major challenges ahead, in particular the increasing bureaucratic burden of conducting clinical trials, which increases costs and decreases efficiency and sample size [103,104]. In addition, obtaining approvals for new drugs and devices is becoming more difficult, even when trials have shown important benefits, because of a reluctance to pay for more expensive but more effective treatments [105]. This latter issue decreases the incentive for industry to invest in clinical trials. There is also an urgent need to ensure that clinicians have the appropriate methodological training and expertise to understand key design issues in clinical trials, and we have attempted to cover many of these issues in this book with the help of a range of expert authors.

References

1. Chan AW, Altman DG. Epidemiology and reporting of randomised trials published in PubMed journals. *Lancet* 2005;365:1159–1162.
2. Hopewell S, Dutton S, Yu LM, Chan AW, Altman DG. The quality of reports of randomised trials in 2000 and 2006: comparative study of articles indexed in PubMed. *BMJ* 2010;340:c723.
3. Greenland S. Randomization, statistics, and causal inference. *Epidemiology* 1990; 1:421–429.
4. Armitage P. The role of randomization in clinical trials. *Stat Med* 1982;1:345–352.
5. Schulz KF, Chalmers I, Hayes RJ, Altman DG. Empirical evidence of bias. Dimensions of methodological quality associated with estimates of treatment effects in controlled trials. *JAMA* 1995;273:408–412.
6. Mega JL, Braunwald E, Mohanavelu S, *et al.*; ATLAS ACS-TIMI 46 study group. Rivaroxaban versus placebo in patients with acute coronary syndromes (ATLAS ACS-TIMI 46): a randomised, double-blind, phase II trial. *Lancet* 2009;374:29–38.
7. Mega JL, Braunwald E, Wiviott SD, *et al.*; ATLAS ACS 2–TIMI 51 Investigators. Rivaroxaban in patients with a recent acute coronary syndrome. *N Engl J Med* 2012; 366:9–19.
8. "Guidance for Institutional Review Boards and Clinical Investigators". Food and Drug Administration. 1999-03-16. http://www.fda.gov/oc/ohrt/irbs/drugsbiologics.html. Retrieved 2007-03-27

9. Collins R, MacMahon S. Reliable assessment of the effects of treatment on mortality and major morbidity, I: clinical trials. *Lancet* 2001;357:373–380.

10. Jolicoeur EM, Ohman EM, Temple R, *et al.*; Working Group Members. Clinical and research issues regarding chronic advanced coronary artery disease part II: Trial design, outcomes, and regulatory issues. *Am Heart J* 2008;155:435–444.

11. Friedman LM, Furberg CD, DeMets DL. *Fundamentals of Clinical Trials*, 3rd edn. New York: Springer, 1998.

12. Rothwell PM. External validity of randomised controlled trials: "to whom do the results of this trial apply?" *Lancet* 2005;365:82–93.

13. Sankoh AJ, D'Agostino RB, Huque MF. Efficacy endpoint selection and multiplicity adjustment methods in clinical trials with inherent multiple endpoint issues. *Stat Med* 2003;22:3133–3150.

14. D'Agostino RB Sr. Controlling alpha in a clinical trial: the case for secondary endpoints (editorial). *Stat Med* 2000;19:763–766.

15. Koch GG. Alpha calculus in a clinical trial: consideration and commentary for the new millennium (discussion). *Stat Med* 2000;19:781–784.

16. Moye LA. Alpha calculus in a clinical trial: consideration and commentary for the new millennium. *Stat Med* 2000;19:767–789.

17. O'Neill RT. Alpha calculus in clinical trials: considerations and commentary for the new millennium (commentary). *Stat Med* 2000;19:785–793.

18. Fisher LD. Carvedilol and the Food and Drug Administration (FDA) approval process: the FDA paradigm and reflections on hypothesis testing. *Controlled Clin Trials* 1999;20:16–39.

19. Buyse M, Molenberghs G. Criteria for the validation of surrogate endpoints in randomized experiments. *Biometrics* 1998;54:1014–1029.

20. D'Agostino RB Jr. The slippery slope of surrogate outcomes (debate). *Curr Control Trials Cardiol* 2000;2:76–78.

21. Polak JF, Pencina MJ, O'Leary DH, D'Agostino RB. Common carotid artery intima-media thickness progression as a predictor of stroke in multi-ethnic study of atherosclerosis. *Stroke* 2011;42:3017–3021.

22. Haakenson C, Akiyama T, Hallstrom A, Sather MR. Masking drug treatments in the Cardiac Arrhythmia Pilot Study (CAPS). FASHP for the CAPS Investigators. *Control Clin Trials* 1996;17:294–303.

23. Echt DS, Liebson PR, Mitchell LB, *et al.*: for the CAST-Investigators: Mortality and morbidity in patients receiving encainide, flecainide, or placebo. *N Engl J Med* 1991;324:781–788.

24. Hulley S, Grady D, Bush T, Furberg C, Herrington D, Riggs B, Vittinghoff E. Randomized trial of estrogen plus progestin for secondary prevention of coronary heart disease in postmenopausal women. Heart and Estrogen/progestin Replacement Study (HERS) Research Group. *JAMA* 1998;280:605–613.

25. Validation of Heart Failure Events in the Antihypertensive and Lipid Lowering Treatment to Prevent Heart Attack Trial (ALLHAT) Participants Assigned to Doxazosin and Chlorthalidone. *Curr Control Trials Cardiovasc Med* 2002;3:10.

26. Piller LB, Davis BR, Cutler JA, *et al.*; The ALLHAT Collaborative Research Group. International Conference on Harmonization: choice of control group in clinical trials. *Fed Register* 1999;64:51767–51780.

27. Pledger G, Hall DB. Active control equivalence studies: do they address the efficacy ssue? In: Peace KE, ed. *Statistical Issues in Drug Research and Development*. New York: Marcel Dekker, 1990:226–238.

28. International Conference on Harmonization: choice of control group in clinical trials. *Fed Register* 1999;64:51767–51780.

29. Temple R, Ellenberg SS. Placebo-controlled trials and active-control trials in the evaluation of new treatments. Part 1: ethical and scientific issues. *Ann Intern Med* 2000;133: 455–463.

30. Schulz KF, Grimes DA. Generation of allocation sequences in randomised trials: chance, not choice. *Lancet* 2002;359:515–519.

31. Taves DR. Minimization—a new method of assigning patients to treatment and control groups. *Clin Pharmacol Ther* 1974;15:443–453.

32. Scott NW, McPherson GC, Ramsay CR, Campbell MK. The method of minimization for allocation to clinical trials. A review. *Control Clin Trials* 2002;23:662–674.

33. Downs M, Tucker K, Christ-Schmidt H, Wittes J. Some practical problems in implementing randomization. *Clin Trials* 2010;7:235–245.

34. Moher D. CONSORT: an evolving tool to help improve the quality of reports of randomized controlled trials. Consolidated Standards of Reporting Trials. *JAMA* 1998;279: 1489–1491.

35. Jüni P, Altman DG, Egger M. Assessing the quality of controlled clinical trials. In: Egger M, Davey Smith G, Altman DG, eds. *Systematic Reviews in Health Care: Meta-analysis in Context*. London: BMJ Books, 2001.

36. Smith DHG, Neutel JM, Lacourciere Y, Kempthorne-Rawson J. Prospective, randomized, open-label, blinded-endpoint designed trials yield the same results as double-blind, placebo-controlled trials with respect to ABPM measurements. *J Hypertens* 2003;21:1291–1298.

37. Hopewell S, Dutton S, Yu LM, Chan AW, Altman DG. The quality of reports of randomised trials in 2000 and 2006: comparative study of articles indexed in PubMed. *BMJ* 2010;340:c723.

38. D'Agostino RB, Massaro JM, Sullivan LM. Non-inferiority trials: design concepts and issues—the encounters of academic consultants in statistics. *Stat Med* 2003;22: 169–186.

39. Guyatt G. Preparing a research protocol to improve chances for success. *J Clin Epidemiol* 2006;59:893–899.

40. Flather M, Delahunty N, Collinson J. Generalizing results of randomized trials to clinical practice: reliability and cautions. *Clin Trials* 2006;3:508–512.

41. Armstrong PW, Furberg CD. Clinical trial data and safety monitoring boards. The search for a constitution. *Circulation* 1995; 91:901–904.

42. Armitage P. Data and safety monitoring in the Concorde and Alpha trials. *Controlled Clin Trials* 1999;20:207–228.

43. DeMets DL, Lan KKG. Interim analysis: the alpha spending function approach. *Stat Med* 194;13:1341–1352.

44. Hollis S, Campbell F. What is meant by intention to treat analysis? Survey of published randomized controlled trials. *BMJ* 1999;319;670–674.

45. Wood AM, White IR, Thompson SG. Are missing outcome data adequately handled? A review of published randomized controlled trials in major medical journals. *Clin Trials* 2004;1:368–376.

46. Montedori, A, Bonacini MI, Casazza G, Luchetta MI, Duca P, Cozzolino F, Abraha I. Modified versus standard intention-to-treat reporting; are there differences in methodological quality, sponsorship, and findings in radnomized trials? A cross-sectional study. *Trials* 2011;12:58.

47. ISIS-2 Collaborative Group. Randomised trial of intravenous streptokinase, oral aspirin, both, or neither among 17,187 cases of suspected acute myocardial infarction: ISIS-2. ISIS-2 (Second International Study of Infarct Survival) Collaborative Group. *Lancet* 1988;2:349–360.

48. Laird NM, Ware JH. Random-Effects Models for Longitudinal Data. *Biometrics* 1982;38:963–974.

49. Liang K-Y, Zeger SL. Longitudinal data analysis using generalized linear models. *Biometrika* 1986;73:13–22.

50. Zeger SL, Liang KY, Albert PS. Models for Longitudinal Data: A Generalized Estimating Equation Approach. *Biometrics* 1988;44:1049–1060.

51. McNemar Q. Note on the sampling error of the difference between correlated proportions or percentages. *Psychometrika* 1947;12:153–157.

52. D'Agostino RB, Lee AFS. Robustness of location estimators under changes of population kurtosis. *J Am Stat Assoc* 1977;72:358:393–396.

53. D'Agostino RB, Chase W, Belanger A. The appropriateness of some common procedures for testing the equality of two independent binomial populations. *Am Stat* 1988;42:198–202.

54. Heeren T, D'Agostino RB. Robustness of the two independent samples t-test when applied to ordinal scaled data. *Stat Med* 1987;6:79–90.

55. Sullivan LM, D'Agostino RB. Robustness of the t test applied to data distorted from normality by floor effects. *J Dent Res* 1992;71;1938–1943.

56. Sullivan LM, D'Agostino RB. Robustness and power of analysis of covariance applied to ordinal scaled data as arising in randomized controlled trials. *Stat Med* 2003;22:1317–1334.

57. Sullivan LM, D'Agostino RB. Robustness and power of analysis of covariance applied to data distorted from normality by floor effects: homogenous regression slopes. *Stat Med* 1996;15:477–496.

58. Kaplan EL, Meier P. Nonparametric estimation from incomplete observations. *J Am Stat Assoc* 1958;53:457–481.

59. Altman DG, Bland JM. Statistics notes: Time to event (survival) data. *BMJ* 1998;317;468–469.

60. Cox D. Regression models and life tables. *J R Stat Soc B* 1972;34:187–220.

61. Guyatt GH, Mills EJ, Elbourne D. In the era of systematic reviews, does the size of an individual trial still matter. *PLoS Med* 2008;5:e4.

62. Schulz KF, Grimes DA. Sample size calculations in randomised trials: mandatory and mystical. *Lancet* 2005;365:1348–1353.

63. Halpern SD, Karlawish JH, Berlin JA. The continuing unethical conduct of underpowered clinical trials. *JAMA* 2002;288:358–362.

64. Chuang-Stein C, Le V, Chen W. Recent advances in the analysis and presentation of safety data. *J Drug Inform Assoc* 2001;35:377–397.

65. Gait JE, Smith S, Brown SL. Evaluation of safety data from controlled clinical trials: the clinical principles explained. *J Drug Inform Assoc* 2000;34:273–287.

66. D'Agostino RB. Editorial: Quantifying the comparison of two groups. *Stat Med* 1999;18:2551–2555.

67. Hansson L, Lindholm LH, Niskanen L, *et al*. Effect of angiotensin-converting-enzyme inhibition compared with conventional therapy on cardiovascular morbidity and mortality in hypertension: the Captopril Prevention Project (CAPPP) randomised trial. *Lancet* 199;353:611–616.

68. Hansson L, Lindholm LH, Ekbom T, *et al*. Randomised trial of old and new antihypertensive drugs in elderly patients: cardiovascular mortality and morbidity the Swedish Trial in Old Patients with Hypertension-2 study. *Lancet* 1999;354:1751–1756.

69. Hansson L, Hedner T, Lund-Johansen P, *et al*. Randomised trial of effects of calcium antagonists compared with diuretics and beta-blockers on cardiovascular morbidity and mortality in hypertension: the Nordic Diltiazem (NORDIL) study. *Lancet* 2000;356:359–365.

70. ALLHAT Officers and Coordinators for the ALLHAT Collaborative Research Group. The Antihypertensive and Lipid-Lowering Treatment to Prevent Heart Attack Trial. Major outcomes in high-risk hypertensive patients randomized to angiotensin-converting enzyme inhibitor or calcium channel blocker vs diuretic: The Antihypertensive and Lipid-Lowering Treatment to Prevent Heart Attack Trial (ALLHAT). *JAMA* 2002;288:2981–2997.

71. Brown MJ, Palmer CR, Castaigne A, *et al*. Morbidity and mortality in patients randomised to double-blind treatment with a long-acting calcium-channel blocker or diuretic in the International Nifedipine GITS study: Intervention as a Goal in Hypertension Treatment (INSIGHT). *Lancet* 2000;356:366–372.

72. Pepine CJ, Handberg EM, Cooper-DeHoff RM, *et al*. INVEST Investigators. A calcium antagonist vs a non-calcium antagonist hypertension treatment strategy for patients with coronary artery disease. The International Verapamil-Trandolapril Study (INVEST): A randomized controlled trial. *JAMA* 2003;390:2859–2861.

73. Dahlof B, Devereux RB, Kjeldsen SE, *et al*. Cardiovascular morbidity and mortality in the Losartan Intervention For Endpoint reduction in hypertension study (LIFE): A randomised trial against atenolol. *Lancet* 2002;359:995–1003.

74. Kjeldsen SE, Dahlof B, Devereux RB, *et al*. Effects of losartan on cardiovascular morbidity and mortality in patients with isolated systolic hypertension and left ventricular hypertrophy: A Losartan Intervention for Endpoint Reduction sub-study (LIFE-ISH) *JAMA* 2002;288:1491–1498.

75. Poulter NR, Wedel H, Dahlöf B, *et al.*; ASCOT Investigators. Role of blood pressure and other variables in the differential cardiovascular event rates noted in the Anglo-Scandinavian Cardiac Outcomes Trial-Blood Pressure Lowering Arm (ASCOT-BPLA). *Lancet* 2005;366:907–913.

76. ONTARGET Investigators, Yusuf S, Teo KK, Pogue J, *et al*. Telmisartan, ramipril, or both in patients at high risk for vascular events. *N Engl J Med* 2008;358:1547–1559.

77. Jamerson K, Weber MA, Bakris GL, *et al.*; ACCOMPLISH Trial Investigators. Benazepril plus amlodipine or hydrochlorothiazide for hypertension in high-risk patients. *N Engl J Med* 2008;359:2417–2428.

78. Turnbull F, Kengne AP, MacMahon S. Blood pressure and cardiovascular disease: tracing the steps from Framingham. *Prog Cardiovasc Dis* 2010;53:39–44.

79. Ninomiya T, Algert C, Arima H, *et al*. Effects of different regimens to lower blood pressure on major cardiovascular events in older and younger adults: meta-analysis of randomised trials. Blood Pressure Lowering Treatment Trialists' Collaboration. *BMJ* 2008;336:1121–1123.

80. Dahlöf B, Sever PS, Poulter NR, *et al.*; ASCOT Investigators. Prevention of cardiovascular events with an antihypertensive regimen of amlodipine adding perindopril as required versus atenolol adding bendroflumethiazide as required, in the Anglo-Scandinavian Cardiac Outcomes Trial-Blood Pressure Lowering Arm (ASCOT-BPLA): a multicentre randomised controlled trial. *Lancet* 2005;366:895–906.

81. Goldstein JL, Brown MS. Progress in understanding the LDL receptor and HMG-CoA reductase, two membrane proteins that regulate the plasma cholesterol. *J Lipid Res* 1984;25:1450–1461.

82. Keys A, Menotti A, Aravanis C, *et al*. The seven countries study: 2,289 deaths in 15 years. *Prev Med* 1984;13:141–154.

83. Frick MH, Elo O, Haapa K, Heinonen OP, *et al*. Helsinki Heart Study: primary-prevention trial with gemfibrozil in middle-aged men with dyslipidemia. Safety of treatment, changes in risk factors, and incidence of coronary heart disease. *N Engl J Med* 1987;317:1237–1245.

84. Endo A. The discovery and development of HMG-CoA reductase inhibitors. *J Lipid Res* 1992;33:1569–1582.
85. Scandinavian Simvastatin Survival Study Investigators. Randomised trial of cholesterol lowering in 4444 patients with coronary heart disease: the Scandinavian Simvastatin Survival Study (4S). *Lancet* 1994;344:1383–1389.
86. Baigent C, Keech A, Kearney PM, *et al.*; Cholesterol Treatment Trialists' (CTT) Collaborators. Efficacy and safety of cholesterol-lowering treatment: prospective meta-analysis of data from 90,056 participants in 14 randomised trials of statins. *Lancet* 2005; 366:1267–1278.
87. Data on Cardiovascular disease 2012. www.who.int
88. ISIS-1 Collaborative Group. Randomised trial of intravenous atenolol among 16 027 cases of suspected acute myocardial infarction: ISIS-1. First International Study of Infarct Survival Collaborative Group. *Lancet* 1986;2:57–66.
89. The MIAMI Trial Research Group.Metoprolol in acute myocardial infarction (MIAMI). A randomised placebo-controlled international trial. *Eur Heart J* 1985;6:199–226.
90. ISIS-2 Collaborative Group. Randomised trial of intravenous streptokinase, oral aspirin, both, or neither among 17,187 cases of suspected acute myocardial infarction: ISIS-2. ISIS-2 (Second International Study of Infarct Survival) Collaborative Group. *Lancet* 1988;2:349–360.
91. GISSI Investigators. Effectiveness of intravenous thrombolytic treatment in acute myocardial infarction. Gruppo Italiano per lo Studio della Streptochinasi nell'Infarto Miocardico (GISSI). *Lancet* 1986;1:397–402.
92. Sørensen JT, Terkelsen CJ, Nørgaard BL, *et al.* Urban and rural implementation of prehospital diagnosis and direct referral for primary percutaneous coronary intervention in patients with acute ST-elevation myocardial infarction. *Eur Heart J* 2011;32:430–436.
93. Peto R, Collins R, Gray R. Large-scale randomized evidence: large, simple trials and overviews of trials. *J Clin Epidemiol* 1995;48:23–40.
94. Peto R, Pike MC, Armitage P, *et al.* Design and analysis of randomized clinical trials requiring prolonged observation of each patient. I. Introduction and design. *Br J Cancer* 1976;34:585–612.
95. Peto R, Pike MC, Armitage P, *et al.* Design and analysis of randomized clinical trials requiring prolonged observation of each patient. II. analysis and examples. *Br J Cancer* 1977;35:1–39.
96. Grouin JM, Coste M, Lewis J. Subgroup analyses in randomized clinical trials: statistical and regulatory issues. *J Biopharm Stat* 2005;15:869–882.
97. Hlatky MA, Owens DK, Sanders GD. Cost-effectiveness as an outcome in randomized clinical trials. *Clin Trials* 2006;3:543–551.
98. Beach JE. Clinical trials integrity: a CRO perspective. *Account Res* 2001;8:245–260.
99. Shuchman M. Commercializing Clinical Trials—Risks and Benefits of the CRO Boom. *N Engl J Med* 2007;357:1365–1368.
100. Morin K, Rakatansky H, Riddick FA Jr, *et al.* Managing conflicts of interest in the conduct of clinical trials. *JAMA* 2002;287:78–84.
101. Goldenberg NA, Spyropoulos AC, Halperin JL, *et al.*; Antithrombotic Trials Leadership and Steering Group. Improving academic leadership and oversight in large industry-sponsored clinical trials: the ARO-CRO model. *Blood* 2011;117:2089–2092.
102. Turer AT, Mahaffey KW, Compton KL, Califf RM, Schulman KA. Publication or presentation of results from multicenter clinical trials: evidence from an academic medical center. *Am Heart J* 2007;153:674–680.
103. Neaton JD, Babiker A, Bohnhorst M, *et al.* Regulatory impediments jeopardizing the conduct of clinical trials in Europe funded by the National Institutes of Health. *Clin Trials* 2010;7:705–718.

104. Halpern SD, Karlawish JH, Berlin JA. The continuing unethical conduct of underpowered clinical trials. *JAMA* 2002;288:358–362.

105. Tsuji K, Tsutani K. Approval of new drugs 1999-2007: comparison of the US, the EU and Japan situations. *J Clin Pharm Ther* 2010;35:289–301.

106. Moher D, Schulz KF, Altman DG. The CONSORT statement: revised recommendations for improving the quality of reports of parallel-group randomized trials. *Ann Intern Med* 2001;134:657–662.

CHAPTER 2

Publishing results of clinical trials and reviewing papers for publication

Tobias Geisler[1] and Marcus D. Flather[2]
[1]University Hospital Tübingen, Tübingen Medical School, Tübingen, Germany
[2]University of East Anglia and Norfolk and Norwich University Hospital, Norwich, UK

General considerations

Writing a scientific article is a way to communicate results of clinical trials to health professionals, researchers, and healthcare providers. It is important to consider the publication policy in the planning phase of a clinical trial, including authorship, contents of the primary publication, and analysis plan. In 2005, the International Committee of Medical Journal Editors (ICMJE) agreed that clinical trials will only be considered for publication if they have been entered into a recognized clinical trials registry [1]. This approach enables the study design and aims to be publicly available, ensures greater transparency of trials, and helps to avoid publication bias by recording trials that are completed but unpublished. In addition, the Food and Drug Administration Modernization Act (FDAMA) requires that notice of a qualifying trial be submitted to http://clinicaltrials.gov/ no later than 21 days after the trial is opened for enrolment. A recent survey shows that *a priori* registration of clinical trials is gradually increasing [2]. The ICMJE accepts publications from studies registered with the following databases:

- National registry of Australia and New Zealand ANZCTR (www.actr.org.au)
- The Dutch trialregister.nl
- The Japanese registry UMIN-CTR (umin.ac.jp)
- The American ClinicalTrials.gov
- The international registry ISRCTN.org

There is an obligation to publish results of clinical trials even if the outcome is unfavorable as these may have an important impact on patient treatment and planning of future trials. By publishing their results, authors commit to certain general rules, including originality of the data, genuine authorship contributions, ethical principles for clinical trials, and disclosure of any potential conflicts of interest. Publication is also a key element of career advancement, and the ability to write clearly and concisely is a necessary attribute of the academic clinician. We recommend that the phrase "write for the reader" should be remembered at all stages of the manuscript preparation process. Some modify this phrase to "write for the reviewer," but the end result of clarity, brevity, and novelty should be present in all scientific reports of clinical trials.

The method of reporting results of randomized clinical trials (RCTs) has a major impact on the understanding of the trial's design, study conduct, analysis, interpretation, and assessment of the validity of results. The Consolidated Standards of Reporting Trials (CONSORT) initiative has been founded to develop common standards and recommendations to avoid problems arising from inadequate reporting of RCTs [3]. This group has developed a 25-point checklist (Table 2.1) [4].

Even though most scientific journals provide a web-based submission process and offer online services and access to articles, the format of scientific articles has remained largely unchanged for many years and is standardized for most types of articles. A scientific paper should adhere to the following format: authorship, title (including an optional running title), short abstract (usually no more than 250 words), and manuscript body consisting of introduction, methods, results, discussion, brief conclusion, references, and tables and figures. Key issues for each section are discussed below.

Authorship

There are generally no restrictions on the number of coauthors stated on a manuscript. Authors should only be included on a paper if they have made a genuine contribution; not because of their reputation. A "true" author will have made an important contribution to the study design, data acquisition, and/or analysis and interpretation of data. Each author should have participated to a sufficient degree in the manuscript preparation to be accountable for substantial parts of the content. All authors should have a significant involvement in drafting the article or revising it critically for important intellectual content and formatting. It is essential that all authors receive the opportunity to approve the final version of the manuscript. The study group has to appoint a lead or "first" author who will normally be responsible for preparing the first draft of the manuscript and subsequent revisions. The lead author will also take responsibility for the integrity of the data on behalf of the group. Journals ask for a corresponding author who is often the lead author and acts as the point of contact for all correspondence relating to the article prior to and after publication. The last position on the author list is conventionally taken by the "senior author," usually someone who has provided substantial guidance to the trial, analysis, and writing of the paper. However, this order is not mandatory and there are national differences in listing authors on a scientific paper.

Table 2.1 Checklist for reporting randomized clinical trials according to CONSORT recommendations (2010). (Reproduced from Schulz *et al.* [4] with permission from BMJ Publishing Group Ltd.)

Section/topic	Item number	Checklist item
Title and abstract		
	1a	Identification as a randomized trial in the title
	1b	Structured summary of trial design, methods, results, and conclusions (for specific guidance see CONSORT for abstracts)
Introduction		
Background and objectives	2a	Scientific background and explanation of rationale
	2b	Specific objectives or hypotheses
Methods		
Trial design	3a	Description of trial design (such as parallel, factorial), including allocation ratio
	3b	Important changes to methods after trial commencement (such as eligibility criteria), with reasons
Participants	4a	Eligibility criteria for participants
	4b	Settings and locations where the data were collected
Interventions	5	Interventions for each group with sufficient detail to allow replication, including how and when they were actually administered
Outcomes	6a	Completely defined prespecified primary and secondary outcome measures, including how and when they were assessed
	6b	Any changes to trial outcomes after the trial commenced, with reasons
Sample size	7a	How sample size was determined
	7b	When applicable, explanation of any interim analyses and stopping guidelines
Randomization:		
Sequence generation	8a	Method used to generate the random allocation sequence
	8b	Type of randomization; details of any restriction (such as blocking and block size)

Table 2.1 (*continued*)

Section/topic	Item number	Checklist item
Allocation concealment mechanism	9	Mechanism used to implement the random allocation sequence (such as sequentially numbered containers), describing any steps taken to conceal the sequence until interventions were assigned
Implementation	10	Who generated the random allocation sequence, who enrolled participants, and who assigned participants to interventions
Blinding	11a	If done, who was blinded after assignment to interventions (e.g., participants, care providers, those assessing outcomes) and how
	11b	If relevant, description of the similarity of interventions
Statistical methods	12a	Statistical methods used to compare groups for primary and secondary outcomes
	12b	Methods for additional analyses, such as subgroup analyses and adjusted analyses
Results		
Participant flow (a diagram is strongly recommended)	13a	For each group, the numbers of participants who were randomly assigned, received intended treatment, and were analysed for the primary outcome
	13b	For each group, losses and exclusions after randomization, together with reasons
Recruitment	14a	Dates defining the periods of recruitment and follow-up
	14b	Why the trial ended or was stopped
Baseline data	15	A table showing baseline demographic and clinical characteristics for each group
Numbers analyzed	16	For each group, number of participants (denominator) included in each analysis and whether the analysis was by original assigned groups
Outcomes and estimation	17a	For each primary and secondary outcome, results for each group, and the estimated effect size and its precision (such as 95% confidence interval)
	17b	For binary outcomes, presentation of both absolute and relative effect sizes is recommended

(*continued*)

Table 2.1 (*continued*)

Section/topic	Item number	Checklist item
Ancillary analyses	18	Results of any other analyses performed, including subgroup analyses and adjusted analyses, distinguishing pre-specified from exploratory
Harms	19	All important harms or unintended effects in each group (for specific guidance see CONSORT for harms)
Discussion		
Limitations	20	Trial limitations, addressing sources of potential bias, imprecision, and, if relevant, multiplicity of analyses
Generalizability	21	Generalizability (external validity, applicability) of the trial findings
Interpretation	22	Interpretation consistent with results, balancing benefits and harms, and considering other relevant evidence
Other information		
Registration	23	Registration number and name of trial registry
Protocol	24	Where the full trial protocol can be accessed, if available
Funding	25	Sources of funding and other support (such as supply of drugs), role of funders

Title

The title should ideally describe the main design and main impact of the article in a short phrase or sentence of no more than 15 words. Some journals and reviewers prefer to avoid titles that leave the interpretation of the main study outcome open (like "Evaluation of . . . ", "Study of . . . ") and instead summarize the main study result in one sentence. A short running title, normally not exceeding 50 letters, is demanded by some journals. Including the study design in the title is helpful for the reader.

Manuscript structure

The manuscript body is composed of the introduction, methods, results, and discussion/conclusions (IMRAD acronym [5]). This is a commonly accepted order and has been adopted by most scientific journals (Figure 2.1) [6]. Some journals prefer slight modifications of the section order or ask for the provision of detailed sections as supplementary material. The main sec-

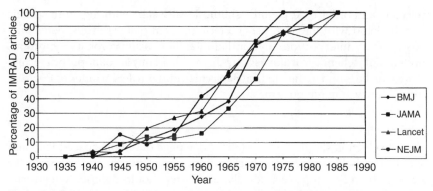

Figure 2.1 Gradual increase in the prevalence of adoption of the IMRAD structure of scientific reports in major journals from 1935 to 1985 (n = 1297). (Reproduced from Sollaci LB and Pereira MG [6].)

tions should aim to answer individual questions, as formulated by Bradford Hill in 1965 [7]:

- Why did you start? (Introduction)
- What did you do? (Methods)
- What did you find? (Results)
- What does it mean? (Discussion).

It is useful to answer the additional question, "What are you going to do about it?" in the discussion section.

Abstract

The abstract is very important as it can interest potential readers; in many cases it is the only part of the paper that is read or accessible as it is retrievable in public electronic databases like PubMed/MEDLINE, Web of Science, Scopus, or Google Scholar. Additionally, up to 65% of the editors' decision to reject or accept a manuscript for review is based on the abstract, and some editors (15–25%) only read the abstract [8–9]. The abstract should be able to "stand alone" and thus should not contain any references, tables or figures. Structured abstracts should be organized according to the IMRAD principle, but there are variations in the section headings from one journal to another (e.g., "background," "aims," or "research setting" may be the preferred title of the first section). Authors are encouraged to check with the particular journal of interest. Structured abstracts should usually not exceed 250 words. Some journals require unstructured abstracts of 150 words or less. The abstract should be concise and the novel aspects of the clinical trial must be made clear to the reader. It should contain essential information about the purpose of the research project, the study design, patient selection, analytical methods, main results, and principal conclusions and clinical implications. Most journals ask for key words (three to six) that aid in searching electronic databases. The selection and order of key words should ideally start with the more specific term and end with the most general term (i.e., antiplatelet drugs, percutaneous coronary intervention, myocardial infarction, acute coronary syndrome, myocardial ischemia, cardiovascular diseases). Examples of appropriate keywords can be found in the Medical Subject Headings (MeSH) index of PubMed (http://www.nlm.nih.gov/mesh).

Introduction

The introduction should be brief (about one page of double-spaced text) and should precisely describe the background, unmet needs, and rationale for starting the research project. Ideally, the writer should describe the specific hypothesis the research project aims to test. It should contain the essential information needed to understand the scientific background to the research project by citing pertinent references and should not go into too much detail (thus avoiding "textbook style," which can be very descriptive).

Methods

The methods section describes the methodological approaches used (including study design, tests and investigations, and statistical analysis). Editors and reviewers will classify the quality of the work mainly by evaluation of the methodology used. A good scientific report can reveal negative or poor results even though appropriate methods have been used, but positive results are rarely reliable if high quality methods have not been used. Therefore, writers should ensure their studies are properly designed and that the methods are presented clearly. Subheadings are recommended within this section, e.g., trial design, ethical considerations and approvals, patient selection, trial procedures, definition of endpoints, and statistical analysis.

Description of study design

Information about specific design issues for RCTs should include:
• Outcomes of interest: efficacy versus effectiveness versus safety
• Hypothesis testing approach: superiority versus non-inferiority versus equivalence
• Randomization and blinding methods: placebo-controlled, active comparator, balanced (1:1) vs. imbalanced (1:n), blinded versus unblinded[#]
• Treatment groups: parallel versus multi-arm parallel, crossover, cluster, or factorial designs
• Setting of the trial: mono- versus multi-center
• Phase of the study (1–4) if appropriate.

[#]The 2010 CONSORT recommendation encourages authors and editors not to differentiate between single- and multiple-blind designs; instead authors should report who was blinded after assignment to interventions (e.g., participants, care providers, outcomes assessors) and how blinding was performed [10].

Patient selection

To understand the selection process in RCTs and to give transparency to any selection bias, a standardized flow diagram is nowadays required by many journals. An example of a flow diagram according to the CONSORT recommendation is provided in Figure 1.2 [4].

Ethical issues

Journals require clear statements about ethical approvals and provision of informed consent, which should be described in the methods section. Adequate disclosure of potential conflicts of interests is also required and is usually considered an ethical issue, although this would usually be inserted at the end of the manuscript. Clinical trials involving investigational products should adhere to the Good Clinical Practice guidelines agreed by the International Conference on Harmonisation (ICH) of Technical Requirements for Registration of Pharmaceuticals for Human Use. Some journals require a particular statement within the submission process or included in the manuscript. It is important to make clear the role of any funding sponsors in the design, data collection, analysis, and publication of data, and whether any approval was required before submission.

Statistical issues

The primary and secondary efficacy and safety endpoints and the rationale underlying the hypotheses for non-inferiority and/or superiority need to be described for randomized trials. Usually, endpoint analysis is described in a separate paragraph integrated in the methods section under the heading "Statistical methods." The section describing statistical methodology should include the sample size estimation (estimated effects size, statistical power, and alpha level) and all statistical tests used to test the main hypothesis as well as any other secondary analysis. Tests that have been applied to compare variables between groups should be specified (e.g., Fisher-Exact test for categorical variables, t-test, Mann–Whitney-U test for continuous variables). A description of any multivariate and regression analyses (i.e., assumptions of linearity and proportional hazards) or survival analyses should be described, including the variables entered in the models.

Results, tables, and figures

The results section can be divided into a description of patient enrolment, completeness of follow-up, compliance with treatment, primary efficacy results, secondary efficacy results, and safety issues. Results should be reported in an objective manner and any interpretation of the data should be avoided at this stage. Each result must be linked to the analytical method used to derive it. The key results should be presented in tables or figures, which need to be presented in numerical order and appropriately cited within the text. Tables are usually preferred to summarize large numerical information of prevalence and effect size in subgroups, e.g., patient demographics. It is advisable not to overload tables with too much information. Redundant presentation of the same information in both table and figure format should be avoided. The choice of figure type is mainly based on the type of statistical analysis. For example, scatterplots can be used to show the correlation of two different variables, bar diagrams for analysis of means, box plots for analysis of medians, Kaplan–Meier curves for survival analysis, and Forest plots for description of multiple treatment effects in meta-analyses or subgroup analyses of RCTs. Effect sizes of the treatment in clinical trials should be reported (or at least sufficient information should be provided to compute them) as they will help to design future studies in the same area and serve as a basis for sample size and power calculations. Journals usually limit the number of tables and figures; in general, four tables and three figures are considered standard.

Discussion

This section offers the possibility to discuss the results in the light of previous publications in the same field. By reading the discussion the reader should be informed whether, from the authors' point of view, the assumed hypothesis was confirmed or rejected, or which main hypothesis was created on the basis of the result. The discussion should go beyond description of previous research activities in this field as presented in the introduction by comparing the current trial results point by point with previous reports. Authors should also declare the limitations of the study, including an evaluation of analytical methods and study design. Following this, an outlook about future unmet needs should be provided to stimulate further research and to address the issues unresolved by the current research. A discussion about the clinical importance of the findings is helpful and informs the reader about the implications for clinical practice. A short summary of the main study results and their implications should be given at the end of the discussion. The structure of the discussion can be summarized in four sections (no more than four pages of double-spaced text):
• Summary of main new findings (short paragraph)
• How do these new findings fit with previous research (place your research into context)?
• Limitations of the study
• Conclusions (including clinical impact) and implications for future research.
    The second section of the Discussion should follow the order of presentation in the Results section, focusing on the new findings of interest.

Database searches

The most frequently used databases are PubMed, Scopus, Web of Science, and Google Scholar. Each database offers several search facilities. Although specific databases like PubMed, Scopus and Web of Science provide a broad, up-to-date and efficient search interface, it has become more and more demanding to quickly identify essential information, owing mainly to the steadily increasing body of biomedical literature. Thus, users are often challenged by extensive lists of search results: over one-third of PubMed queries result in 100 or more citations. As a consequence, the National Center for Biotechnology Information (NCBI) has made attempts to enhance standard PubMed searches by suggesting more specific queries [11,12]. Google Scholar, Scopus, and Web of Science offer rating of articles by citation index, which can serve as a relative parameter for the importance of the article. Scopus is limited to articles published after 1995. PubMed and Google Scholar offer free access, whereas Scopus and Web of Science require licenses liable to charges [13]. Many universities have an arrangement with Science Direct to provide free articles to their members using the individual's university log in.

References

Citation of references is essential to back-up statements and to refer to specific methodological approaches. Style of citation of original articles should follow the particular journal requirement. There are two main styles of citing. The Harvard style cites the first author and publication year in the manuscript text, and usually provides a reference index in alphabetical order and order according to publication year at the end of the manuscript. In contrast, the numbered reference style (Vancouver style) enumerates references within the text in order of their appearance. The numbers are then linked to a reference index at the end of the manuscript. Format of references (i.e., numbers of cited authors, position of publication year, etc.) varies among the different journals, but most frequently follows the following examples:

• Original article citation: Seaman AJ, Griswold HE, Reaume RB, Ritzmann L. Long-term anticoagulant prophylaxis after myocardial infarction. *N Engl J Med.* 1969;281(3):115–9.

• Book citations: Libby P, Bonow RO, Mann DL, Zipes DP, eds. *Braunwald's Heart Disease: A Textbook of Cardiovascular Medicine.* 8th ed. Saunders, 2007.

Thirty references is a reasonable maximum for most manuscripts for publication and should include the most up-to-date literature.

Reviewing a submitted article for a journal

The following section will focus on the peer review of scientific manuscripts, but many of the principles can be applied also to the review of research grant proposals and books. Although peer review can slow down the publication process, it represents the basis for a good scientific report and peer-reviewed articles are usually considered to be of a higher scientific standard than non–peer-reviewed articles [14]. It is an honor to be invited to be a peer reviewer because this recognizes the reviewer as an expert in the particular field and offers him/her the possibility of being updated on current research activities by groups working in the same or a similar scientific field. Peer review is considered a duty to the rest of the scientific community and may be undertaken without remuneration. Some journals provide an open peer review system, which offers the authors knowledge of who has reviewed their work and provides more transparency, but has the potential to limit honest criticism. In a randomized trial to evaluate the effects of open peer review, identification of reviewers did not influence the quality of the review, the recommendation for publication, or the time taken for the review; however, it significantly increased the likelihood of reviewers declining to review [15].

Most journals commission two experts to review the manuscript, but up to six reviewers can be assigned. Some editors circulate all comments to each individual reviewer, which allows a comparison of her/his own comments with those of others and in general improves the individual reviewing technique. The quality of critical reviews varies widely, not only among journals but also within a particular journal. Writing a good review is challenging and time consuming. Reviews need to be brief and provide constructive comments to the authors in a systematic fashion with the main aim of improving the manuscript. There are some checklists available that can be used to systematically detect lapses in a manuscript [16]. However, they are rarely applied in practice. Most journals ask the reviewer to declare any competing interest that might relate to the manuscript. Potential reviewers who have a bias against the author or author group should not accept the invitation to review the manuscript from the competing group. It is also the reviewer's duty to report any suspected plagiarism.

The following suggestions give some idea of the approach, structure, and elements of a scientific review. The tone of the review should always be constructive, even if the manuscript is poorly written or the reviewer does not agree with the correctness of the results or the way they are presented. Journal editors usually screen out poor articles which are then not distributed for peer review. In general, journals offer the possibility to submit separate, confidential comments to the editors which can address these concerns. "A detailed appraisal for the author . . . should be divided into major and minor comments, with annotations given according to page and paragraph" (*The Lancet*). Comments should be concise and an individual review should probably be about 250 words or less. The comments should in particular address the adequacy of the choice of study type and methods, including statistical methods to draw conclusions from the results, the novelty and generalizability of the results, and the integrity of the data. The editorial team may also point out journal-specific formatting issues. It is recommended to focus on different major aspects in at least two subsequent reading steps. In the first step, the reviewer might focus on trying to understand the main scientific question and getting an idea of the main hypothesis and the study design. Also, obvious problems with the science, methodology, presentation, and ethics should be formulated. On the first reading, open questions should be noted in the text and their explanation should be checked in the context of the whole content of the manuscript at the second reading. Some journals like the *British Medical Journal* offer checklists and online training packages to guide reviewers to good and systematic scientific review (e.g., http://resources.bmj.com/bmj/reviewers/training-materials). The main quality aspects to evaluate in a scientific manuscript are given in Table 2.2.

Table 2.2 Considerations for reviewing a submitted article for a journal (from *BMJ* guidance for reviewers, http://resources.bmj.com/bmj/reviewers/peer-reviewers-guidance).

Main quality issues	Questions used to judge quality
Integrity of the data and novelty of the results	Does the work add enough to what is already in the published literature? If so, what does it add?
Generalizability	Does this work matter to clinicians, researchers, policymakers, educators, or patients? Can the results be applied to more general populations? Is the size and complexity of study interventions representative for general health environments?
Appropriateness of the study design	Is the overall design of the study appropriate and adequate to answer the research question? Is the patient selection correct and appropriate?
Scientific value of hypothesis and validity of study results	Is a research question clearly defined and appropriately answered? Are there flaws in the randomization process? Is the treatment compliance adequate?
Adequateness of methods	Are the methods sufficiently described? Are the methods appropriate and presented in a clear way to allow the results to be reproduced? Is the main outcome measure clear? Are randomized trials, systematic reviews, observational studies, health economics studies reported in line with the appropriate reporting statement or checklist (available at http://www.equator-network.org/)?
Ethical issues, plagiarism, publication fraud	Was the study ethical (this may go beyond simply whether the study was approved by an ethics committee or IRB)? If the research involved human subjects, was the study performed in accordance with the Declaration of Helsinki? Have substantial parts of the manuscript or the study results been published elsewhere by the same author group (duplicate submission) or by a different author group (plagiarism)?
Language style, formatting, and presentation of the data	Is the language style adequate, concise and clear enough to be understood by the addressed readership? Is the title of the manuscript clear and adequate to describe the main result of the manuscript? Are figures presented in a sufficient quality (e.g., adequate resolution, sharp text in annotations of graph axes, distinct coloring of curves)? Are tables clearly arranged and condense, without redundant information?
Adequateness of citation	Are citations in the correct format as required by the journal? Is the order of authors, title and publication details correct? Are the results of cited references adequately interpreted?

Integrity of the data and novelty of the results

The reviewer should determine the importance of the hypothesis being tested and how well the study tests this hypothesis. In an analysis of 529 publications widely cited as evidence for a change in medical practice or cardiorespiratory medicine and surgery, about 40% did not in fact give results that have subsequently proved to be important in diagnosis or therapy [17]. Even if results are negative they may generate a novel hypothesis that deserves further investigation.

Generalizability

Generalizability is the validity of applying study results to other patient populations and whether they can be translated to the routine clinical setting. Limited generalizability should not be a principal criterion to decline a manuscript; however, it should be adequately acknowledged as a limitation of the manuscript. Evaluation of generalizability of results of RCTs demands a careful review of eligibility criteria, study setting and procedures, and main outcome measure. Of note, the healthcare environment and treatment compliance presented in clinical trials should be applied to general populations with caution (external validity). The size of a study population and the complexity of treatment additionally influence the generalizability of results. Hence, larger trials of less complex treatment interventions can be transferred more easily than small studies of more complex interventions [18].

Appropriateness of the study design

Randomized trials generally test specific hypotheses, but the results inevitably generate new hypotheses to be tested. For a hypothesis to be tested, the study must be adequately powered (sufficient number of outcome events). However, if a study is hypothesis confirmative, it will generally be better designed and better powered than previous studies dealing with a similar research question.

Scientific value of hypothesis and validity study results

The scientific value of a study is mainly based on the importance of the question being addressed and the clartity and reliability of the results. The reviewer needs to evaluate if the methods are described sufficiently clearly to allow for internal validation of the study results, i.e., whether the study has been conducted appropriately and to a high standard. If the results are unclear, the reviewer must judge whether the study was designed poorly, or analysis of data was poor. These defects usually mean that the manuscript is not acceptable for publication [19].

Adequateness of methods

The methods section is the most important indicator of the quality of the manuscript; it should provide a blueprint for readers to be able to reproduce the study. Therefore, the reviewer should pay particular attention to the methodology being used to generate the results, and to the completeness and clarity of the description of the methods.

Ethical issues, plagiarism, and publication fraud

Reviewers need to check for statements in the manuscript about appropriate ethical and regulatory approvals. The clinical trial registration number should be provided and the study should have been registered before enrolment of the first patient.

Publication fraud may encompass duplicate publication and plagiarism [20]. Plagiarism is the adoption of major parts of a published scientific paper or identical study design by another author groups. As the number of scientific publications continues to increase worldwide, so has the number of duplicate publications and plagiarism, although the rate of duplicate scientific manuscripts varies between countries (Figure 2.2) [20].

Journals usually demand a separate statement of unique submission by the authors. Programs like eTBLAST exist to check for duplicity of parts of the manuscript, but these are currently not applied as a matter of routine [21]. Unethical duplicity of publication does not include updates of clinical trials or longitudinal cohort studies that provide new data.

Language style, formatting, and presentation of data

Figures should clearly describe important study results, be of adequate quality, and not contain too much information. They should depict one key message rather than multiple results. Different styles of figures can be applied (e.g., graphs, diagrams, Forest plots), but there are some favorite figure styles depending on the results (i.e., box plots and interquartile ranges for comparisons of non-parametric data; bar diagrams and standard deviation/error for parametric data comparison). Legends should clearly describe the key result in one or two sentences rather than using non-specific formulations (i.e., "Figure x: Comparison of parameter A with parameter B").

Adequateness of citation

Citation of references is frequently a major flaw as either the references are in the wrong format or the order of authors, title or publication details is incorrect. Additionally, references can be misinterpreted in the context of the study results. Usually, the reviewers do not have sufficient time to screen every reference or check the key results of every publication for correct interpretation. Thus, it is recommended to make some general check of references.

Recommendation to accept or decline the manuscript

It is up to the journal editor to accept or decline a manuscript for publication, but reviewers have a major influence on this process. The reviewer should be aware of his/her role as an advisor and many journals ask the reviewer to give a preliminary recommendation. The decision can be categorized into five types:
- Immediate rejection
- Authors may resubmit as a new manuscript (major revisions needed)
- Editorial invitation to resubmit with major revision

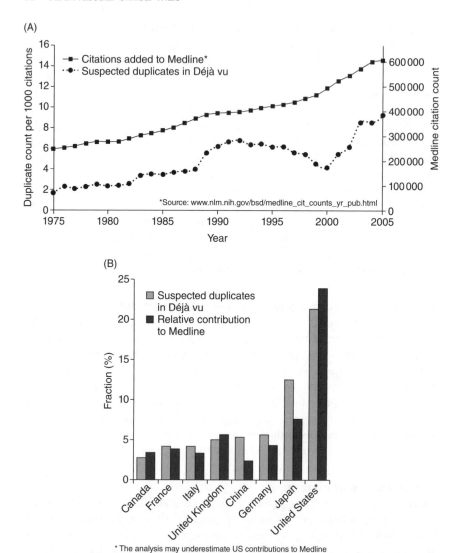

Figure 2.2 Trends of duplicate biomedical publications throughout the last decades (A) and nationwide distribution (B). (Reproduced from Errami M, Garner H [21], with permission.)

- Provisionally accept with minor revisions
- Final acceptance.

Many journals circulate all the reviewers' comments to all reviewers, and this is a useful way to check the consistency of your own review with others, and also to see if your review agrees with the Editor's decision to accept or reject a manuscript. Overall, the review process is an important method of quality assurance which requires the dedication and time of those involved.

References

1. De Angelis C, Drazen JM, Frizelle FA, *et al.* Clinical trial registration: a statement from the International Committee of Medical Journal Editors. *Ann Intern Med* 2004;141: 477–478.
2. Reveiz L, Krleza-Jerić K, Chan AW, de Aguiar S. Do trialists endorse clinical trial registration? Survey of a Pubmed sample. *Trials* 2007;8:30.
3. Moher D, Schulz KF, Altman DG. The CONSORT statement: revised recommendations for improving the quality of reports of parallel-group randomised trials. *Lancet* 2001;357:1191–1194.
4. Schulz KF, Altman DG, Moher D, for the CONSORT Group. CONSORT 2010 Statement: updated guidelines for reporting parallel group randomised trials. *BMJ* 2010;340:c332.
5. Huth EJ. Structured abstracts for papers reporting clinical trials. *Ann Intern Med* 1987;106:626–627.
6. Sollaci LB, Pereira MG. The introduction, methods, results, and discussion (IMRAD) structure: a fifty-year survey. *J Med Libr Assoc* 2004;92:364–367.
7. Hill B. The reason for writing. *Br Med J* 1965;2:870.
8. Schroter S, Barratt H. Editorial decision making based on abstracts. *Eur Sci Edit* 2004; 30:8–9.
9. Groves T, Abbasi K. Screening research papers by reading abstracts. *BMJ* 2004; 329:470–471.
10. Moher D, Hopewell S, Schulz KF, *et al.* "CONSORT 2010 explanation and elaboration: updated guidelines for reporting parallel group randomised trials". *BMJ* 2010;340:c869.
11. Lu Z, Wilbur WJ, McEntyre JR, *et al.* Finding query suggestions for PubMed. *AMIA Annu Symp Proc* 2009;2009:396–400.
12. Lu Z. PubMed and beyond: a survey of web tools for searching biomedical literature. *Database (Oxford)* 2011 Jan 18;2011:baq036. Print 2011.
13. Falagas ME, Pitsouni EI, Malietzis GA, Pappas G. Comparison of PubMed, Scopus, Web of Science, and Google Scholar: strengths and weaknesses. *FASEB J* 2008;22:338–342.
14. Armstrong JS. Peer review for journals: Evidence on quality control, fairness, and innovation. *Sci Eng Ethics* 1997;3:63–84.
15. van Rooyen S, Godlee F, Evans S, Black N, Smith R. Effect of open peer review on quality of reviews and on reviewers' recommendations: a randomised trial. *BMJ* 1999;318: 23–27.
16. Seals DR, Tanaka H. Manuscript peer review: a helpful checklist for students and novice referees. *Adv Physiol Educ* 2000;23:52–58.
17. Comroe JH Jr, Dripps RD. Scientific basis for the support of biomedical science. *Science* 1976;192:105–111.
18. Flather M, Delahunty N, Collinson J. Generalizing results of randomized trials to clinical practice: reliability and cautions. *Clin Trials* 2006;3:508–512.
19. Regehr G. Presentation of results. *Acad Med* 2001;76:940–942.
20. DeMaria AN. Duplicate publication: insights into the essence of a medical journal. *J Am Coll Cardiol* 2003;41:516–517.
21. Errami M, Garner H. A tale of two citations. *Nature* 2008;451:397–399.

CHAPTER 3

Management of chronic coronary artery disease

Sabu Thomas[1] and William E. Boden[2]
[1]University of Rochester School of Medicine, Rochester, NY, USA
[2]Albany Medical Center, Albany, NY, USA

Introduction

Ischemic heart disease (IHD) is not only protean in its manifestations but is also rampant in modern society. In the US alone, the prevalence of chronic coronary heart disease (CHD) is estimated at 13 million cases, of which 6.5 million cases represent stable angina pectoris. Chronic stable angina is the major presentation in nearly half of all CHD patients [1,2]. The economic burden of chronic CHD is therefore significant, resulting in estimated annual direct and indirect costs in excess of US$150 billion [3]. Despite the sustained decline in age-specific case fatality rates from coronary artery disease (CAD) over the past several decades, IHD is now the leading cause of death worldwide. It is expected that this rate of rise will continue to accelerate over the coming decade as a consequence of the epidemic rise in obesity, type 2 diabetes, and the metabolic syndrome, which may increase the risk of developing premature CAD in younger generations. The World Health Organization has projected thatthe global number of deaths from CAD will increase by 46% from 7.6 million in 2005 to 11.1 million in 2020.

This chapter will outline the basic categories of CHD, definitions, and pathophysiology, with a particular emphasis on medical and invasive approaches to therapy.

Definition and classification

Stable angina refers to discomfort in the chest, neck, arms, and jaw that is precipitated typically by physical or emotional stress and is relieved by rest or nitroglycerin. It usually occurs in patients with significant obstruction in one or more coronary arteries, but can occur in patients without overt obstruction—in these instances, coronary spasm or variant angina has been

Cardiovascular Clinical Trials: Putting the Evidence into Practice, First Edition.
Edited by Marcus D. Flather, Deepak L. Bhatt, and Tobias Geisler.
© 2013 Blackwell Publishing Ltd. Published 2013 by Blackwell Publishing Ltd.

implicated. Impaired microvascular perfusion due to obstructive plaque can result in a mismatch between myocardial oxygen supply and demand, which contributes to the development and progression of angina [4,5].

Stable angina classically manifests as precordial or substernal chest discomfort that may radiate to the neck or jaw. It usually presents as a sensation of squeezing or heaviness, which lasts up to 15 minutes and abates when the stressor is gone, the patient rests, or the patient uses sublingual nitroglycerin. Anginal equivalents include exertional dyspnea, excessive fatigue, diaphoresis, and fainting, and these are more common in the elderly and female patients. Atypical presentations such as inframammary pain, palpitations or sharp stabbing pain are more common in females as well. Diabetic patients may present with atypical pain, dyspnea or even no symptoms at all. Often, angina is described incorrectly as "chest pain." The term "angina," however, derives from a neologism of two Latin words "*angor animi,*" which literally translates as "fear of life being extinguished," according to Heberden's original description in 1768. Had Heberden been trying to convey the term "chest pain," he would more likely have used the Latin term "*dolor pectoris.*"

Almost 40 years ago, Campeau published a functional classification system to stratify the severity of angina pectoris, which became widely known and accepted as the Canadian Cardiovascular Society (CCS) angina grading scale. Angina severity is classified on this ordinal scale from I to IV (Table 3.1) [5,6]. Angina pectoris on this scale ranges from mild (class I: angina occurring only during strenuous or prolonged physical activity) to severe (class IV: inability to perform any activity without angina, or angina at rest) and includes the full spectrum of angina from "chronic stable" to "unstable." This system of grading the severity of angina pectoris has gained widespread clinical acceptance, most notably because of its simplicity.

Pathophysiology

An imbalance between the oxygen demands of the myocardium during exertion and the reduced coronary blood flow due to stenosed epicardial coronary arteries is the principal factor resulting in angina pectoris in CHD

Table 3.1 Canadian Cardiovascular Society Classification of Angina Pectoris. (Reproduced from Campeau [92] with permission from Wolters Kluwer Health.)

Classification	Description
Class I	No angina with ordinary physical activity Angina with prolonged and more than usual exertion
Class II	Early onset-limitation of ordinary activity
Class III	Marked limitation of ordinary activity even when walking one to two blocks
Class IV	Angina at rest/inability to carry out physical activity without chest discomfort

[7]. Adrenergic stresses from physical or emotional stimuli or infection can result in increases in heart rate and subsequently lead to increases in demand ischemia and angina. Coronary blood flow is the most important determinant of myocardial oxygen supply. Numerous factors influence the epicardial and subendocardial blood flow. Limitations on blood flow may be due to atherosclerosis in either the epicardial coronary arteries or microvasculature. As atherosclerosis progresses, there is progressive plaque deposition in the wall of the artery. As atherosclerosis worsens, the plaque may cause hemodynamic obstruction to coronary blood flow and this can result in angina [8]. Stenoses of less than 70–80% may not cause spontaneous or exercise-induced angina or ischemia since the microvasculature has the capacity to dilate and increase subendocardial perfusion in response to increasing demand. When stenoses exceed 70% however, downstream dilation is maximized and this can trigger spontaneous or exercise-induced angina episodes 25–30 seconds after the onset of the ischemic cascade [9]. Approximately half of all stable CAD patients experience episodes of silent myocardial ischemia and these are particularly prevalent in patients with diabetes [9].

Medical management of myocardial ischemia

Lifestyle changes

Intensive multifactorial risk reduction has been shown to reduce the rate of coronary luminal narrowing and decrease hospitalizations for cardiac events [10]. A diet low in saturated fat and with appropriate restriction of carbohydrate consumption is encouraged [1]. Epidemiological studies have also consistently demonstrated the benefits associated with modest alcohol intake, which may lower the likelihood of developing coronary events and reduce the progression of CAD [1]. Smoking cessation and weight control should be encouraged in all patients [1]. In diabetic patients, achieving a glycosylated hemoglobin (HbA1C) of less than 7% with good control of blood pressure (<140/80 mmHg) may reduce the rates of secondary events [1]. Regular exercise is encouraged and can promote ischemic preconditioning, which can provide additional protection during recurring bouts of ischemia. A trial comparing percutaneous coronary intervention (PCI) with graded regular aerobic exercise in patients with single-vessel CAD showed that 20 minutes of daily exercise was associated with improved maximal myocardial oxygen uptake, lower costs, and fewer rehospitalizations for angina pectoris as compared with PCI during 1-year follow-up [11]. All patients should be encouraged to participate in a comprehensive cardiac rehabilitation program.

Antiplatelet agents

In high-risk patients, the use of aspirin was associated with a significantly reduced risk (by 22%) of non-fatal myocardial infarction (MI), stroke, and vascular death [12]. Long-term aspirin at a dose of 81–325 mg is recommended in all patients with stable angina who do not have evidence of aspirin resistance or allergy [1]. In the case of true aspirin allergy, clopidogrel is recommended. In the CAPRIE (Clopidogrel versus Aspirin in Patients at Risk of Ischaemic Events) study, the use of clopidogrel alone was associated with an 8.7% relative reduction in vascular death, ischemic stroke, and MI [13]. The use of dual antiplatelet therapy with aspirin (75–162 mg daily) and clopidogrel (75 mg daily) was not significantly more effective than aspirin alone, as demonstrated in the CHARISMA (Clopidogrel for High Atherothrombotic Risk and Ischemic Stabilization, Management, and Avoidance) trial which looked at a composite endpoint of MI, stroke, or death from cardiovascular causes in patients with stable CHD or multiple cardiovascular risk factors [14].

ACE inhibitors

The use of angiotensin converting enzyme inhibitors (ACE-Is) in patients with stable angina and diabetes, previous MI, and evidence of left ventricular (LV) systolic dysfunction (LV ejection fraction [LVEF] <40%) is considered a class IA recommendation [15]. The TREND (Trial on Reversing Endothelial Dysfunction) demonstrated that treatment with quinapril improved endothelial function in patients who did not have severe hyperlipidemia or heart failure [16]. The HOPE (Heart Outcomes Prevention Evaluation) trial showed that ramipril reduced cardiovascular death, MI, and stroke in patients with vascular disease in the absence of heart failure [17]. In contrast, the PEACE (Prevention of Events with ACE inhibition) trial showed that in patients with stable heart disease and preserved LV function receiving standard therapy, the addition of trandolapril added no incremental mortality benefit [18].

Controversy exists over the best ACE-I to use in patients with CAD. It is thought that tissue-specific agents such as quinapril, ramipril, perinopril, and trandolapril may have high lipophilicity and better ACE-binding capacity. Tissue-specific ACE-Is are thought to penetrate the endothelial wall better and achieve better degrees of ACE inhibition that may impede atherogenesis. In patients who cannot tolerate ACE-Is, angiotensin-receptor blockers are thought to be as effective as ACE-Is in high-risk patients [19–21].

Statins

There is an overwhelming breadth of clinical trial data in support of statins for both primary and secondary prevention in stable CAD. These trials have demonstrated the benefit of statins in reducing death, MI, and stroke. The role of statins in these patients continues to evolve with aggressive efforts to lower low density lipoprotein (LDL) levels to less than 70 mg/dL. This is driven by a consistent and positive relationship between LDL cholesterol and the risk of CHD [22]. Statins have been shown to achieve LDL reductions in the range of 30–60%, promote plaque stabilization in acute coronary syndrome (ACS) patients [23], improve endothelial dysfunction, and promote regression of atherosclerotic plaque [24]. The anti-inflammatory effects of statins are reflected in the reduction seen in C-reactive protein (CRP) levels [25]. Intensive (LDL <70 mg/dL) compared with moderate (LDL <100 mg/dL) lipid lowering has been shown to reduce the progression of atherosclerosis not only in native vessels, but also in graft vessels after coronary artery bypass graft (CABG) surgery [26]. Higher doses of statins may increase the incidence of adverse effects and of elevated serum aminotransferases, and increase the risk of muscle injury.

The role of high density lipoprotein-cholesterol (HDL-C) is increasingly being recognized because of the strong inverse relationship between low HDL and the risk of developing cardiac events. Low HDL-C is a strong independent predictor of CHD risk with levels less than 35 mg/dL associated with an eight-fold higher risk than HDL-C greater than 65 mg/dL [27]. Combination therapy with extended-release niacin and a statin offers the best strategy for controlling mixed dyslipidemia with increased LDL and low HDL [28]. Whether niacin reduces the residual risk in patients already at target LDL levels by raising low HDL levels further was studied in the recently published AIM-HIGH (Atherothrombosis Intervention in Metabolic syndrome with low HDL/high triglycerides: impact on Global Health outcomes) trial [29]. Investigators randomized 3414 patients to receive extended-release niacin (1.5–2 g/ day) or placebo in addition to simvastatin, with the option to use ezetimibe to maintain LDL levels between 40 and 80 mg/dL (1.03–2.07 mmol/L). The primary endpoint was a composite of death from CHD, non-fatal MI, ischemic stroke, hospitalization for an ACS, or symptom-driven coronary or cerebral revascularization. The trial was stopped early due to a lack of efficacy. While niacin did increase HDL levels significantly from a median HDL-C of 35 mg/dL (0.91 mmol/L) to 42 mg/dL (1.08 mmol/L), it lowered the triglyceride and LDL-C levels further. There was no significant difference in the occurrence of the primary endpoint in the niacin group compared with the placebo group (HR, 1.02; 95% CI, 0.87–1.21; p = 0.79). Whether clinical event reduction can be demonstrated with niacin and statin therapy must await the results of the ongoing HPS-2 THRIVE (Treatment of HDL to Reduce the Incidence of Vascular Events) trial, which is underway in over 25 000 CHD patients in the UK, China, and Scandinavia, and is scheduled to conclude in 2013. In addition, it remains unclear whether higher risk patients than those enrolled in AIM-HIGH would benefit from combination dyslipidemic therapy with niacin and a statin [30].

Inhibition of cholesterol absorption
Ezetimibe is the first of a class of agents that inhibit the absorption of cholesterol from the intestine [31,32]. When combined with statins, it inhibits both cholesterol synthesis and absorption, resulting in complementary effects that lower LDL-C. This leads to an 18–24% reduction in LDL-C beyond the reduction expected with statins alone [33,34]. Ezetimibe also leads to significantly greater reductions in CRP when combined with statins [25]. Definitive clinical outcomes data are presently lacking until the IMPROVE-IT trial is completed and published.

Beta-blockers

Beta-blockers are given a class IA recommendation for the initial therapy of patients with prior MI [1]. However, the fewer data for patients without a prior MI have led the American College of Cardiology (ACC)/American Heart Association (AHA) to give beta-blockers a class IB recommendation for these patients. Beta-blockers reduce heart rate and contractility, and myocardial oxygen demand. Reduction in heart rate increases diastolic filling time during which the coronaries receive blood flow. This enhances myocardial tissue perfusion. Beta-blockers can be non-selective (e.g., propranolol), selective (e.g., atenolol and metoprolol), have intrinsic sympathomimetic activity (pindolol, acebutolol) or have alpha-blocking properties (labetolol or carvedilol) [35–37]. All beta-blockers have been studied for the treatment of stable angina [38,39]. Beta-blockers have been shown to improve survival in patients with previous MI, primary angioplasty for acute ST elevation MI, and heart failure from LV systolic dysfunction. There are no randomized controlled trials (RCTs) demonstrating survival benefit or reduction in the rates of coronary events in patients with stable angina only. All beta-blockers are equally effective in alleviating angina pectoris, although optimal doses may vary. Important side effects of beta-blockers include: bradycardia, bronchoconstriction, fatigue, depression, impotence, and worsening of peripheral vascular disease. The combination of beta-blockers and nitrates is more effective than either agent alone [40,41].

Calcium channel blockers

Calcium channel blockers promote coronary and peripheral vasodilation by blocking the entry of calcium into the myocardial and vascular smooth muscle cells. Dihydropyridine-type calcium channel blockers (amlodipine, nicardipine, nifedipine) have a greater effect on vascular smooth muscle cells and are particularly effective in reducing systemic arterial blood pressure. Despite earlier concerns, the results of a meta-analysis indicate that the use of these drugs for hypertension does not increase morbidity and mortality [42]. Nondihydropyridine calcium channel blockers like verapamil and diltiazem affect conduction through the atrioventricular node and have a negative chronotropic action. All calcium channel blockers have been shown to be effective in chronic stable angina [43,44]. Dihydropyridines reduce the frequency of angina episodes, improve exercise duration, and reduce the need for nitroglycerin. Verapamil, diltiazem, and short-acting nifedipine are effective in vasospastic angina [45]. Short-acting nifedipine has an increased incidence of cardiovascular events and is not recommended for patients with ACS or unstable angina [46].

Nitrates

Nitroglycerin preparations were the first antianginal agents and have been in use for more than 150 years. Their mechanism of action is the reduction of myocardial oxygen demand through increased venous capacitance which leads to decreased LV volume/preload; they also dilate coronary arteries and favorably enhance subendocardial perfusion [47]. Sublingual nitroglycerin has been used to treat the acute onset of anginal symptoms as well as to act as a prophylaxis for angina symptoms prior to activities known to cause angina. Isosorbide dinitrate and its active metabolite isosorbide mononitrate are used as an oral preparation for the longer-term control of angina [48]. Extended-release preparations like transdermal nitrate patches and isosorbide mononitrate offer the convenience of once-daily regimens. Due to the development of tachyphylaxis, none of the nitrate preparations provides truly 24-hour prophylaxis [49]. To prevent nitrate tolerance, a 12-hour nitrate-free interval is often required. Combining nitrates with hydralazine, folic acid, and antioxidants like vitamin E may reduce the development of nitrate tolerance [50,51]. Nitrates are generally well tolerated. Their most common side effects include facial flushing and headache. Nitrates should be avoided within 24 hours of taking phosphodiesterase inhibitors (such as sildenafil) as hypotension may ensue.

Newer agents

Ranolazine
Ranolazine is a late sodium current inhibitor that has an antianginal and anti-ischemic effect without eliciting any changes in heart rate or blood pressure [52,53]. During ischemia, there is an exaggerated late inward sodium current, which leads to increased intracellular sodium and this in turn leads to intracellular calcium overload. With the increase in intracellular calcium, there is an increase in diastolic LV stiffness, which compresses intramyocardial vessels, causing reduced coronary blood flow. By preventing the abnormal increase in late inward sodium, the downstream effects of increased left ventricular stiffness are prevented, thereby leading to less ischemia [52]. In chronic stable angina, the use of ranolazine improves exercise duration, time to angina onset, and time to ST depression compared with placebo [54]. Ranolazine is also effective in patients with diabetes, leading to reduced angina episodes per week and a reduction in HbA1C from baseline in a post-hoc analysis of the CARISA (Combination Assessment of Ranolazine in Stable Angina) trial [55].

As a result of its multiple effects on transmembrane ion currents ranolazine causes a slight prolongation of the QT interval; however, to date no clinical consequences, including torsade de pointes, have been reported [56]. In the recently published MERLIN trial, ranolazine therapy was found to be safe and well tolerated in 6500 patients, including those at high risk with ACS [57]. While this study did not show a reduction in the composite primary outcome of death, MI, or recurrent myocardial ischemia, ranolazine did demonstrate a reduction in the secondary endpoint of recurrent MI. Ranolazine can be used in combination with calcium channel blockers, beta-blockers, or nitrates. Dosing is initiated at 50 mg twice daily and increased to a maximum dose of 1000 mg b.i.d. based on clinical symptoms. The most common side effects are dizziness and nausea. Concomitant administration of potent inhibitors of

CYP3A4 such as macrolides or protease inhibitors should be avoided as this can cause excess QT prolongation.

Fasudil

Fasudil is an orally available Rho-kinase inhibitor that increases the time to ST segment depression and improves exercise duration. Rho kinase in the myocardial cell triggers vasoconstriction through accumulation of phosphorylated myosin. Fasudil, like ranolazine, does not affect the heart rate or blood pressure and is generally well tolerated [58].

Trimetazidine

Trimetazidine is a metabolic modulator and partial fatty acid oxidation inhibitor that has proven to be beneficial for combination therapy in patients with stable angina by decreasing the number of weekly angina attacks [59]. There is less oxygen demand when the glucose pathway is used compared with the free fatty acid pathway. Trimetazidine inhibits beta-oxidation and shifts the equilibrium toward increased use of glucose, thus improving oxygen utilization.

Ivabradine

Ivabradine is a heart rate lowering medication that acts on SA node cells by specifically inhibiting the If current is a dose-dependent manner. Ivabradine was found to be non-inferior to beta-blockers in the INITIATIVE study for the reduction of angina [60]. The BEAUTIFUL (Morbidity-Mortality Evaluation of the If Inhibitor Ivabradine in Patients With Coronary Artery Disease and Left Ventricular Dysfunction) trial, which included CHD patients with LV dysfunction in its enrolment, demonstrated that while there was no long-term reduction in clinical events with ivabradine, it did improve angina compared with placebo [61].

Nicorandil

Nicorandil activates the ATP-sensitive K^+ channels which play an important role in ischemic preconditioning. It also promotes dilation of the coronary resistance arterioles. Its nitrate moiety dilates epicardial coronary vessels and systemic veins. When added to standard therapy in the IONA trial, nicorandil was associated with a significant improvement in CAD death, non-fatal MI, or unplanned hospital admission for cardiac chest pain [62].

Non-pharmacological antianginal approaches

Non-pharmacological antianginal strategies include enhanced external counterpulsation (EECP), transmyocardial laser revascularization (TMR), and spinal cord stimulation (SCS). EECP has been shown to reduce the frequency and severity of angina in randomized trials. It promotes coronary collateral formation and may improve endothelial function [63]. TMR involves laser to create channel into the myocardium, which promotes angiogenesis. It improves angina class in patients with class IV angina symptoms [64]. Both EECP and TMR are FDA approved for the treatment of chronic stable angina. SCS causes the release of endogenous opiates, redistributes myocardial blood flow, and decrease neurotransmission of painful stimuli. In patients with class III/IV angina, SCS may provide equivalent symptom relief to CABG [65]. However, none of these strategies is routinely used, but if available in tertiary centers all may be used to palliate symptoms in selected patients with resistant symptoms and poor quality of life.

Role of myocardial revascularization

Comparing percutaneous coronary intervention with medical therapy

Revascularization strategies, including percutaneous coronary intervention (PCI) with balloon angioplasty with or without stenting and CABG surgery represent important therapies that have been shown to improve symptoms and in certain subsets of patients improve survival [66–68]. Since the advent of PCI in 1977, remarkable evolution of these technologies has shifted treatment largely away from an initial pharmacological approach to one that focuses on an anatomically-driven management strategy. Despite this, there are relatively few RCTs comparing PCI to medical therapy in patients with stable CHD and these have involved fewer than 5000 patients in total. The majority of these trials recruited patients predominantly with single-vessel disease and were completed prior to routine use of coronary stenting and contemporary aggressive preventive medical therapy. Overall, the results of trials completed before 2005 supported superior control of angina, improved exercise capacity, and improved quality of life in patients treated with PCI compared with medical therapy. However, none of these trials demonstrated a reduction in death or MI with PCI (predominantly angioplasty) compared with medical therapy for patients with chronic stable angina [69,70]. Better outcomes have been demonstrated in some trials for high-dose atorvastatin compared to percutaneous transluminal coronary angioplasty (PTCA) alone and, with usual (less aggressive) care (AVERT [Atorvastatin VErsus Revascularization Treatment] trial) [71], and for exercise training plus medical therapy compared to PCI with stenting plus medical therapy [11].

There are now multiple contemporary RCTs that address the large group of stable IHD patients. In 2007, the COURAGE (Clinical Outcomes Utilizing Revascularization and Aggressive druG Evaluation) trial was designed to determine whether PCI coupled with optimal medical therapy (OMT) reduces the risk of death or MI in patients with stable CAD, as compared with OMT alone [72]. Such a "strategy trial" had not been conducted previously. COURAGE enrolled 2287 patients with objective evidence of MI and significant CAD from 50 centers in the US and Canada between 1999 and 2004; 1149 patients were assigned to PCI with OMT and 1138 to OMT alone [72]. The primary outcome was all-cause mortality or non-fatal MI during a 2.5–7.0-

year (median 4.6-year) follow-up. Overall, there were no significant differences in the composite primary outcome between the two management strategies, nor were any significant differences in other outcomes such as stroke or hospitalization for ACS. The main study findings indicated that, *as an initial management strategy in patients with stable CAD*, PCI with OMT did not reduce death, MI, or other major cardiovascular events when compared to OMT alone. The findings from COURAGE, along with the previous randomized trials of PCI versus medical therapy, reinforce the importance of preventive pharmacotherapy and lifestyle modification for secondary prevention of major cardiovascular events in patients with stable CHD. CAD is a systemic problem that clearly requires systemic treatment. Flow-limiting lesions cause angina and ischemia, but may not necessarily be the lesions predisposing to death, MI, and ACS. OMT is directed toward stabilizing so-called vulnerable plaques that are frequently mild angiographically and non-obstructive.

Comparisons of CABG with medical therapy

While individual RCTs have failed to show a significant reduction in overall death or MI for CABG compared with medical therapy, certain subsets of patients with left main stem coronary disease or three-vessel CAD *and* depressed LV function (LVEF <50%) appear to benefit from CABG surgery. However, a meta-analysis of these trials involving about 2500 patients who were followed for about 10–12 years indicated that an initial strategy of routine CABG surgery compared to initial medical therapy significantly reduced the risk of mortality by about 25% at 7 years, with the largest benefits being observed in those with left main disease and those with three-vessel CAD. Furthermore, at 1 year, there was little difference in mortality between those allocated to CABG surgery versus medical therapy, but the benefits of CABG surgery over medical therapy steadily emerged over the next 3–5 years. Thereafter, however, there was a diminution in the benefits of CABG surgery, perhaps as a result of late occlusion of saphenous vein grafts, progression of disease in the native coronary arteries, and increasing rates of CABG surgery in those in the medical group with high-risk anatomy/severe symptoms ("crossovers"). Very few patients in these trials received arterial grafts (which would likely improve the long-term results of CABG surgery), or routine therapy with aspirin to prevent graft occlusion, or lipid-lowering drugs to mitigate late graft disease progression [73]. Therefore, with improvements in operative techniques, more routine use of antiplatelet agents, and more aggressive risk factor management over the last decade, the benefits of modern-day CABG surgery may be larger and more durable compared to the results observed in the trials when surgery was performed about two or three decades earlier. Alternatively, medical therapy has also improved dramatically over the past decade and, even if the relative differences persist, the absolute benefit of CABG surgery over medical therapy may have diminished.

The results of all the trials comparing CABG with medical therapy indicate that a greater severity of ischemia, a greater extent of disease, and the presence of LV dysfunction favor a greater magnitude of survival benefit from surgical over medical therapy. CABG prolongs survival in patients with significant left main CAD irrespective of symptoms, in patients with multivessel CAD and impaired LV function, and in patients with three-vessel CAD that includes the proximal left anterior descending (LAD) coronary artery. As such, current treatment guidelines recommend CABG for patients with certain anatomic subsets of disease, regardless of the severity of symptoms or LV dysfunction.

Comparisons of PCI with CABG surgery for multivessel coronary artery disease

At least nine published studies have compared PCI with CABG in patients with multivessel CAD. Notably, these trials have excluded patients with significant left main CAD and those with impaired LV systolic function. Despite the heterogeneity of the trials in regard to study design and patient characteristics, the results are generally comparable and provide a consistent perspective on CABG and PCI in selected patients with multivessel CAD. A major limitation is that the majority of these trials were conducted before the widespread use of stents and other advances in PCI technology, as well as newer adjunctive medical therapy.

The BARI (Bypass Angioplasty Revascularization Investigation) trial (n = 1829) is among the largest of the completed RCTs of percutaneous balloon angioplasty and CABG surgery. At 5 years, there was no overall difference in survival rates between the two groups, nor any difference in the incidence of MI. CABG was associated with a greater initial improvement in angina and with a diminished frequency of repeat revascularization procedures compared with PCI. A significant survival advantage was observed in patients with previously treated diabetes who underwent CABG rather than angioplasty. More recently, two novel pieces of data have emerged regarding revascularization in diabetic patients. First, the BARI investigators reported that the survival benefit of CABG persisted at 10 years; second, in a collaborative, patient-level meta-analysis of 10 PCI versus CABG trials (n = 7812), there was a significant 30% reduction in total mortality with CABG in the subset of 1233 diabetic patients—a finding that persisted even after exclusion of the original BARI trial [74]. Similarly, recent data from the BARI-2D trial of 2368 diabetic patients with CAD who were randomized to prompt revascularization versus delayed/no revascularization and OMT showed no significant difference between prompt revascularization (PCI or CABG) versus OMT for the trial primary endpoint of total mortality [75]. Importantly, PCI or CABG was prespecified before randomization, typically with patients manifesting more severe CAD being allocated to CABG. Thus, the BARI-2D results replicate the principal finding of the COURAGE trial—that an initial strategy of PCI provides no incremental clinical benefit over intensive medical therapy, and an "OMT-first" instead of a "PCI-first" strategy seems justifiable in many diabetic patients with coronary disease.

Among those who remain symptomatic despite intensive treatment, or who have substantial ischemia or extensive CAD, revascularization is appropriate and either PCI or CABG is a reasonable choice, depending on the anatomic complexity of disease. If the goal of revascularization is to reduce long-term clinical events (especially MI), BARI-2D reinforces other current scientific evidence supporting the benefits of CABG surgery over PCI, especially in diabetic patients and those with multivessel CAD. The cardioprotective superiority of CABG is postulated to result from bypass grafts to the mid-coronary vessels that not only treat culprit lesions (even those that are anatomically complex), but also afford prophylaxis against new proximal disease development, whereas stents only treat suitable stenotic segment(s) with no benefit against *de novo* disease.

In another recent landmark trial (SYNTAX [SYNergy between PCI with TAXUS and Cardiac Surgery]), 1800 patients with three-vessel or left main CAD were randomly assigned to undergo CABG or PCI (in a 1:1 ratio) [76]. For these patients, the local cardiac surgeon and interventional cardiologist determined that equivalent anatomic revascularization could be achieved with either treatment. Rates of major adverse cardiac or cerebrovascular events (i.e., death from any cause, stroke, MI, or repeat revascularization) at 12 months were significantly higher in the PCI group (17.8% vs 12.4% for CABG; $p = 0.002$), in large part because of an increased rate of repeat revascularization (13.5% vs 5.9%; $p < 0.001$). At 12 months, the rates of death and MI were similar between the two groups, although stroke was significantly more likely to occur with CABG (2.2% vs 0.6% with PCI; $p = 0.003$). Thus, based on these 1-year findings, the SYNTAX authors concluded that CABG remains the standard of care for patients with three-vessel or left main CAD.

Prognosis with optimal management

Despite the enormous growth in PCI and CABG for addressing symptomatic CHD, the prevalence of angina pectoris continues to increase. Of 1620 consecutive patients in an NHLBI registry who underwent PCI, 26% continued to report angina despite receiving more than one antianginal medication [77]. The ARTS trial found that despite optimal revascularization with either PCI or CABG, 80% of the patients in the PCI group and 60% of the patients in the CABG group continued to experience angina severe enough to necessitate antianginal medications at the end of follow-up [8]. Thus, revascularization continues to result in residual ischemia and an ongoing need for medical therapy. Furthermore, there are now data from two prospective, randomized trials (COURAGE and BARI-2D) in over 4600 patients with stable IHD (with or without diabetes) showing that the long-term prognosis (4–5-year follow-up) with multifaceted medical therapy, aggressive secondary prevention, and lifestyle intervention is very favorably influenced. In the medically-treated COURAGE cohort, the annualized rate of all-cause mortality or MI was 3.8% per year, in spite of the fact that all patients had documented ischemia and over two-thirds had multivessel CAD. This underscores what can be achieved using contemporary OMT, and that such treatment may reduce the subsequent clinical events by reducing the propensity for plaque rupture that is the proximate cause in the majority of patients with IHD.

CHARISMA trial

The CHARISMA trial compared dual antiplatelet therapy with clopidogrel plus aspirin versus aspirin monotherapy in a widely heterogeneous population of patients (n = 15603) with established atherothrombotic disease or atherothrombotic risk factors [14]. The "symptomatic" group included patients with documented CAD, cerebrovascular disease (CVD), or symptomatic peripheral arterial disease (PAD). The "asymptomatic" group included patients with multiple cardiac risk factors, such as hypertension, hypercholesterolemia, diabetes, or smoking, but without clinical manifestations of a documented ischemic syndrome in one or more vascular beds.

In the overall population there was no significant benefit associated with the addition of clopidogrel to aspirin in reducing the composite primary endpoint of MI, stroke, or death. On the other hand, there was a significant 1% RRR with clopidogrel compared with placebo in the principal prespecified secondary endpoint of MI, stroke, death from cardiovascular causes or hospitalization for unstable angina, transient ischemic attack (TIA) or a revascularization procedure (16.7% vs 17.9; $p = 0.04$).

The rate of the primary safety endpoint of severe bleeding (according to the GUSTO definition) was not significantly different between the two treatment arms (1.7% in the clopidogrel group vs. 1.3% in the placebo group; $p = 0.09$). The rate of moderate bleeding, however, was 2.1% in the clopidogrel group compared with 1.3% in the placebo group (relative risk, 1.62; $p < 0.001$).

Results for the prespecified subgroups showed that combination therapy in the asymptomatic group (n = 3284), which comprised 21% of the entire study population, was associated with a non-significant (but unexpected) 20% relative increase in primary events ($p = 0.2$), a 40% increase in severe bleeding, a 40% increase in cardiovascular death ($p = 0.04$), and a 30% increase in all-cause mortality ($p = 0.01$) [14]. Conversely, in the symptomatic group (n = 12153), which comprised 77% of the entire study population (1% of patients could not be classified precisely as symptomatic or asymptomatic), dual clopidogrel plus aspirin therapy yielded the opposite result, with a significant 12% RRR in primary events compared with aspirin alone ($p = 0.046$). There was no significant increase in severe bleeding ($p = 0.39$) and no significant effect on cardiovascular death in the symptomatic subgroup [14].

In the overall trial analysis, the potential harm in asymptomatic patients (primary prevention) versus benefit in the symptomatic group (secondary prevention) combined to show an overall lack of benefit in a widely heterogeneous population at risk for atherothrombosis. In essence, the benefit associated with dual antiplatelet therapy observed in the 77% of patients with established vascular disease was negated by the unexpectedly higher event rate with aspirin plus clopidogrel in the 21% of asymptomatic patients. Thus, these divergent results for the subgroups provoked a debate regarding the analysis and interpretation of the trial subgroup data [14,78,79].

Putting CHARISMA into therapeutic perspective

As the debate over dual antiplatelet therapy for secondary prevention continues, it should once again be re-emphasized that clopidogrel plus aspirin has proven efficacy and superiority over aspirin alone in various important patient populations. Additional analyses of the CHARISMA trial data and results of ongoing trials should identify other patient (sub)populations that are most likely to benefit from dual antiplatelet therapy beyond aspirin alone.

For any given clinical situation in which a practitioner is challenged to apply the results of an RCT to an individual patient at the bedside, it is important to remember that the individual being treated may not represent the "average" patient reflected in the overall results of a given clinical trial. It is precisely for this fundamental reason that investigators conduct further analyses on identifiable subsets of patients within the larger pool of trial participants. The biological and clinical variability, as well as the complexity of the disease process and associated comorbidities of patients, is unquestionable. It is axiomatic then that treatment effects may vary among individual patients.

However, an entire study's findings should not be completely dismissed if they do not provide a "one size fits all" conclusion applicable to all patients. There is a scientific and ethical obligation to try to identify subgroup populations for whom a specific treatment might be more or less effective, or for that matter harmful. The need to detect even modest differences in patient outcomes that are of significant value to clinical practice thus, at times, collides with the statistical limitations of doing so. Meaningful information from such subgroup analyses may be limited by low statistical power or multiplicity of testing. For this reason, readily-available guidelines are in place to provide direction for proper execution of subgroup analyses in such a way as to minimize erroneous findings.

In summary, scrupulous adherence to these guidelines and basic principles of sound statistical analysis were observed in the CHARISMA trial. As noted previously, the investigators advised appropriate caution and restraint in interpretation of their subgroup analyses because the possibility remains that these significant results occurred by the play of chance only. Accordingly, physicians are left to consider how best to interpret the somewhat conflicting results of an important trial such as CHARISMA that will likely never be replicated, and will clearly not result in a change in clinical practice guidelines. Nevertheless, patients with atherothrombotic disease continue to fare poorly, with an unacceptably high rate of residual mortality and morbidity, despite optimal treatment with existing evidence-based therapies. It is in the context of this imperative to optimize clinical outcomes for our patients that we must weigh clinical decisions to treat or not to treat—at times, based on imperfect data from well-designed and well-conducted RCTs such as CHARISMA.

Table 3.2 Cardiovascular outcomes in the COURAGE trial.

Outcome	PCI + OMT (n = 1149)	OMT (n = 1138)	HR (95% CI)	P-value
Cardiac death	39 (3.4%)	44 (3.9%)	0.87 (0.56–1.33)	0.51
Cardiac death/MI	172 (15%)	162 (14.2%)	1.07 (0.86–1.33)	0.62
Cardiac death/MI/ACS	270 (23.5%)	257 (22.6%)	1.07 (0.91–1.27)	0.60
Cardiac death/MI/stroke	188 (16.4%)	173 (15.2%)	1.10 (0.89–1.35)	0.45
Cardiac death/MI/ACS/stroke	313 (27.2%)	305 (26.8%)	1.05 (0.89–1.22)	0.51
MI/stroke	160 (13.9%)	139 (12.2%)	1.16 (0.93–1.46)	0.23
Total MI	147 (12.8%)	126 (11.1%)	1.14 (0.90–1.44)	0.48
Total MI: Spontaneous	109 (10.4%)	113 (9.5%)	0.91 (0.70–1.18)	0.46
Total peri-PCI MI	37 (3.4%)	11 (1.0%)	3.57 (1.83–6.96)	<0.001
Total peri-CABG MI	1	2		
Total ACS	136 (11.8%)	125 (11.0%)	1.08 (0.85–1.38)	0.52
Total stroke	22 (1.9%)	14 (1.2%)	1.56 (0.80–3.05)	0.19

ACS, acute coronary syndrome; CABG, coronary artery bypass graft; HR, hazard ratio; MI, myocardial infarction; OMT, optimal medical therapy; PCI, percutaneous coronary intervention.

COURAGE trial

The COURAGE trial was designed to determine whether PCI coupled with OMT reduces the risk of death or non-fatal MI in patients with stable CAD, as compared with OMT alone [72,80]. Such a robust "strategy trial" had not been conducted since the advent of angioplasty in 1977, although there were 11 prior studies that compared PCI *in apposition to*—not *in combination with*—OMT [81]. COURAGE enrolled 2287 patients with objective evidence of MI and significant CAD from 50 US and Canadian centers. Between 1999 and 2004, 1149 patients were assigned to PCI with OMT and 1138 to OMT alone. The primary outcome was all-cause mortality or non-fatal MI during a 2.5–7.0-year (median 4.6-year) follow-up. The major clinical outcomes are summarized in Table 3.2. There were 211 primary events in the PCI group and 202 events in the medical therapy group. The 4.6-year cumulative primary event rates were 19.0% and 18.5% in the PCI and medical therapy groups, respectively (HR in the PCI group compared with the medical therapy group, 1.05; 95% CI, 0.87–1.27; p = 0.62). Comparing the PCI and medical therapy groups, there were no differences in death, MI, or stroke (20.0% vs 19.5%; HR, 1.05; 95% CI, 0.87–1.27; p = 0.62); hospitalization for ACS (12.4% vs 11.8%; HR, 1.07; 95% CI, 0.84–1.37; p = 0.56); or MI (13.2% vs 12.3%; HR, 1.13; 95% CI, 0.89–1.43; p = 0.33) [72]. Thus, the main study findings indicate that, *as an initial management strategy in patients with stable CAD*, PCI did not reduce death, MI, or other major cardiovascular events when added to OMT.

Importantly, the Kaplan–Meier life-table curves for the primary outcome measure of death or MI were virtually superimposable for the two randomized groups over the initial 4.5 years of follow-up (HR, 1.05; 95% CI, 0.87–1.27). In fact, the 95% CI excludes a potential benefit of PCI of greater than 13%, which means that there is only a 5% chance that a death or MI reduction with PCI is 13% or greater (i.e., only a 5% probability that the absolute risk reduction of PCI is no greater than 2.47% [4.6-year median death/ MI rate for PCI = 0.19 x 0.13 = 0.0247]) [72]. This means it is exceedingly unlikely that a true PCI benefit has been missed.

Additionally, cause-specific cardiac outcomes from the COURAGE trial have recently been published [82]. The major cardiovascular outcomes are summarized in Table 3.2. The composite of cardiac death or MI occurred in 172 patients (15%) in the PCI group and in 162 patients (14.2%) in the OMT group (HR, 1.07; 95% CI, 0.86–1.33; p = 0.62). This hazard ratio was identical to the trial primary outcome measure of all-cause mortality or MI that was published previously [72]. The composite of cardiac death, MI or ACS occurred in 270 patients (23.5%) in the PCI group and in 257 patients (22.6%) in the OMT group (HR, 1.07; 95% CI, 0.91–1.27; p = 0.60). The time to first event for the composite of cardiac death, MI, ACS, or stroke was observed in 313 patients (27.2%) in the PCI group as compared with 305 patients (26.8%) in the OMT group (HR, 1.05; 95% CI, 0.89–1.22; p = 0.51). Overall, all composite cardiovascular outcomes showed no significant between-group differences [82], and paralleled closely the primary and secondary composite outcomes of the trial as a whole, including all-cause mortality.

Thus, the main study findings [72] and recent cause-specific outcomes [82] indicated that, *as an initial management strategy in patients with stable CAD*, PCI did not reduce death, MI, or other major cardiovascular events when added to OMT. When these findings were first presented and published in 2007, there was intense controversy and criticism of the main study findings, although it now appears that there has been greater acceptance of the trial results and their therapeutic implications.

Intensity of optimal medical therapy and importance of achieving treatment targets

Most cardiovascular clinical trials test a single intervention. COURAGE tested a comprehensive set of lifestyle and pharmacological interventions as part of OMT with or without PCI in patients with stable IHD. Unlike earlier studies that employed only modest anti-ischemic therapy as the comparator, COURAGE sought to utilize aggressive medical therapy of each important drug class (e.g., aspirin, beta-blockers, ACE-Is, statins, etc.) that had been proven to be of clinical benefit in individual, placebo-controlled RCTs. In COURAGE, these pharmacological agents were used in the aggregate and applied equally to the PCI and OMT groups so as not to deprive the PCI arm of the putative benefits associated with intensive secondary prevention. No other trial has attempted such a comprehensive treatment approach in stable IHD patients, nor attempted to incorporate guideline-driven best practice to achieve and maintain multiple treatment targets during long-term follow-up.

All patients, regardless of treatment assignment, received equivalent lifestyle and pharmacological interventions for secondary prevention and angina therapy. Most medications were provided at no cost. Therapy was administered by nurse case managers according to protocols to achieve predefined lifestyle and risk factor goals. Among the 2287 patients who were followed for a median 4.6 years, there were no significant differences between treatment groups in percent of patients achieving therapeutic goals [72]. At baseline 23% of subjects smoked, and this fell to 19% during the trial. Food choices and level of physical activity improved, but body mass index remained unchanged at approximately $29 \, kg/m^2$. Medication use changed from baseline to 60 months as follows: antiplatelet agents 97% to 96%; beta-blockers 85% to 88%; renin-angiotensin system inhibitors 61% to 72%; and statins 89% to 93%. Systolic blood pressure fell from 130 mmHg to 123 mmHg. LDL-C cholesterol fell from 101 mg/dL at baseline to 71 mg/dL at 60 months of follow-up. Thus, aggressive secondary prevention and guideline-driven therapy [72] was applied equally and intensively to both treatment groups in COURAGE by nurse case managers using treatment protocols. As such, OMT as used in COURAGE represents a model for secondary prevention in clinical practice.

A notable strength of the COURAGE trial was the hypothesis that a combination of PCI directed at focal flow-limiting stenoses causing chronic angina and ischemia, combined with disease-modifying therapies such as statins, renin-angiotensin system inhibitors, and beta-blockers as a fundamental part of OMT, would be inherently superior to OMT alone in reducing prognostically-important clinical endpoints during long-term follow-up. Intuitively, the combination of both a *focal* and *systemic* approach to CAD management would be plausibly expected to mitigate cardiac events better than a systemic approach alone in stable IHD patients with extensive angiographic CAD, significant inducible ischemia, and appreciable clinical comorbidity. The clinical and non-invasive stress test findings and coronary angiographic features of the study group are summarized in Table 3.2, and highlight the fact that this was not a low-risk population. On the contrary, the median 4.6-year composite rate of death or MI was 19%, and the composite rate for cardiovascular death, MI, stroke, and hospitalization for ACS was 27%. These findings are consistent with at least an "intermediate-risk" profile [72,80].

It has been argued by some critics that the "OMT" as used in COURAGE was "too good" and cannot be replicated in routine clinical practice [83]. Contrary to the perception that the COURAGE investigators and study coordinators went to extraordinary lengths to ensure that patients complied with OMT or were seen at multiple time intervals to reinforce protocol adherence, after the first year of follow-up (during which patients were seen at 3-month intervals), follow-up visits between years 1 and 7 were scheduled only at 6-month intervals. Investigators and coordinators worked closely with referring physicians to underscore the importance of maintaining medical therapy and lifestyle changes and treating patients to multiple treatment targets. Indeed, in most busy clinical cardiology practices today (either office- or hospital-based), the use of physician extenders such as nurse practitioners and/or physician assistants can provide an important, additional source of manpower to replicate the approach that was used in COURAGE to achieve treatment adherence and therapeutic targets for blood pressure, lipids, and glycemic control.

A recent thoughtful review by several interventional cardiology opinion leaders makes the following statement about the importance of OMT as used in COURAGE: "In trials of patients with stable CAD, no reduction in death or MI have been observed, and these limitations of PCI in this clinical setting need to be emphasized. OMT forms the cornerstone of management for any patient with CAD" [84].

Angina relief and improved quality of life

Rates of angina were consistently lower in the PCI patients as compared with the medical therapy patients during follow-up, and rates of subsequent revascularization were likewise lower. However, there was a substantial increase in freedom from angina in the medically treated patients as well, most of which had taken place by 1 year but with a further improvement to 5 years [72]. To what extent this reflects a benefit of specific antianginal medications (such as nitrates and beta-blockers) and to what extent it may reflect an effect of disease-modifying therapies such as statins and inhibitors of the renin-angiotensin system on coronary stenoses is unclear.

In addition, whether PCI can provide an incremental quality-of-life (QOL) benefit over OMT in patients with chronic angina due to stable IHD was largely unknown before the COURAGE trial. A comprehensive, prospective assessment of QOL was imbedded in the trial proper; angina-specific health status (Seattle Angina Questionnaire [SAQ]) and overall physical and mental function (RAND-36) were assessed at baseline and sequentially during follow-up [85]. Clearly, how patients regard their own health and functioning is critical, and both the SAQ and RAND-36 are patient-reported health outcomes instruments. Based on the SAQ analysis, there was significantly better angina control with PCI for the first 12–24 months across the key domains of physical limitation, anginal frequency, and QOL. While the differences between treatment arms were statistically significant, the clinical differences were substantially smaller than the within-group benefits noted for both arms. The SAQ data were likewise supported by the RAND-36, which, as a general health questionnaire, showed less consistent benefit of PCI + OMT, because not all scales on the RAND-36 showed incremental benefit of PCI + OMT. Somewhat unexpectedly, there was rapid improvement in health status for almost all measures in both groups by 1–3-months of follow-up. Importantly, there was a significant and rapid improvement in SAQ scores in OMT patients who did *not* cross over to PCI + OMT. However, the small group of patients who crossed over early from OMT to PCI + OMT (only 16.5% of OMT patients crossed over during the first year of follow-up) had remarkably low SAQ scores at baseline, and rapid and dramatic improvement in their scores [85].

What this indicates can be summarized as follows: COURAGE demonstrated that an initial strategy of PCI added to OMT in patients with stable CAD relieved angina to a greater extent than an initial strategy of OMT alone for a period of approximately 24 months. Since the overall COURAGE trial results did not show that the addition of PCI to OMT reduced cardiovascular events [72,81], these important QOL findings [85] permit physicians to engage in an evidence-based discussion with patients about the expected clinical and health status benefits of initial versus deferred PCI when added to OMT. If PCI is deferred, physician and patient alike can be confident that the risk of MI or death is not increased. This should foster a patient-centered approach that considers both the incidence of clinical events as well as health-related QOL to help guide the decision about timing and need for PCI.

Reducing myocardial ischemia

A substudy of the COURAGE trial evaluated the effectiveness of PCI as an adjunct to OMT using myocardial perfusion imaging (MPI) [86]. Of 2287 patients, 314 underwent MPS before treatment and 6–18 months thereafter. At follow-up, the reduction in ischemia was greater with PCI + OMT than with OMT alone (-2.7% vs -0.5%; $p < 0.0001$), and more patients in the PCI + OMT group exhibited reduction in ischemia of 5% or greater (33% vs 19%; $p = 0.0004$). However, ischemia reduction did not lower the risk of death or MI after adjustment for other baseline inequalities and relevant covariates. These findings are consistent with those of Mahmarian *et al.*, showing that intensive medical treatment was comparable to revascularization with respect to cardiac events even in high-risk stable postinfarction patients with ischemic perfusion defects [87]; however, both trials were non-randomized and under-powered for this purpose. While two other trials have reported a reduction in risk (including mortality) using PCI in asymptomatic patients with exercise-induced MI [88,89], the intensity of medical therapy was not as rigorous as in COURAGE [72].

More recently, a meta-analysis by Schomig *et al.* purports to show a signifi-cant long-term survival advantage with PCI "in patients with stable coronary artery disease," based on a pooled analysis of 17 randomized trials comparing a PCI-based invasive strategy with medical treatment in 7513 patients [90]. While the odds ratio for all-cause death was 0.80 (95% CI, 0.64–0.99), indica-tive of a 20% relative mortality reduction, five of the 17 trials included in this so-called meta-analysis were either acute MI trials or post-MI trials. In a follow-up analysis and reinterpretation of the Schomig meta-analysis, Wijeysundera and Ko performed a "corrected meta-analysis" and demon-strated that, after the appropriate removal of these five acute or post-MI trials, there was no evidence for a mortality reduction with PCI as compared with OMT—highlighting what they described was an "apples and oranges" com-parison [91].

Has clinical practice changed post COURAGE?

COURAGE has begun to shift thinking and change clinical practice in the US, as well as worldwide. While no one trial is likely to lead to profound change, there is reason to believe that COURAGE will reorient our decision-making "set point" away from what has been a largely routine procedural approach to initial patient management for stable CAD. Additionally, the recent results of the BARI-2D trial [75] in 2368 type 2 diabetics replicate the principal finding of the COURAGE trial—that an initial strategy of PCI provides no incremental clinical benefit over intensive medical therapy, and an "OMT-first" instead of a "PCI-first" strategy seems justifiable in many diabetic patients with coronary disease. Among those who remain symptomatic despite intensive treatment, or who have substantial ischemia or extensive CAD, revascularization is appropriate and either PCI or CABG is a reasonable choice, depending on the anatomic complexity of disease.

Thus, there are now two contemporary randomized trials of OMT versus PCI in over 4600 stable IHD patients [72,75] showing that OMT as an initial management strategy is the equal of PCI. Together with the 11 randomized trials of chronic stable angina patients prior to COURAGE, comprising 2950 patients [81], there are now outcome data on 7605 patients from 13 trials supporting the clinical benefit of OMT.

The results of both COURAGE and now BARI-2D emphasize that, over the past 20 years, there have been profound advances in PCI, CABG surgery, and OMT. Is it likely these trial results will change clinical practice? PCI use in the US remains high (1.2 million procedures/year) and 75% involve drug-eluting stents [3]. As healthcare reform looms on the horizon, physicians increasingly will need to make informed, evidence-based treatment decisions that improve not only patients' symptoms, but clinical outcomes as well. Both COURAGE and BARI-2D indicate that, for many patients with stable IHD (with or without diabetes), and certainly those with less severe anatomic CAD, OMT rather than any intervention is an excellent first-line strategy. When revascularization is indicated, both BARI-2D and other studies currently support CABG surgery as the preferred approach, while PCI may be considered in patients who need revascularization for symptom relief or less extensive anatomic CAD [34].

Lastly, while the results of any randomized trial must be individualized to specific patients, a "multidisciplinary team approach" to clinical decision-making can ensure that all therapeutic options (OMT, PCI or CABG) are fully and transparently discussed so that patients are offered the most appropriate evidence-based treatment recommendations. The leading interventional cardiologists in the previously-cited authoritative review [84] wrote: "The 'convenient' approach to treat what is there [with PCI] has become ingrained and is part of both patients' and physicians' expectations. The consequence of this approach may be the lost opportunity to discuss all the therapeutic options in a less urgent setting and with all the information at hand" [84].

Conclusions

In summary, there are three appropriate treatment approaches for patients with chronic stable angina: PCI, CABG surgery, and OMT. Selection of the most appropriate treatment requires a full understanding of the potential risks and benefits of each treatment approach. In patients with stable symptoms, an initial approach of aggressive medical therapy is supported by existing ACC/AHA clinical practice guidelines. For patients whose angina or QOL is not adequately controlled with OMT, revascularization with either PCI or CABG surgery should be considered.

References

1. Fraker TD Jr, Fihn SD, Gibbons RJ, *et al.* 2007 chronic angina focused update of the ACC/AHA 2002 guidelines for the management of patients with chronic stable angina: a report of the American College of Cardiology/American Heart Association Task Force on Practice Guidelines Writing Group to develop the focused update of the 2002 guidelines for the management of patients with chronic stable angina. *J Am Coll Cardiol* 2007; 50:2264–2274.

2. Pepine CJ, Abrams J, Marks RG, Morris JJ, Scheidt SS, Handberg E. Characteristics of a contemporary population with angina pectoris. TIDES Investigators. *Am J Cardiol* 1994;74:226–231.

3. Rosamond W, Flegal K, Friday G, *et al.* Heart disease and stroke statistics–2007 update: a report from the American Heart Association Statistics Committee and Stroke Statistics Subcommittee. *Circulation* 2007;115:e69–171.

4. Panting JR, Gatehouse PD, Yang GZ, *et al.* Abnormal subendocardial perfusion in cardiac syndrome X detected by cardiovascular magnetic resonance imaging. *N Engl J Med* 2002;346:1948–1953.

5. Abrams J. Clinical practice. Chronic stable angina. *N Engl J Med* 2005;352:2524–2533.

6. Sangareddi V, Chockalingam A, Gnanavelu G, Subramaniam T, Jagannathan V, Elangovan S. Canadian Cardiovascular Society classification of effort angina: an angiographic correlation. *Coron Artery Dis* 2004;15:111–114.

7. O'Rourke RA, ed. *Diagnosis and Management of Patients with Chronic Ischemic Heart Disease.* 10 ed: McGraw Hill, 2001.

8. Serruys PW, Unger F, Sousa JE, *et al.* Comparison of coronary-artery bypass surgery and stenting for the treatment of multivessel disease. *N Engl J Med* 2001;344:1117–1124.

9. Cohn PF, Fox KM, Daly C. Silent myocardial ischemia. *Circulation* 2003;108:1263–1277.

10. Haskell WL, Alderman EL, Fair JM, *et al.* Effects of intensive multiple risk factor reduction on coronary atherosclerosis and clinical cardiac events in men and women with coronary artery disease. The Stanford Coronary Risk Intervention Project (SCRIP). *Circulation* 1994;89:975–990.

11. Hambrecht R, Walther C, Mobius-Winkler S, *et al.* Percutaneous coronary angioplasty compared with exercise training in patients with stable coronary artery disease: a randomized trial. *Circulation* 2004;109:1371–1378.

12. Collaborative meta-analysis of randomised trials of antiplatelet therapy for prevention of death, myocardial infarction, and stroke in high risk patients. *BMJ* 2002;324:71–86.

13. CAPRIE Steering Committee. A randomised, blinded, trial of clopidogrel versus aspirin in patients at risk of ischaemic events (CAPRIE). *Lancet* 1996;348:1329–1339.

14. Bhatt DL, Fox KA, Hacke W, *et al.* Clopidogrel and aspirin versus aspirin alone for the prevention of atherothrombotic events. *N Engl J Med* 2006;354:1706–1717.

15. Fraker TD Jr, Fihn SD, Gibbons RJ, *et al.* 2007 chronic angina focused update of the ACC/AHA 2002 Guidelines for the management of patients with chronic stable angina: a report of the American College of Cardiology/American Heart Association Task Force on Practice Guidelines Writing Group to develop the focused update of the 2002 Guidelines for the management of patients with chronic stable angina. *Circulation* 2007; 116:2762–2772.

16. Mancini GB, Henry GC, Macaya C, *et al.* Angiotensin-converting enzyme inhibition with quinapril improves endothelial vasomotor dysfunction in patients with coronary artery disease. The TREND (Trial on Reversing ENdothelial Dysfunction) Study. *Circulation* 1996;94:258–265.

17. Yusuf S, Sleight P, Pogue J, Bosch J, Davies R, Dagenais G. Effects of an angiotensin-converting-enzyme inhibitor, ramipril, on cardiovascular events in high-risk patients. The Heart Outcomes Prevention Evaluation Study Investigators. *N Engl J Med* 2000; 342:145–153.

18. Braunwald E, Domanski MJ, Fowler SE, *et al.* Angiotensin-converting-enzyme inhibition in stable coronary artery disease. *N Engl J Med* 2004;351:2058–2068.

19. Dickstein K, Kjekshus J. Effects of losartan and captopril on mortality and morbidity in high-risk patients after acute myocardial infarction: the OPTIMAAL randomised trial. Optimal Trial in Myocardial Infarction with Angiotensin II Antagonist Losartan. *Lancet* 2002;360:752–760.

20. Pfeffer MA, McMurray JJ, Velazquez EJ, *et al.* Valsartan, captopril, or both in myocardial infarction complicated by heart failure, left ventricular dysfunction, or both. *N Engl J Med* 2003;349:1893–1906.

21. Yusuf S, Teo KK, Pogue J, *et al.* Telmisartan, ramipril, or both in patients at high risk for vascular events. *N Engl J Med* 2008;358:1547–1559.

22. Pekkanen J, Linn S, Heiss G, *et al.* Ten-year mortality from cardiovascular disease in relation to cholesterol level among men with and without preexisting cardiovascular disease. *N Engl J Med* 1990;322:1700–1707.

23. Cannon CP, Braunwald E, McCabe CH, *et al.* Intensive versus moderate lipid lowering with statins after acute coronary syndromes. *N Engl J Med* 2004;350:1495–1504.

24. Corti R, Fayad ZA, Fuster V, *et al.* Effects of lipid-lowering by simvastatin on human atherosclerotic lesions: a longitudinal study by high-resolution, noninvasive magnetic resonance imaging. *Circulation* 2001;104:249–252.

25. Ridker PM, Cannon CP, Morrow D, *et al.* C-reactive protein levels and outcomes after statin therapy. *N Engl J Med* 2005;352:20–28.

26. The effect of aggressive lowering of low-density lipoprotein cholesterol levels and low-dose anticoagulation on obstructive changes in saphenous-vein coronary-artery bypass grafts. The Post Coronary Artery Bypass Graft Trial Investigators. *N Engl J Med* 1997; 336:153–162.

27. Gordon T, Castelli WP, Hjortland MC, Kannel WB, Dawber TR. High density lipoprotein as a protective factor against coronary heart disease. The Framingham Study. *Am J Med* 1977;62:707–714.

28. Gordon DJ, Probstfield JL, Garrison RJ, *et al.* High-density lipoprotein cholesterol and cardiovascular disease. Four prospective American studies. *Circulation* 1989;79:8–15.

29. Boden WE, Probstfield JL, Anderson T, *et al.* Niacin in patients with low HDL cholesterol levels receiving intensive statin therapy. *N Engl J Med* 2011;365:2255–67.

30. Treatment of HDL to Reduce the Incidence of Vascular Events HPS2-THRIVE. *Clinicaltrials.gov* 2010.

31. Sudhop T, Lutjohann D, Kodal A, *et al.* Inhibition of intestinal cholesterol absorption by ezetimibe in humans. *Circulation* 2002;106:1943–1948.

32. Kosoglou T, Meyer I, Veltri EP, *et al.* Pharmacodynamic interaction between the new selective cholesterol absorption inhibitor ezetimibe and simvastatin. *Br J Clin Pharmacol* 2002;54:309–319.

33. Pearson TA, Denke MA, McBride PE, Battisti WP, Brady WE, Palmisano J. A community-based, randomized trial of ezetimibe added to statin therapy to attain NCEP ATP III goals for LDL cholesterol in hypercholesterolemic patients: the ezetimibe add-on to statin for effectiveness (EASE) trial. *Mayo Clin Proc* 2005;80:587–595.

34. Bays HE, Ose L, Fraser N, et al. A multicenter, randomized, double-blind, placebo-controlled, factorial design study to evaluate the lipid-altering efficacy and safety profile of the ezetimibe/simvastatin tablet compared with ezetimibe and simvastatin mono-therapy in patients with primary hypercholesterolemia. *Clin Ther* 2004;26:1758–1773.

35. Jackson G, Schwartz J, Kates RE, Winchester M, Harrison DC. Atenolol: once-daily cardioselective beta blockade for angina pectoris. *Circulation* 1980;61:555–560.

36. Weiss R, Ferry D, Pickering E, *et al*. Effectiveness of three different doses of carvedilol for exertional angina. Carvedilol-Angina Study Group. *Am J Cardiol* 1998;82:927–931.

37. Kaski JC, Rodriguez-Plaza L, Brown J, Maseri A. Efficacy of carvedilol (BM 14,190), a new beta-blocking drug with vasodilating properties, in exercise-induced ischemia. *Am J Cardiol* 1985;56:35–40.

38. Furberg B, Dahlqvist A, Raak A, Wrege U. Comparison of the new beta-adrenoceptor antagonist, nadolol, and propranolol in the treatment of angina pectoris. *Curr Med Res Opin* 1978;5:388–393.

39. Jackson G, Harry JD, Robinson C, Kitson D, Jewitt DE. Comparison of atenolol with propranolol in the treatment of angina pectoris with special reference to once daily administration of atenolol. *Br Heart J* 1978;40:998–1004.

40. Waysbort J, Meshulam N, Brunner D. Isosorbide-5-mononitrate and atenolol in the treat-ment of stable exertional angina. *Cardiology* 1991;79 (Suppl 2):19–26.

41. Krepp HP. Evaluation of the antianginal and anti-ischemic efficacy of slow-release isosorbide-5-mononitrate capsules, bupranolol and their combination, in patients with chronic stable angina pectoris. *Cardiology* 1991;79 (Suppl 2):14–18.

42. Alderman MH, Cohen H, Roque R, Madhavan S. Effect of long-acting and short-acting calcium antagonists on cardiovascular outcomes in hypertensive patients. *Lancet* 1997;349:594–598.

43. Weiner DA, Klein MD. Verapamil therapy for stable exertional angina pectoris. *Am J Cardiol* 1982;50:1153–1157.

44. Subramanian VB, Bowles MJ, Davies AB, Raftery EB. Calcium channel blockade as primary therapy for stable angina pectoris. A double-blind placebo-controlled compari-son of verapamil and propranolol. *Am J Cardiol* 1982;50:1158–1163.

45. Chahine RA, Feldman RL, Giles TD, *et al*. Randomized placebo-controlled trial of amlodipine in vasospastic angina. Amlodipine Study 160 Group. *J Am Coll Cardiol* 1993;21:1365–1370.

46. Furberg CD, Psaty BM, Meyer JV. Nifedipine. Dose-related increase in mortality in patients with coronary heart disease. *Circulation* 1995;92:1326–1331.

47. Kaski JC, Plaza LR, Meran DO, Araujo L, Chierchia S, Maseri A. Improved coronary supply: prevailing mechanism of action of nitrates in chronic stable angina. *Am Heart J* 1985;110:238–245.

48. Abrams J. Nitroglycerin and long-acting nitrates in clinical practice. *Am J Med* 1983; 74:85–94.

49. Thadani U. Nitrate tolerance, rebound, and their clinical relevance in stable angina pectoris, unstable angina, and heart failure. *Cardiovasc Drugs Ther* 1997;10:735–742.

50. Gogia H, Mehra A, Parikh S, *et al*. Prevention of tolerance to hemodynamic effects of nitrates with concomitant use of hydralazine in patients with chronic heart failure. *J Am Coll Cardiol* 1995;26:1575–1580.

51. Gori T, Burstein JM, Ahmed S, *et al*. Folic acid prevents nitroglycerin-induced nitric oxide synthase dysfunction and nitrate tolerance: a human in vivo study. *Circulation* 2001; 104:1119–1123.

52. Belardinelli L, Shryock JC, Fraser H. Inhibition of the late sodium current as a potential cardioprotective principle: effects of the late sodium current inhibitor ranolazine. *Heart* 2006;92 (Suppl 4):iv6–iv14.

53. Nash DT, Nash SD. Ranolazine for chronic stable angina. *Lancet* 2008;372:1335–1341.
54. Chaitman BR, Pepine CJ, Parker JO, *et al.* Effects of ranolazine with atenolol, amlodipine, or diltiazem on exercise tolerance and angina frequency in patients with severe chronic angina: a randomized controlled trial. *JAMA* 2004;291:309–316.
55. Timmis AD, Chaitman BR, Crager M. Effects of ranolazine on exercise tolerance and HbA1c in patients with chronic angina and diabetes. *Eur Heart J* 2006;27:42–48.
56. Antzelevitch C, Belardinelli L, Zygmunt AC, *et al.* Electrophysiological effects of ranolazine, a novel antianginal agent with antiarrhythmic properties. *Circulation* 2004;110: 904–910.
57. Morrow DA, Scirica BM, Karwatowska-Prokopczuk E, *et al.* Effects of ranolazine on recurrent cardiovascular events in patients with non-ST-elevation acute coronary syndromes: the MERLIN-TIMI 36 randomized trial. *JAMA* 2007;297:1775–1783.
58. Vicari RM, Chaitman B, Keefe D, *et al.* Efficacy and safety of fasudil in patients with stable angina: a double-blind, placebo-controlled, phase 2 trial. *J Am Coll Cardiol* 2005;46:1803–1811.
59. Chazov EI, Lepakchin VK, Zharova EA, *et al.* Trimetazidine in Angina Combination Therapy–the TACT study: trimetazidine versus conventional treatment in patients with stable angina pectoris in a randomized, placebo-controlled, multicenter study. *Am J Ther* 2005;12:35–42.
60. Tardif JC, Ford I, Tendera M, Bourassa MG, Fox K. Efficacy of ivabradine, a new selective I(f) inhibitor, compared with atenolol in patients with chronic stable angina. *Eur Heart J* 2005;26:2529–2536.
61. Fox K, Ford I, Steg PG, Tendera M, Ferrari R. Ivabradine for patients with stable coronary artery disease and left-ventricular systolic dysfunction (BEAUTIFUL): a randomised, double-blind, placebo-controlled trial. *Lancet* 2008;372:807–816.
62. Effect of nicorandil on coronary events in patients with stable angina: the Impact Of Nicorandil in Angina (IONA) randomised trial. *Lancet* 2002;359:1269–1275.
63. Bonetti PO, Barsness GW, Keelan PC, *et al.* Enhanced external counterpulsation improves endothelial function in patients with symptomatic coronary artery disease. *J Am Coll Cardiol* 2003;41:1761–1768.
64. Allen KB, Dowling RD, Fudge TL, *et al.* Comparison of transmyocardial revascularization with medical therapy in patients with refractory angina. *N Engl J Med* 1999;341: 1029–1036.
65. Mannheimer C, Eliasson T, Augustinsson LE, *et al.* Electrical stimulation versus coronary artery bypass surgery in severe angina pectoris: the ESBY study. *Circulation* 1998;97: 1157–1163.
66. Rihal CS, Raco DL, Gersh BJ, Yusuf S. Indications for coronary artery bypass surgery and percutaneous coronary intervention in chronic stable angina: review of the evidence and methodological considerations. *Circulation* 2003;108:2439–2445.
67. Hoffman SN, TenBrook JA, Wolf MP, Pauker SG, Salem DN, Wong JB. A meta-analysis of randomized controlled trials comparing coronary artery bypass graft with percutaneous transluminal coronary angioplasty: one- to eight-year outcomes. *J Am Coll Cardiol* 2003;41:1293–1304.
68. Berger PB, Sketch MH Jr, Califf RM. Choosing between percutaneous coronary intervention and coronary artery bypass grafting for patients with multivessel disease: what can we learn from the Arterial Revascularization Therapy Study (ARTS)? *Circulation* 2004;109:1079–1081.
69. Hueb W, Soares PR, Gersh BJ, *et al.* The medicine, angioplasty, or surgery study (MASS-II): a randomized, controlled clinical trial of three therapeutic strategies for multivessel coronary artery disease: one-year results. *J Am Coll Cardiol* 2004;43:1743–1751.

70. Bucher HC, Hengstler P, Schindler C, Guyatt GH. Percutaneous transluminal coronary angioplasty versus medical treatment for non-acute coronary heart disease: meta-analysis of randomised controlled trials. *BMJ* 2000;321:73–77.

71. Pitt B, Waters D, Brown WV, *et al.* Aggressive lipid-lowering therapy compared with angioplasty in stable coronary artery disease. Atorvastatin versus Revascularization Treatment Investigators. *N Engl J Med* 1999;341:70–76.

72. Boden WE, O'Rourke RA, Teo KK, *et al.* Optimal medical therapy with or without PCI for stable coronary disease. *N Engl J Med* 2007;356:1503–1516.

73. Yusuf S, Zucker D, Chalmers TC. Ten-year results of the randomized control trials of coronary artery bypass graft surgery: tabular data compiled by the collaborative effort of the original trial investigators. Part 2 of 2. *Online J Curr Clin Trials* 1994;Doc No 144.

74. Hlatky MA, Bravata DM. Stents or surgery? New data on the comparative outcomes of percutaneous coronary intervention and coronary artery bypass graft surgery. *Circulation* 2008;118:325–327.

75. Frye RL, August P, Brooks MM, *et al.* A randomized trial of therapies for type 2 diabetes and coronary artery disease. *N Engl J Med* 2009;360:2503–2515.

76. Serruys PW, Morice MC, Kappetein AP, *et al.* Percutaneous coronary intervention versus coronary-artery bypass grafting for severe coronary artery disease. *N Engl J Med* 2009;360:961–972.

77. Holubkov R, Laskey WK, Haviland A, *et al.* Angina 1 year after percutaneous coronary intervention: a report from the NHLBI Dynamic Registry. *Am Heart J* 2002;144:826–833.

78. Lagakos SW. The challenge of subgroup analyses–reporting without distorting. *N Engl J Med* 2006;354:1667–1669.

79. Pfeffer MA, Jarcho JA. The charisma of subgroups and the subgroups of CHARISMA. *N Engl J Med* 2006;354:1744–1746.

80. Boden WE, O'Rourke R A, Teo KK, *et al.* The evolving pattern of symptomatic coronary artery disease in the United States and Canada: baseline characteristics of the Clinical Outcomes Utilizing Revascularization and Aggressive DruG Evaluation (COURAGE) trial. *Am J Cardiol* 2007;99:208–212.

81. Katritsis DG, Ioannidis JP. Percutaneous coronary intervention versus conservative therapy in nonacute coronary artery disease: a meta-analysis. *Circulation* 2005;111:2906–2912.

82. Boden WE, O'Rourke RA, Teo KK, *et al.* Impact of optimal medical therapy with or without percutaneous coronary intervention on long-term cardiovascular end points in patients with stable coronary artery disease (from the COURAGE Trial). *Am J Cardiol* 2009;104:1–4.

83. Kereiakes DJ, Teirstein PS, Sarembock IJ, *et al.* The truth and consequences of the COURAGE trial. *J Am Coll Cardiol* 2007;50:1598–1603.

84. Holmes DR Jr, Gersh BJ, Whitlow P, King SB, 3rd, Dove JT. Percutaneous coronary intervention for chronic stable angina: a reassessment. *JACC Cardiovasc Interv* 2008;1:34–43.

85. Weintraub WS, Spertus JA, Kolm P, *et al.* Effect of PCI on quality of life in patients with stable coronary disease. *N Engl J Med* 2008;359:677–687.

86. Shaw LJ, Berman DS, Maron DJ, *et al.* Optimal medical therapy with or without percutaneous coronary intervention to reduce ischemic burden: results from the Clinical Outcomes Utilizing Revascularization and Aggressive Drug Evaluation (COURAGE) trial nuclear substudy. *Circulation* 2008;117:1283–1291.

87. Mahmarian JJ, Dakik HA, Filipchuk NG, *et al.* An initial strategy of intensive medical therapy is comparable to that of coronary revascularization for suppression of scinti-

graphic ischemia in high-risk but stable survivors of acute myocardial infarction. *J Am Coll Cardiol* 2006;48:2458–2467.

88. Davies RF, Goldberg AD, Forman S, *et al.* Asymptomatic Cardiac Ischemia Pilot (ACIP) study two-year follow-up: outcomes of patients randomized to initial strategies of medical therapy versus revascularization. *Circulation* 1997;95:2037–2043.

89. Erne P, Schoenenberger AW, Burckhardt D, *et al.* Effects of percutaneous coronary interventions in silent ischemia after myocardial infarction: the SWISSI II randomized controlled trial. *JAMA* 2007;297:1985–1991.

90. Schomig A, Mehilli J, de Waha A, Seyfarth M, Pache J, Kastrati A. A meta-analysis of 17 randomized trials of a percutaneous coronary intervention-based strategy in patients with stable coronary artery disease. *J Am Coll Cardiol* 2008;52:894–904.

91. Wijeysundera HC, Ko DT. Does percutaneous coronary intervention reduce mortality in patients with stable chronic angina: are we talking about apples and oranges? *Circ Cardiovasc Qual Outcomes* 2009;2:123–126.

92. Campeau L. Letter: Grading of angina pectoris. *Circulation* 1976;54:522–523.

CHAPTER 4

Acute coronary syndromes (ST elevation and non-ST elevation)

Tobias Geisler,[1] Deepak L. Bhatt,[2] and Marcus D. Flather[3]
[1]University Hospital Tübingen, Tübingen Medical School, Tübingen, Germany
[2]VA Boston Healthcare System; Brigham and Women's Hospital and Harvard Medical School, Boston, MA, USA
[3]University of East Anglia and Norfolk and Norwich University Hospital, Norwich, UK

Definition and pathophysiology

Acute coronary syndromes (ACS) are caused by partial or total coronary artery occlusion leading to transient or persistent myocardial ischemia, with a typical presentation of retrosternal chest pain, sweating, and nausea. ACS are classically subdivided into unstable angina, non–ST-elevation and ST-elevation myocardial infarction (NSTEMI and STEMI) depending on the electrocardiogram (EKG) at presentation and results of biomarkers and cardiac enzymes.

The most common underlying disease is coronary atherosclerosis, leading to the development of coronary plaques, with plaque rupture triggering the acute event by causing coronary thrombosis. However, other rare etiologies have to be considered (e.g., embolism, dissection, spasm, plaque erosion, acute stress-induced cardiomyopathy). ACS may be the first manifestation of coronary artery disease (CAD) or may repeatedly occur in patients with a known history of CAD. Platelets play a pivotal role in the development of acute myocardial ischemia. As a consequence of exposure of the extracellular matrix at the site of a coronary lesion, a cascade triggered by platelet activation and aggregation leads to the formation of a platelet- and fibrin-rich thrombus. Thus, platelets represent a major pharmacological target to break this cascade and to reduce the extent of ischemia.

In most cases, ACS present with acute chest pain (angina pectoris) which has to be distinguished from other causes of chest pain (e.g., pulmonary embolism, aortic dissection/rupture, esophageal spasm). Unstable angina can be caused by significant coronary stenosis that does allow sufficient blood

Cardiovascular Clinical Trials: Putting the Evidence into Practice, First Edition.
Edited by Marcus D. Flather, Deepak L. Bhatt, and Tobias Geisler.
© 2013 Blackwell Publishing Ltd. Published 2013 by Blackwell Publishing Ltd.

flow to preserve myocardial perfusion, but increasingly causes symptoms of chest pain without any discernible trigger and of random frequency. Unstable angina is associated with a high imminent risk of developing MI in which perfusion is reduced, causing necrosis of myocardial tissue. Patients with STEMI often present with an occluding thrombus in one proximal coronary branch, whereas in NSTEMI the culprit artery is usually partially occluded, allowing a minimal flow, or there may be collateral flow via related arteries. In STEMI, thrombus can disappear over time due to embolization or local fibrinolysis, making angiographic confirmation difficult in some cases, particularly if angiography is delayed for any reason.

Epidemiology and healthcare costs

ACS are a major cause of premature mortality and morbidity and globally result in millions of hospitalizations annually. ACS consume large amounts of healthcare resources and have a major negative economic and social impact through days lost at work, support for disability, and coping with the psychological consequences of illness.

The mean annual incidence of hospital admission for an acute MI is 1900 per 1 million population in European countries [1]. In the US, about 1.3 million people each year are affected by unstable angina/NSTEMI and about 400 000 by STEMI. About 4% of US citizens admitted to hospital with unstable angina/NSTEMI die within 30 days and 8% develop reinfarction. In 2006 more than 6 million patients were seen in US emergency departments with acute chest pain, highlighting the large annual number of patients with suspected ACS and the need for effective diagnostic and therapeutic guidelines [2]. The estimated cost of a typical ACS admission in the US (hospital stay 5 days with coronary angiography and percutaneous coronary intervention) is about US$15000, amounting to an annual healthcare cost of about US$15 billion; in addition there is the ongoing cost of care for ACS patients.

Diagnosis

The development of diagnostic algorithms in the setting of chest pain units that include sensitive cardiac biomarkers and non-invasive imaging techniques has led to more accurate detection of small amounts of myocardial necrosis and more rapid and reliable diagnosis of myocardial ischemia. These improvements have led to new early medical and interventional approaches to reduce myocardial ischemia. Acute MI is now defined if one of the following European Society of Cardiology, American College of Cardiology, American Heart Association and World Heart Federation (ESC/ACCF/AHA/ WHF) Task Force criteria is met [3,4]:
• Detection of a rise of cardiac biomarkers (>99th percentile) together with either symptoms of ischemia, EKG changes indicative of new ischemia, or imaging evidence of newly occurring regional wall motion abnormality
• Sudden unexpected death due to a cardiac cause

Table 4.1 Clinical classification of different types of myocardial infarction according to the joint ESC/ACC/AHA/WHF Task Force definition [3,4].

Type 1
Spontaneous myocardial infarction (MI) related to ischemia due to a primary coronary event such as plaque erosion and/or rupture, fissuring, or dissection

Type 2
MI secondary to ischemia due to either increased oxygen demand or decreased supply, e.g., coronary artery spasm, coronary embolism, anemia, arrhythmias, hypertension, or hypotension

Type 3
Sudden unexpected cardiac death, including cardiac arrest, often with symptoms suggestive of myocardial ischemia, accompanied by presumably new ST elevation, or new left bundle branch block, or evidence of fresh thrombus in a coronary artery by angiography and/or at autopsy, but death occurring before blood samples could be obtained, or at a time before the appearance of cardiac biomarkers in the blood

Type 4a
MI with percutaneous coronary intervention (PCI)

Type 4b
MI associated with stent thrombosis as documented by angiography or at autopsy

Type 5
MI associated with coronary artery bypass graft (CABG)

- Pathological findings of an acute MI (e.g., angiographic confirmation of a newly occluded coronary artery).

The clinical classification of acute MI has been further described as shown in Table 4.1.

A typical history of ACS often goes hand in hand with recurrent episodes of chest pain, which are characterized by dynamic alterations over time and an increase in frequency and duration or decreased levels of exercise leading to chest pain. However, nausea, vomiting, shortness of breath, palpitations, sweating, and anxiety are also commonly associated with ACS. The typical presentation of ACS with cardiac chest pain is often modified in the elderly, patients with diabetes, and women. For example, women tend to present with fewer symptoms and atypical chest pain, which may delay diagnosis or lead to inappropriate discharge of these patients from the emergency department [5]. The clinical difference between unstable angina and acute MI is often characterized by the persistence of chest pain at rest with acute MI and reversible or intermittent chest pain with unstable angina. The magnitude of angina can be described using the Braunwald classification (Table 4.2) [6,7]. Symptoms and onset can differ in NSTEMI and STEMI, mainly due to the different pathophysiologies characterized by either complete occlusion in STEMI versus incomplete or complete occlusion in the presence of good collateral flow in non–ST-elevation ACS.

Table 4.2 Braunwald classification of unstable angina [6,7].

Severity		Develops in presence of extracardiac condition that intensifies myocardial ischemia (secondary UA)	Develops in the absence of extracardiac condition (primary UA)	Develops within 2 weeks after acute myocardial infarction (postinfarction UA)
I	New onset of severe angina or accelerated angina; no pain at rest	IA	IB	IC
II	Angina at rest within past month but not within prior 48 h (angina at rest, subacute)	IIA	IIB	IIC
III	Angina at rest within 48 h (angina at rest, acute)	IIIA	IIIB Troponin negative IIIB Troponin positive	IIIC

UA, unstable angina.

Examination

In patients with ACS a rapid diagnosis is crucial. An accurate, abbreviated history is essential in the management of suspected ACS: nature of symptoms, time of symptom onset, previous cardiac history, associated risk factors, comorbidities, and medication use. Due to the urgent nature of the condition, a history has to be assessed in 5–10 minutes during which time the patient may also be undergoing an EKG and blood tests. Patients presenting with ACS are usually very anxious and a reassuring and informative manner is essential in the early stages of assessment.

Investigation

Routine immediate tests in the emergency room include an EKG and routine blood tests to detect elevations in cardiac markers and heart muscle damage, and to assess hematology, electrolytes, and renal and liver function. Chest X-rays are routinely performed to help rule out pulmonary edema or other pulmonary abnormalities, including pneumothorax or other differential diagnoses such as aortic aneurysm or aortic dissection. The EKG provides valuable diagnostic information, but a normal EKG does not exclude ACS, as the event can cause dynamic EKG changes that might not be captured by a single recording [8].

Risk scores have been developed to evaluate the future risk for death or recurrent MI in patients with ACS. The Thrombolysis in Myocardial Infarction

(TIMI) and GRACE scores have shown good prognostic accuracy [9,10]. Scores can help assign patients to more intensive therapy versus a more conservative approach.

Electrocardiography

STEMI is typically defined as an ST elevation of greater than 1 mm in two contiguous limb leads and greater than 2 mm in precordial leads or new left bundle branch block [11]. Not every STEMI results in the development of Q-waves in subsequent EKGs and likewise Q-waves can develop as a result of NSTEMI. In patients with symptoms consistent with myocardial ischemia but non-diagnostic EKG findings, EKGs should be repeated every 15–30 minutes to detect dynamic changes [12]. NSTEMI is often characterized by ST depression of 0.5 mV or greater in chest or limb leads or T-wave inversion of 0.3 mm or greater. Continuous EKG monitoring can help to detect episodes of "silent" ischemia and arrhythmias.

Cardiac markers

Standard diagnostic biomarkers are creatine kinase-MB (CK-MB) and cardiac troponin, although older markers like creatine kinase, lactate dehydrogenase or myoglobin are still used for the diagnosis and evaluation of time course and extent of ischemia in the setting of MI.

Cardiac troponin assays have a high sensitivity (>90%) and high specificity (>80%) to detect myocardial damage; however, they may have a false-negative time window of up to 6 hours after onset of ischemia (Figure 4.1). Troponin is found in both cardiac and skeletal muscle, but the specific subunits of tro-

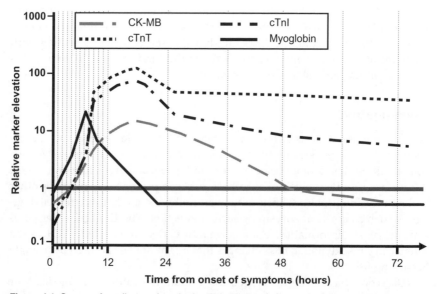

Figure 4.1 Course of cardiac markers in the early phase of myocardial infarction [22,23].

ponin differ between types of muscle. There are two major types of cardiac troponins: T (cTnT) and I (cTnI). Troponin T binds to tropomyosin, interlocking it to form a troponin—tropomyosin complex, whereas troponin I binds to actin in thin myofilaments to keep the troponin—tropomyosin complex in place. While cTnI tests measure only cardiac troponin, cTnT tests may cross-react with troponin from other muscle tissue, resulting in false-positive findings in the absence of heart damage. Cross-reaction with skeletal muscle TnT was a particular problem in early immunoassays, but this has been minimized in newer cardiospecific assays [13]. cTnI has been reported to be a more sensitive marker of minor cardiac muscle damage [14], but the outcome prediction is fairly similar between both assays [15]. The documentation of a dynamic pattern is required to distinguish background increased troponin levels as these can occur in the setting of other diseases. Thus, cTnT background levels in particular are elevated in patients with chronic renal disease [16] and chronically elevated troponin levels can be a sign of myocardial damage in structural heart disease [17,18]. Recently developed "high sensitivity" troponin assays may improve the early detection of acute MI in patients with a high pre-test probability of MI (i.e., in the setting of chest pain units) [19–21]. Raised troponin can occur in a variety of non-cardiac settings, including acute infection, intensive care, and post trauma, and in these cases it is essential to obtain a clinical opinion to understand the primary cause of the raised troponin.

Role of imaging techniques

A number of imaging tests are available to stratify patients according to risk at the time of an acute coronary event. These tests have been evaluated for their role in the early diagnosis of ACS.

Echocardiography

Echocardiography has been included in early diagnostic algorithms for ACS in chest pain centers. With advances in imaging techniques and development of high-resolution portable systems, echocardiography has become a valuable non-invasive tool to obtain immediate information about a number of cardiac abnormalities underlying ACS, thus contributing to the initial diagnosis as well as to the further risk estimation of the patient. This includes wall motion abnormalities, left and right ventricular function, heart valve disorders, pericardial effusion, and dissection of the ascending aorta and detection of intracardiac thrombi. With the use of 3D and contrast echocardiography, the sensitivity to detect wall motion abnormalities has been increased. Additionally, stress echocardiography has been applied with sufficient accuracy to rule out ACS in patients with chest pain and negative findings on EKG and laboratory tests.

Echocardiography is not considered a routine tool for the early diagnosis of ACS, but patients should undergo echocardiography routinely during a hospital admission for ACS as part of their cardiac assessment and future risk stratification.

Myocardial perfusion imaging

Radionuclide myocardial perfusion imaging (MPI) may be of value for evaluating patients who have persistent chest pain suggestive of ACS, but a negative pre-test probability (normal or near-normal EKG, initial cardiac markers below the reference value). Exercise MPI with thallium-201 (Tl-201) was considered to be a reliable tool to differentiate low- versus high-risk post-infarct patients who might benefit from subsequent revascularization therapy in the thrombolytic era [24]. This has changed, however, since primary percutaneous coronary intervention (PCI) is widely available in most specialist centers, allowing for short revascularization times and increased prognostic benefit of early revascularization. Stress MPI with Tl-201 or technetium (Tc)-99m agents, such as sestamibi and tetrofosim, still has some value in estimating myocardium at risk after coronary ischemia and in assessing the final infarct size, and in those centers where early angiography may not be available [25]. In some studies, stress MPI has been performed safely 2–4 days after infarction [26]. The INSPIRE (adenosINe Sestamibi Post-InfaRction Evaluation) trial included 728 stable patients who survived MI to investigate whether high-risk patients could be identified from the initial left ventricular (LV) perfusion defect [27]. Myocardial perfusion was assessed in all patients by single photon emission computed tomography (SPECT) using adenosine Tc-99m sestamibi as the radionuclide. The study showed that a combination of MPI and LV function assessment was a reliable predictor of major adverse events at 1 year. Thus, it is considered, although not directly documented, that the integration of perfusion and function yields superior risk stratification after ACS. Cardiac positron emission tomography (PET) imaging has developed from a research tool into an applicable clinical imaging modality. However, current guidelines for the management of ACS patients do not include PET in routine diagnostic algorithms.

Whether "fused" scans (the combination of MPI and coronary computed coronary angiography) can provide additional useful information in ACS patients will be evaluated in upcoming clinical trials [28].

Computed tomography angiography

Coronary computed tomography angiography (CTA) has been included in the diagnostic algorithms of chest pain centers. CTA may be able to evaluate coronary calcification, extent of coronary stenoses, myocardial perfusion, and ventricular function in ACS, and may help to differentiate ACS from other life-threatening cardiovascular diseases, such as aortic dissection and pulmonary embolus. These features and the use of a rapid scanning method have the potential to make CTA a suitable tool to triage patients with chest pain in the emergency department, especially in those patients with low-to-moderate enzyme and EKG scores. In the ROMICAT (Rule Out Myocardial Infarction using Computer Assisted Tomography) trial, CTA showed a high negative predictive value, suggesting the capability to obviate further tests if the CTA is negative in patients presenting with chest pain, negative initial troponin, and a normal EKG [29].

Magnetic resonance imaging

Magnetic resonance imaging (MRI) can yield important information in the "diagnostic gap" during the first hours after onset of ischemia in ACS. It excels in being able to evaluate perfusion, viability, function, and morphology [30]. The first prospective trial evaluating MRI in patients with acute chest pain demonstrated additional diagnostic gain from wall motion assessment and coronary imaging compared with conventional risk stratification by cardiac markers and EKG (sensitivity and specificity for detecting ACS were 84% and 85%, respectively, for MRI) [31]. However, MRI can fail to detect transient pathologies due to dynamic changes in perfusion, wall motion abnormalities, and ventricular stunning during ACS. Adenosine stress MRI has also been demonstrated to serve as a superior prognostic risk marker compared with classical risk factors in post-ACS patients [32].

Management

General measures

The introduction of chest pain centers has helped to improve diagnostic algorithms to detect myocardial ischemia and provide timely anti-ischemic treatment. Additionally, they are cost-effective by triaging low-risk patients towards early discharge and further follow-up in the outpatient clinic [33]. Typically, patients are provided with oxygen and pain relief with opiates or other effective analgesics as part of their early general care.

Antithrombotic therapies

Oral antiplatelet therapy

Since platelet activation leading to thrombus formation is a key pathophysiological process in ACS, antiplatelet treatment is essential to improve the short- and long-term prognosis. Antiplatelet therapy with aspirin (generally 300 or 325 mg) and a thienopyridine (clopidogrel 300 or 600 mg) given as a loading dose as soon as NSTE-ACS is diagnosed is standard practice in many centers. Some centers avoid upstream thienopyridine therapy before coronary anatomy has been determined in order to prevent bleeding in those patients who have an indication for coronary artery bypass graft (CABG) surgery. However, post-hoc analysis of trials investigating the effect of upstream clopidogrel treatment in ACS patients undergoing subsequent CABG surgery did not find an increased perioperative bleeding risk; instead they found reduced ischemic events, potentially supporting the safety of upstream ADP-receptor blockade with clopidogrel [34]. According to recent guidelines, novel $P2Y_{12}$ blockers (prasugrel, ticagrelor) are preferred in some settings of ACS and after exclusion of contraindications against each of the substance. In patients undergoing stent implantation (bare metal stents [BMS] or drug-eluting stents [DES]) during PCI for NSTE-ACS and STEMI, clopidogrel 75 mg/day, prasugrel 10 mg/day or ticagrelor 180 mg/day (class IA evidence) should be given for at least 12 months [35]. If the individual bleeding risk outweighs the anticipated antiplatelet benefit, earlier discontinuation of the P2Y$_{12}$-receptor blocker should be considered (class IA evidence) [12]. Patients with medically managed unstable angina and NSTEMI should be treated with clopidogrel or ticagrelor for optimally up to 1 year [36,37].

A new class of oral antiplatelet drugs targets the main thrombin receptor on platelets (protease-activated receptor, PAR-1), thus preventing thrombin-induced platelet activation. Two substances belonging to this group (voraxapar [SCH 530348] and atopaxar [E5555]) have been under investigation in clinical trials for their effect as additional antiplatelet treatment in ACS patients. Voraxapar (40 mg loading dose followed by 2.5 mg daily maintenance dose) in addition to standard therapy failed to reduce the primary efficacy endpoint (combination of cardiovascular death, MI, stroke, hospitalization for ischemia, and urgent revascularization), but led to a significantly higher rate of major bleeding events in the TRACER (Thrombin Receptor Antagonist for Clinical Event Reduction in Acute Coronary Syndrome) trial that enrolled 12 944 NSTE-ACS patients [38]. The LANCELOT-ACS (Lessons from Antagonizing the Cellular Effect of Thrombin—Acute Coronary Syndrome) trial investigated atopaxar in different doses for its safety on top of standard therapy. A total of 603 unstable angina or non-STEMI patients were randomized to placebo or a 400-mg loading dose of atopaxar followed by a daily dose of 50, 100, or 200 mg for 12 weeks. An analysis combining all patients treated with atopaxar showed a numerically but not significantly higher incidence of any CURE bleeding, compared with placebo (3.1% vs. 2.2%; p = 0.63). Additionally, there was no significant difference of CURE major bleeding (1.8% vs. 0%; p = 0.12). The study also showed a 34% relative reduction in the incidence of Holter-detected ischemia 48 hours following the 400-mg loading dose. The trial, however, was not powered for differences in ischemic clinical endpoints [39].

Additional antiplatelet therapy

The rationale for general periprocedural administration of glycoprotein (GP) IIb/IIIa inhibitors in the era of high-dose thienopyridine is a topic for discussion. In the ISAR-REACT-2 (Intracoronary Stenting and Antithrombotic-Regimen Rapid Early Action for Coronary Treatment 2) trial the benefit of peri-interventional GP inhibition with abciximab was restricted to higher risk non–ST-elevation ACS patients presenting with significant elevation of cardiac markers [40]. Additionally, GP inhibitor treatment showed a benefit mainly in patients with ACS undergoing PCI [41] rather than in conservatively treated patients [42]. However, there was no significant difference in risk of death, recurrent MI, or urgent target vessel revascularization (TVR) between the tirofiban and placebo arms at 30 days. The bleeding risk associated with GP IIb/IIIa inhibitors is noteworthy and the net clinical benefit of heparin and GP inhibitor treatment has been shown to be lower compared to single treatment with the direct thrombin inhibitor bivalirudin in high-risk non–ST-elevation ACS and STEMI patients undergoing primary PCI [43–45].

The issue of timing of GP inhibitor administration is a further issue to be addressed. Recent studies have evaluated the benefits of prehospital and preangiography administration of GP IIb/IIIa inhibitors. The ON-TIME 2 (Ongoing Tirofiban in Myocardial Infarction Evaluation) study evaluated the effects of early provisional treatment with tirofiban given to STEMI patients in the ambulance. A high-dose bolus of tirofiban was associated with increased ST-segment resolution and better clinical outcome after PCI [46]. The FINESSE (Facilitated Intervention With Enhanced Reperfusion Speed to Stop Events) trial randomized patients with a new STEMI in a double-blind, double-dummy fashion to one of three treatment strategies: primary PCI; facilitated PCI with abciximab alone; or facilitated PCI with reteplase/abciximab. Study enrollment was difficult and was stopped prematurely. At 90 days there was no difference in the primary composite endpoint of all-cause mortality/rehospitalization for congestive heart failure, resuscitated ventricular fibrillation more than 48 hours after randomization, or cardiogenic shock [47]. According to the results of the EARLY-ACS and ACUITY-timing trials, there is currently no evidence of a benefit of upstream GP IIb/IIIa antagonism in NSTE-ACS patients who receive guideline adherent dual antiplatelet and anticoagulation before PCI [48–50].

Current practice guidelines support the selective use of GP IIb/IIIa inhibitors in STEMI patients undergoing primary PCI who show a large thrombus burden or have not received adequate thienopyridine loading (class IIa/b; see Table 4.2) [12]. Routine upstream administration is not supported (class III; see Table 4.2). There has been no evidence that the route of administration (intravenous versus intracoronary) results in a different outcome of ACS [51]. However, intracoronary application may be preferred in some situations when a large thrombus burden is visible and may be associated with improved myocardial perfusion [52,53].

Anticoagulant therapy

Anticoagulant therapy should be added to antiplatelet therapy as soon as possible after ACS patients present. In patients who are selected for an invasive strategy, regimens with established efficacy include enoxaparin and unfractionated heparin (UFH) (class IA evidence), bivalirudin or fondaparinux (class IB evidence) [12,35].

These recommendations are based on the results of important randomized clinical trials. The design and main results of the key trials investigating the role of anticoagulants in ACS are briefly discussed below.

The low weight molecular heparin (LMWH) enoxaparin was compared to standard heparin treatment of ACS in two major trials. The SYNERGY (Superior Yield of the New strategy of Enoxaparin, Revascularisation, and GlYcoprotein inhibitors) trial randomized 10000 high-risk patients with ACS to enoxaparin (1 mg/kg subcutaneously every 12 hours) or UFH (60 U/kg bolus then 12 U/kg/h adjusted to an aPTT of 50–70 seconds). An early invasive strategy within a median of 21 hours from randomization was achieved in 90% of the study patients, and 47% and 19% underwent PCI and CABG, respectively; 57% of the patients were treated with GP IIb/IIIa inhibitors. The primary endpoint of death or MI at 30 days was not significantly different between the two treatment arms. However, there was a significant increase in TIMI major bleeding in the enoxaparin arm (9.1% vs 7.6; p = 0.008). In terms of efficacy, enoxaparin failed to show superiority over UFH, but non-inferiority criteria were met [54].

The EXTRACT-TIMI 25 (Enoxaparin and Thrombolysis Reperfusion for Acute Myocardial Infarction Treatment—Thrombolysis in Myocardial Infarction 25) trial randomized 20506 patients with STEMI who were scheduled to undergo fibrinolysis to either enoxaparin (until hospital discharge or for a maximum of 8 days, whichever came first) or UFH for at least 48 hours. The primary endpoint of death or non-fatal recurrent MI was significantly reduced in those patients who received enoxaparin (9.9% vs 12.0%; p < 0.001). This was primarily driven by a 33% reduction in the rate of non-fatal MI in the enoxaparin group, as there was no significant difference in mortality between the two arms. Treatment with enoxaparin was associated with a higher bleeding rate (2.1% vs 1.4%; p < 0.001), but the net clinical benefit remained in favor of LMWH treatment (relative risk reduction for the combination of MI, death, and major bleeding 14%; p < 0.001) [55].

The OASIS 5 (Fifth Organization to Assess Strategies in Acute Ischemic Syndromes) trial was a randomized, double-blind, multicenter study evaluating the safety and efficacy of the factor Xa inhibitor fondaparinux compared with LMWH enoxaparin in patients with unstable angina and NSTEMI. Fondaparinux is a synthetic pentasaccharide that acts through specific inhibition of the coagulation factor Xa via antithrombin. The OASIS 5 trial included 20078 patients recruited at 576 sites in 41 countries. Patients were randomized to either fondaparinux 2.5mg (n = 10057) or enoxaparin 1mg/kg twice daily (n = 10021). All patients received standard treatment with aspirin, clopidogrel, and GP IIb/IIIa inhibitors, according to local practice. Both study drugs were administered for an average of 5 days. Fondaparinux was non-inferior to enoxaparin in terms of the primary efficacy endpoint (combination of death, MI, refractory ischemia at 9 days) and associated with fewer overall and major bleeding events, resulting in a substantial net clinical benefit in favor of fondaparinux [56]. In addition there was a significant reduction in all-cause mortality in the fondaparinux group. These benefits appeared to be consistent whether or not patients underwent PCI [57]. Notably, rates of guide catheter thrombosis were greater in patients receiving fondaparinux (0.9% vs 0.4%; p = 0.01). The benefit of adjunctive heparin treatment in NSTE-ACS patients undergoing PCI was further investigated in the FUTURA-OASIS-8 trial. This was a prospective, randomized, double-blind trial that enrolled 3235 patients of whom 2046 were randomized to administration of standard-dose heparin (n = 1002) or low-dose heparin (n = 1024) as an adjunctive antithrombotic regimen at the time of PCI. Rates of guide catheter thrombosis were not significantly different between the two groups (0.1% vs 0.5%; p = 0.15) and were numerically smaller compared with the historical OASIS-5 fondaparinux-alone arm (0.9%). Although a systematic randomized trial is lacking, the findings of the FUTURA-OASIS-8 and the earlier OASIS-5 trial suggest that adjunctive UFH at the time of PCI reduces the risk of guide catheter thrombosis without increasing major bleeding events [58].

The OASIS-6 trial tested the efficacy and safety of fondaparinux in 12 092 STEMI patients who were randomized to fondaparinux (2.5 mg once daily given for up to 8 days) or standard care (placebo for those in whom UFH was not indicated or UFH for up to 48 hours followed by placebo for up to 8 days). The primary endpoint consisted of the composite of death or reinfarction at 30 days; it was significantly reduced in the fondaparinux treatment arm (9.7 vs 11.2; HR, 0.86; 95% CI, 0.77–0.96; p = 0.008). There was a trend towards fewer major bleeding episodes at day 9 under fondaparinux compared to control (UFH/placebo) (1.0 vs 1.3), although these effects were non-significant (p = 0.13). However, there was no benefit seen in the subgroup of 3789 patients undergoing primary PCI [59].

Taken together, these results suggest that fondaparinux provides a net clinical benefit in NSTE-ACS patients compared with enoxaparin, and in STEMI patients who are not treated with primary PCI compared with usual care.

The direct thrombin inhibitor bivalirudin was compared to heparin and GP IIb/IIIa inhibitor treatment in ACS patients in the ACUITY and HORIZON AMI trials. The ACUITY trial involved 13 819 patients with moderate- to high-risk ACS (NSTEMI) who all underwent cardiac catheterization within 72 hours and received percutaneous or surgical revascularization. Patients were randomized to one of three treatment arms: bivalirudin plus routine GP IIb/IIIa inhibition; UFH or enoxaparin plus routine GP IIb/IIIa inhibition; or bivalirudin alone, with GP IIb/IIIa inhibition only given as bailout (~7% of patients in the bivalirudin treatment arm received a bailout GP IIb/IIIa blocker). When bivalirudin alone was compared with UFH/enoxaparin plus a GP IIb/IIIa blocker, there was a mild but non-significant increase in ischemic events after 30 days fulfilling the prespecified criteria for non-inferiority (efficacy endpoint death, MI or unplanned revascularization 7.8 vs 7.3; p = 0.011 for non-inferiority). However, bivalirudin was associated with a significant decrease in major bleeding events (3.0 vs 5.7; p < 0.001) and a significantly higher net clinical benefit (combined ischemic and bleeding events 10.1 vs 11.7; p = 0.015) [60].

In the ISAR-REACT-4 trial, 1721 patients with acute NSTEMI undergoing PCI were randomized to receive abciximab plus UFH (861 patients) or bivalirudin (860 patients). The study tested whether abciximab and heparin are superior to bivalirudin with respect to the primary composite endpoint of death, large recurrent MI, urgent TVR, or major bleeding within 30 days of follow-up. Secondary endpoints were the composite of death, any recurrent MI, or urgent TVR (efficacy endpoint) and major bleeding (safety endpoint) within 30 days of follow-up. The primary endpoint was no different between patients in the abciximab bivalirudin arms (10.9% vs. 11.0%; p = 0.94). Additionally there were no significant differences in the secondary efficacy endpoints. However, major bleeding occurred more frequently (4.6%) in the abciximab-treated patients as compared with 2.6% of patients treated with bivalirudin (RR, 1.84; 95% CI, 1.10–3.07; p = 0.02) [46].

The HORIZONS AMI trial included 3602 patients with STEMI (symptom onset <12 hours) from 123 centers in 11 countries. Patients were randomized in a 1:1 fashion to UFH 60 U/kg IV, with subsequent boluses targeting an activated clotting time (ACT) of 200–250 seconds, plus a GP IIb/IIIa inhibitor (abciximab or eptifibatide), or to bivalirudin monotherapy (0.75 mg/kg bolus; infusion of 1.75 mg/kg/h stopped at the end of the procedure) plus provisional GP IIb/IIIa inhibitors (~7% of patients in the bivalirudin-treated group received a GP IIb/IIIa inhibitor in the cath lab). With bivalirudin there was a significant 24% reduction in net adverse clinical events and a 40% reduction in major bleeding at 30 days. MACE, defined as all-cause death, re-infarction, ischemic TVR, or stroke, was no different between the two groups, but in an analysis of individual event rates, bivalirudin treatment was associated with a substantial reduction of cardiac deaths (1.8 vs 2.9; p = 0.035) [61].

Current guidelines support the use of bivalirudin in patients with STEMI undergoing primary PCI irrespective of prior UFH use (class IB evidence) and especially in those who have a high bleeding risk (class IIaB evidence) [12]. In NSTEMI patients, bivalirudin is the recommended anticoagulant in patients who are managed with an early invasive strategy (<72 hours) [35].

The role of long-term oral thrombin inhibition (direct thrombin inhibition, oral factor Xa inhibition) in ACS on top of dual antiplatelet therapy has been investigated in a number of recent clinical trials. RE-DEEM was a phase 2 trial comparing four doses of the oral direct thrombin inhibitor dabigatran etexilate (50, 75, 110, and 150 mg b.i.d.) with placebo, in addition to dual antiplatelet treatment, in 1861 patients with STEMI (60%) or high-risk NSTEMI (40%). PCI was performed in 54% of the patients. Results showed that International Society on Thrombosis and Haemostasis (ISTH) major bleeding rates increased moderately with higher dabigatran doses (p for trend <0.001), occurring in 0.8%, 0.3%, 2%, and 1.2%, respectively, with increasing dabigatran, compared with 0.5% with placebo. The trial was not powered for efficacy endpoints and the overall event rate of cardiovascular death, non-fatal MI, or stroke was low [62].

The APPRAISE-2 (Apixaban for Prevention of Acute Ischemic Events 2) trial was a double-blind, placebo-controlled trial involving 7392 patients with a recent ACS and at least two additional risk factors for recurrent ischemic events. Patients were randomly assigned to the oral factor Xa inhibitor apixaban 5 mg twice daily or placebo. During a median follow-up of 241 days, the primary efficacy outcome (composite of cardiovascular death, MI, or ischemic stroke) occurred with a similar frequency in the apixaban and placebo groups (HR, 0.95; p = 0.51). In an interim analysis, the primary safety endpoint of major bleeding, as defined by the TIMI classification, occurred significantly more often among those given apixaban (HR, 2.59; p = 0.001), with a higher incidence of intracranial and fatal bleeding events. These results led to a premature termination of the trial by the Data and Safety Monitoring Board (DSMB) due to safety reasons [63].

Another oral factor Xa inhibitor, rivaroxaban, has been tested in ACS patients. After an initial dose finding study [64], the ATLAS-TIMI 51 trial randomized 15 526 patients within 7 days after hospital admission for an ACS (NSTE-ACS and STEMI) to standard therapy plus either placebo or rivaroxaban in one of two doses (2.5 or 5 mg) twice daily. The incidence of the composite primary endpoint (death, MI, or stroke) was significantly lower among patients receiving rivaroxaban (combined dose groups) compared with patients receiving placebo (8.9% vs 10.7%) at a mean follow-up of 13 months. Compared with placebo, rivaroxaban at either dose was associated with significant increases in major bleeding (2.1% vs 0.6%) and intracranial hemorrhage (0.6% vs 0.2%). Notably, the 2.5 mg twice daily dose was associated with a significant reduction of cardiovascular and overall mortality without an excess of fatal bleeding [65].

Other treatments

Beta-blockers are used routinely in the treatment of ACS as they decrease oxygen demand due to the reductions in heart rate, contractility, and blood pressure, and can lead to relief of ischemic chest pain. Furthermore, they can be beneficial in lowering the threshold for developing automaticity and ventricular fibrillation [66,67] and show a proven long-term benefit in patients with prior MI by suppressing adverse ventricular remodeling and improving ventricular function [68,69].

Current guidelines recommend beta-blockers for patients with unstable angina/NSTEMI unless contraindicated [70]. Treatment should begin within a few days of the event, if not initiated acutely, and should be continued indefinitely (class IB evidence). Patients with unstable angina/NSTEMI with moderate or severe LV failure should receive beta-blocker therapy with a gradual titration scheme (class IB evidence) [35].

In STEMI patients, oral administration of beta-blockers, if not contraindicated, should be initiated promptly (class IA evidence). Early intravenous beta-blockade should be avoided in patients with an increased risk* for cardiogenic shocks (class IIIA evidence) [71]. The latter recommendation was mainly based on the observation of a higher rate of early cardiogenic shock in patients who were allocated to the metoprolol treatment arm in the COMMIT/CCS-2 (Clopidogrel and Metoprolol in Myocardial Infarction Trial/Second Chinese Cardiac Study) [72]. COMMIT-CCS-2 was a randomized, double-blind, 2 × 2 factorial trial involving 45 852 patients with STEMI randomized to daily, oral treatment with clopidogrel 75 mg plus aspirin 162 mg (n = 22 960); or daily aspirin plus placebo (n = 22 891) and intravenous metoprolol followed by oral administration (22 928); or placebo (n = 22 923) for up to 4 weeks. Although the addition of metoprolol

---

*Risk factors for cardiogenic shock were defined as age >70 years, systolic blood pressure <120 mmHg, sinus tachycardia >110 bpm or heart rate <60 bpm, and increased time since onset of symptoms of STEMI.

significantly reduced the relative risk of recurrent MI and ventricular fibrillation by 18% and 17%, respectively, it significantly increased the relative risk of cardiogenic shock by 30%. These events mainly occurred during the first day of treatment (i.e., subsequent to intravenous treatment) and the event-rate was much larger in high-risk individuals.

A meta-analysis including 13 024 patients with ACS revealed that initiation of statin therapy within 14 days following the onset of a coronary event does not reduce major adverse events over up to 4 months follow-up, thus not suggesting a short-term benefit [73]. Another meta-analysis of 13 randomized trials has also analyzed the effects of early intensive statin therapy in a total of 17 963 ACS patients; early, intensive statin therapy significantly reduced death and cardiovascular events beyond 4 months of treatment, indicating their long-term positive impact [74]. However, many centers routinely give higher-dose statins early in the course of ACS as there do not appear to be any adverse effects.

Reperfusion therapy

Early reperfusion in STEMI and high-risk NSTE-ACS is clearly associated with improved outcome, and time between symptom onset and re-establishment of revascularization correlates with the extent of myocardial damage and mortality [75,76]. PCI is the favored treatment in patients with STEMI and in high-risk patients with NSTE-ACS. In general, the indication and timing for coronary angiography and PCI depends on the underlying risk profile of an individual patient. Guidelines support immediate primary PCI in patients with STEMI [12], and an early invasive strategy (<72 hours) in moderate- and high-risk patients with NSTE-ACS [35,63].

Fibrinolytic therapy may be the first treatment of choice in STEMI patients if immediate primary PCI cannot be performed (i.e., in facilities that do not offer PCI), but early transfer to a cath lab is recommended for high-risk patients (i.e., large MI or hemodynamic or electrical instability or persistence of symptoms)[†] independently of the success of fibrinolytic therapy (CARESS-in-AMI and TRANSFER-AMI trials) [12,77,78]. The first medical contact-to-balloon time in STEMI patients should be less than 90 minutes; however, mortality advantages of primary PCI compared with fibrinolytic therapy have been observed with longer times [79].

No additional benefit between immediate, early (<24 hours), and delayed (>24 hours) invasive management has been observed in the overall study cohorts of moderate- to high-risk NSTEMI patients if treated with guideline-adherent antithrombotic therapy (ABOARD and TIMACS studies) [80,81], but the data also indicate that NSTEMI patients at highest risk (i.e. defined by the GRACE score) do benefit from early PCI by risk reduction of major adverse events.

[†]Further high risk features of STEMI are: extensive ST-segment elevation, new-onset left bundle branch block, previous MI, Killip class >2, LVEF 35% or less, systolic blood pressure <100 mmHg, heart rate >100 bpm.

Appraisal of selected clinical trials that have changed the management of acute coronary syndromes

Clinical trials have fundamentally changed medical and interventional treatment regimens of ACS and we discuss some examples that have led to improved antiplatelet treatment strategies in ACS (Table 4.3).

CURE trial

Trial design
The CURE (Clopidogrel in Unstable angina to prevent Recurrent Events) trial compared clopidogrel versus placebo in patients with unstable angina or NSTEMI (Table 4.3). The primary hypothesis of superiority of clopidogrel was tested in a randomized, double-blind, placebo-controlled fashion. Patients were treated with a 300-mg loading dose of clopidogrel followed by a 75-mg maintenance dose or by matching placebo for the duration of follow-up (average treatment duration 9 months). All patients received aspirin (ASA) 75–325 mg daily at the discretion of the treating physician. The primary outcome measure was the composite of cardiovascular death, MI, or stroke. Secondary endpoints were the combination of cardiovascular death, MI, stroke, or refractory ischemia. Safety endpoints were the occurrence of major bleeds.

Eligibility
Patients hospitalized for ACS were included in this study. They had to have myocardial ischemia either documented by typical EKG changes or elevated cardiac necrosis markers. Mainly centers favoring a conservative approach for management of ACS were involved. Patients were excluded from the study if they had contraindications against antithrombotic or antiplatelet therapy, if there was an indication for use of oral anticoagulant, if they had severe heart failure, or if they had recently undergone PCI or been recently treated with GP IIb/IIIa inhibitors.

Main results
Clopidogrel treatment was associated with a 20% relative risk reduction (RRR) in the overall patient cohort (n = 12562 patients). This was to a large extent influenced by the reduction of rate of MI. The benefit occurred early, within a few hours after randomization, and persisted for the duration of the follow-up. Clopidogrel treatment was associated with a higher rate of major and minor bleeding. The risk of fatal bleeding was not significantly increased; however, more patients in the active comparator arm suffered from bleeding requiring blood transfusion. Bleeding in patients undergoing CABG was similar between the clopidogrel and placebo arms if clopidogrel was discontinued at least 5 days before the operative procedure. There was a trend towards more postoperative bleeding events in patients who had received clopidogrel within 5 days before CABG [82].

Table 4.3 Overview of design and results of selected clinical trials that have changed the management of ACS.

Trial	Patient population	Study design	Centers	Patient number	Treatment groups	Outcome measures	Results
CURE	ACS with or without ST-segment elevation	Prospective, randomized, double blind	482 centers, 28 countries	12 562 (n = 1313 clopidogrel, n = 1345 placebo)	Clopidogrel 300 mg + ASA 75–325 mg/day followed by 75 mg/day Placebo + ASA 75–325 mg/day	Primary: composite of CV death, non-fatal MI or stroke Safety: life-threatening and major bleeding	Primary: 9.3% of patients receiving clopidogrel vs 11.4% of patients receiving placebo (HR, 0.8; 95% CI, 0.72–0.90; P < 0.001) Safety: 3.7% of patients receiving clopidogrel vs 2.7% of patients receiving placebo (HR, 1.4; 95% CI, 1.1–1.7; P < 0.001); life-threatening bleeding 2.2% vs 1.8% (P = 0.13), respectively
PCI-CURE	Substudy of CURE			2658 (n = 1313 clopidogrel, n = 1345 placebo)			
TRITON-TIMI-38	ACS with or without ST-segment elevation	Prospective, randomized, double blind	707 centers, 30 countries	13 608 (n = 6813 prasugrel, n = 6795 clopidogrel)	Prasugrel (60-mg loading dose followed by 10-mg once a day) Clopidogrel (300-mg loading dose followed by 75 mg/day)	Primary: composite of CV death, non-fatal MI, or non-fatal stroke Safety: Major bleeding	Primary: 9.9% of patients receiving prasugrel vs 12.1% of patients receiving clopidogrel (HR, 0.81; 95% CI, 0.73–0.90; p < 0.001) Safety: 2.4% of patients receiving prasugrel vs 1.8% of patients receiving clopidogrel (HR, 1.32; 95% CI, 1.03–1.68; p = 0.03)

Study	Condition	Design	Centers	N	Intervention	Endpoints	Results
PLATO	ACS with or without ST-segment elevation	Prospective, randomized, double blind	862 centers, 43 countries	18624 (n = 9333 ticagrelor, n = 9291 clopidogrel)	Ticagrelor (180-mg loading dose followed by 90mg twice a day) Clopidogrel and placebo (300–600-mg loading dose or continuation with maintenance dose followed by 75mg/day)	Primary: composite of CV death, MI, or stroke Safety: Major bleeding	Primary: 9.8% of patients receiving ticagrelor vs 11.7% of patients receiving clopidogrel (HR, 0.84; 95% CI, 0.77–0.92; p < 0.001) Safety (major bleed): 11.6% of patients receiving ticagrelor vs 11.2% of patients receiving clopidogrel (HR, 1.19; 95% CI, 1.02–1.38; p = 0.43)
PLATO Invasive	Substudy of PLATO						
CURRENT-OASIS 7	ACS with or without ST-segment elevation managed with an early invasive strategy (as early as possible within 72h)	Multicenter, international, randomized, 2 × 2 factorial design	597 hospitals 39 countries	25087 PCI subset: 17232	High-dose regimen of clopidogrel (600-mg loading dose, followed by 150mg/day on days 2–7, followed by 75mg/day from days 8–30) vs the standard dose regimen (300-mg loading dose followed by 75mg/day from days 2–20) High-dose ASA (300–325mg/day) vs low-dose ASA (75–100mg)	Primary: composite of CV death, MI, or stroke at 30 days Safety: Major bleeding	Primary (preliminary results presented at ESC hotline): Overall group 600 vs 300mg 4.4% vs 4.2% (HR, 0.94; 95% CI 0.83–1.06; p = 0.304) PCI subset: 600mg vs 300mg 4.5% vs 3.9% (HR, 0.85; 95% CI, 0.74–0.99; p = 0.034) Safety: major bleeding 600mg vs 300mg 2.5% vs 2.0% (HR, 1.25; 95% CI, 1.05–1.47; p = 0.01). No difference in TIMI major bleeding between the study groups

ACS, acute coronary syndromes; ASA, acetylsalicylic acid; CV, cardiovascular; HR, hazard ratio; MI, myocardial infarction; PCI, percutaneous coronary intervention; TIMI, thrombolysis in myocardial infarction.

Results of the PCI substudy

The PCI cohort in the CURE trial comprised 2658 patients of whom 1313 were treated with clopidogrel and 1345 with placebo. Patients were further evaluated according to timing of PCI and categorized into the following groups: very early (<72 hours after randomization [n = 535]), early (≥72 hours after randomization, but during hospitalization [n = 1195]), and late (after initial hospital discharge [n = 928]).

There was a significantly lower rate of cardiovascular events in patients treated with clopidogrel compared with placebo, and an even more pronounced effect in those undergoing very early and early PCI (<48 hours, RRR 47%; <72 hours, RRR 41%). Bleeding rates were similar among the groups [83].

Interpretation and implications for clinical practice

The benefit of therapy with clopidogrel in addition to aspirin in patients with ACS and in the subgroup of patients undergoing PCI was consistent and significant.

The benefit of clopidogrel treatment in the PCI group was irrespective of the timing of intervention. The combination of an early interventional approach (<24 hours) and dual antiplatelet therapy, however, was associated with the lowest absolute event rates.

From the perspective of cost-effectiveness, clopidogrel treatment was significantly associated with reduction of hospitalization costs (incremental cost-effectiveness ratio [ICER] on the basis of the Framingham Heart Study US$6318 per life-year gained [LYG] with clopidogrel) [84].

The study had important clinical implications. Following publication of the results of the CURE trial and the PCI-CURE trial, a dual antiplatelet approach including a theinopyridine and aspirin for the treatment of ACS was translated into clinical practice throughout cardiac care units worldwide and was finally implemented in treatment guidelines.

TRITON-TIMI-38 trial

Prasugrel is a novel, third-generation thienopyridine, blocking the $P2Y_{12}$-ADP receptor on platelets in the same way as clopidogrel. In contrast, prasugrel provides a faster onset of action and less variability of platelet responsiveness due to fewer metabolization steps, leading to higher plasma levels and faster availability of the active metabolite.

Trial design

The TRITON-TIMI-38 (Trial to Assess Improvement in Therapeutic Outcomes by Optimizing Platelet Inhibition with Prasugrel—Thrombolysis in Myocardial Infarction) trial was a randomized, double-blind study to test the hypothesis that prasugrel is more effective than clopidogrel in preventing major ischemic events in patients undergoing PCI for ACS (ST elevation and non-ST elevation). The trial included 13608 patients who were randomly assigned to receive either prasugrel (60mg LD, 10mg MD) or clopidogrel (300mg LD, 75mg MD) (Table 4.3). Patients were on aspirin treatment for the duration of the study (median 14.5 months). The primary endpoint of the study was the composite of the rate of death from cardiovascular causes, non-fatal MI, or non-fatal stroke. Key safety endpoints were TIMI major bleeding unrelated to CABG, non–CABG-related TIMI life-threatening bleeding, and TIMI major or minor bleeding [85].

Eligibility

Patients with non-ST elevation ACS were included if ischemic symptoms occurred less than 72 hours prior to randomization and if they had a TIMI risk score of 3 or greater, and either ST-segment deviation of 1 mm or more or elevated levels of a cardiac biomarker of necrosis. Patients with ST elevation were included in the study if symptom onset was within the previous 12 hours and primary PCI was planned or within 14 days of medical treatment when cardiac anatomy was known. The main exclusion criteria were thienopyridine use within 5 days prior to enrolment, increased risk of bleeding, thrombocytopenia, or intracranial pathological findings in the patient history.

Main results

Patients were randomized to prasugrel (n = 6813) or to clopidogrel (n = 6795). PCI was performed in 91% of the patients, of whom 95% received a stent (equally distributed between DES and BMS). At a median of 14.5 months the primary endpoint was reached in 9.9% of the prasugrel group versus 12.1% of the clopidogrel group (HR, 0.81; 95% CI, 0.73–0.90; p < 0.001). A landmark analysis, a form of post-hoc survival analysis that uses a fixed time after randomization to assess the response in treatment groups [86], showed that prasugrel treatment was associated with benefits as early as 3 days after randomization. There was a further incremental benefit of prasugrel after day 3 until the end of follow-up. Additionally, prasugrel reduced the incidence of probable and definite stent thrombosis by 52% during follow-up (HR, 0.48; 95% CI, 0.36–0.64; p < 0.001).

The stronger antiplatelet effect of prasugrel translated into a significant increase in the key safety bleeding endpoint and all other bleeding endpoints (non–CABG-related TIMI major bleeding 2.4% vs. 1.8%; p = 0.03) (Table 4.3). The net clinical benefit was in favor of the prasugrel arm: for every 1000 patients treated, 23 MIs were prevented at the expense of six major non–CABG-related bleeds. There were certain patient subgroups who showed no net clinical benefit (patients aged 75 years or older and patients weighing <60 kg) or even harm (patients with prior stroke or transient ischemic attack) from prasugrel treatment (Figure 4.2).

Interpretation and implications for clinical practice

In patients with high-risk ACS, prasugrel significantly reduced the rate of ischemic events in the short and long term when compared with clopidogrel given as a 300-mg loading dose followed by a 75-mg maintenance dose. The higher efficacy correlated with an increased risk of bleeding, although the net

Bleeding Risk Subgroups

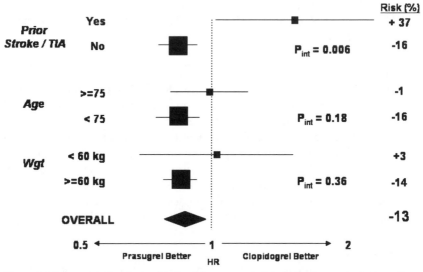

Figure 4.2 Subgroups of patients showing little or no net clinical benefit or potential harm from prasugrel treatment.

clinical benefit remained in favor of prasugrel in the overall study cohort. Some subgroups did not appear to gain a benefit from prasugrel treatment or were potentially harmed as documented by an excess of bleeding. Limitations of the study were the relative under-dosing of the active comparator (e.g., 300 mg), and the fact that the majority (72%) of the patients in the clopidogrel arm received the study medication at the time of PCI and were not sufficiently preloaded, which is routine clinical practice in many centers. Furthermore, the excess of recurrent MI in the clopidogrel group was mostly due to an increase in cardiac enzymes rather than clinically overt infarction.

In July 2009, the US Food and Drug Administration (FDA) approved prasugrel for clinical use during PCI in the setting of ACS based on the TRITON data, stating that the efficacy of prasugrel outweighs the bleeding risk due to the low frequency of fatal bleeding. It recommended prasugrel after careful weighing of the individual patient's bleeding risk. Consideration should be given to lowering the maintenance dose of prasugrel to 5 mg in patients who weigh less than 60 kg, bearing in mind that the effectiveness and safety of the 5 mg dose have not been prospectively studied to date. The FDA further provided a general warning for the use of prasugrel in patients aged 75 years or older due a higher risk of bleeding in these patients [87]. In the UK, the National Institute of Health and Clinical Excellence (NICE) has supported the use of prasugrel for STEMI patients, diabetics with ACS undergoing PCI, and those with stent thrombosis [88].

PLATO trial

Ticagrelor is a cyclopentyl-triazolo-pyrimidine, similar to adenosine triphosphate (ATP), that is orally active and reversibly inhibits the $P2Y_{12}$ receptor on platelets with a rapid onset of action (peaking of plasma levels and achievement of maximum antiplatelet effects in 1–3 hours). Compared with clopidogrel, ticagrelor provides a faster onset and offset of antiplatelet action, and a greater inhibition after loading and in the maintenance dosing phase [89].

Trial design

The PLATO (A Study of Platelet Inhibition and Patient Outcomes) trial tested the hypothesis that the reversible $P2Y_{12}$ receptor antagonist ticagrelor is superior to clopidogrel in a broad spectrum of patients with ACS. A total of 18 624 patients in 43 countries were randomly assigned to receive ticagrelor (a 180-mg loading dose followed by a 90-mg twice daily maintenance dose) or clopidogrel (a 300–600-mg loading dose followed by a 75-mg daily maintenance dose) [90]. The primary endpoint was the composite of death from cardiovascular causes, MI, or stroke within 1 year.

Eligibility

Patients were eligible if they were admitted to hospital for ACS (non-ST elevation and ST elevation) with symptom onset within the previous 24 hours. For individuals with NSTE-ACS at least two of the following criteria had to be met: changes on EKG consistent with ischemia; positive biomarkers of myocardial necrosis or one of several risk factors (age ≥60 years; previous MI or CABG; CAD with stenosis of ≥50% in at least two vessels; previous ischemic stroke/transient ischemic attack, carotid stenosis of at least 50%, or cerebral revascularization; diabetes mellitus; peripheral arterial disease; or chronic kidney disease).

Patients were excluded from the study if they had any contraindication to clopidogrel; received fibrinolytic therapy within the previous 24 hours, were in need of oral anticoagulation therapy, were at increased risk of bradycardia, and/or received concomitant therapy with a strong cytochrome P-450 3A inhibitor or inducer.

Main results

The primary endpoint occurred in 11.7% of patients treated with clopidogrel vs 9.8% of patients randomized to ticagrelor, representing a highly significant benefit (HR, 0.84; CI, 0.77–0.92; p = 0.001). Overall major bleeding events were similar between the treatment groups; however, ticagrelor was associated with a significantly higher incidence of fatal intracerebral bleeds (0.1% vs 0.01%; p = 0.02) and non–CABG-related bleeds independently of bleeding definition (non-CABG bleeds PLATO criteria: 4.5% vs 3.8%; p = 0.03. TIMI criteria: 2.8% vs 2.2%; p = 0.03) (Table 4.3). Concerning predescribed side effects associated with ticagrelor, dyspnea probably caused by transient bronchoconstriction (HR, 1.84; 95% CI, 1.68–2.02; p < 0.001) and ventricular pauses (p = 0.01) occurred more frequently in the ticagrelor arm. Increased uric acid as well as elevated creatinine were more often found in patients treated with ticagrelor (p = 0.001 for both). Benefits of ticagrelor were also observed in the large subset of patients undergoing PCI in the study (72% of the PLATO population) which were summarized in the PLATO Invasive study. The primary efficacy endpoint was reduced regardless of whether patients in the comparator arm were treated with 300- or 600-mg loading doses (HR 0.85 and 0.83, respectively) [91].

Interpretation and implications for clinical practice

The overall results of the PLATO and PLATO Invasive study show that reversible $P2Y_{12}$ blockade with rapid onset is associated with a lower rate of ischemic events in the short and long term in ACS patients, regardless of an invasive or conservative approach. As compared with clopidogrel, ticagrelor was associated with an increased frequency of non–CABG-related bleeding, but there was a numerical trend towards lower bleeding rates with ticagrelor in patients undergoing CABG. This result supports an important advantage of reversible platelet inhibition with ticagrelor in ACS patients scheduled for surgery. Ticagrelor therapy may be of particular benefit in those patients whose coronary anatomy is unknown. The promising trial results are likely to have a major impact on future treatment guidelines and change the present landscape of oral antiplatelet therapy in high-risk ACS patients. The drug has still to be evaluated by the regulatory authorities and direct comparisons with prasugrel are not currently available.

CURRENT-OASIS 7 trial

Trial design

The CURRENT-OASIS (Clopidogrel optimal loading dose Usage to Reduce Recurrent EveNTs/Optimal Antiplatelet Strategy for Intervention) trial tested two hypotheses: clopidogrel given at a higher loading dose and higher maintenance dose, and aspirin given at a higher daily dose have an effect on the primary outcome of cardiovascular death, MI, or stroke at 30 days in patients with non-ST and ST-elevation ACS. One secondary outcome measure was the incidence of major bleeding, defined by trial-specific criteria (CURRENT bleeding definition) (Table 4.3). The trial used a 2×2 factorial randomized design. Treatment was double-blinded to either one of two different clopidogrel dosing regimens (300-mg loading dose followed by 75 mg maintenance dose, or a 600-mg loading dose followed by 150 mg daily for 7 days and a 75-mg daily maintenance dose thereafter) [92]. Aspirin in two different doses (300–325 mg q.d. or 75–100 mg q.d.) was provided in an open-label way.

Eligibility

Patients were included if they had a proven NSTEMI or STEMI or ischemic symptoms suspected to represent a non–ST-segment elevation ACS (unstable angina or NSTEMI) and planned to be managed with an early invasive strat-

egy with intent to perform a PCI no later than 72 hours after randomization. Additionally, at least one of the following criteria had to be met:
• EKG changes compatible with new ischemia (ST depression of at least 1 mm or transient ST elevation or ST elevation of ≤1 mm or T-wave inversion of >3 mm in at least two contiguous leads), or
• Elevated cardiac enzymes (e.g., CK-MB) or biomarkers (troponin I or T) above the upper limit of normal.

Patients were excluded if they were aged under 18 years; were treated with oral anticoagulants within the last 10 days with an INR of greater than 1.5 or anticoagulant treatment was planned during the hospitalization period; had received clopidogrel greater than 75 mg within 24 hours before randomization; showed any contraindication to the use of clopidogrel and/or ASA; or had active bleeding or significant increased risk of bleeding, and/or uncontrolled hypertension.

Main results
A total of 24 769 patients were included in the study. Of the enrolled patients, 70.8% had unstable angina/NSTEMI and 29.2% had STEMI. All patients underwent angiography and a subgroup of 17 232 patients underwent PCI and formed a cohort for post-hoc analysis. When stratifying patients according to low- versus high-dose aspirin, there was no significant difference in the primary endpoint in the overall study cohort or in patients undergoing PCI compared with those who did not. Similarly, higher dose clopidogrel had no effect in the overall study population on the composite endpoint or on single efficacy endpoints. There was a significantly higher incidence of the primary bleeding endpoint (CURRENT major bleeding) in the higher dose clopidogrel group. However, there was neither a significant difference in TIMI major bleeding nor in CABG-related bleeding (Table 4.3). In the PCI subset of patients, there was a significant reduction in the risk of ischemic events at 30 days, particularly a 37% relative reduction in MI, in patients who received the double dose of clopidogrel. Risk of bleeding was not increased between the two clopidogrel dosing arms (PCI subset). In Kaplan—Meier analysis, curves for the cumulative primary endpoint began to diverge early with ongoing separation of curves beyond the first week of therapy, suggesting that both higher loading dose and higher maintenance dose given for 6 days contributed to the outcome in this treatment arm (PCI subset). Additionally, there was a notable reduction in the rate of definite stent thrombosis, according to the Academic Research Consortium criteria in the higher clopidogrel treatment arm undergoing PCI (1.2% vs. 0.7%; p < 0.001; 42% RRR).

Interpretation and implications for clinical practice
The key results of the CURRENT-OASIS trial have three major implications:
• In patients with ACS undergoing PCI, a post-randomization subset, treatment with high loading dose and double-dose clopidogrel for 6 days instead of standard dose is likely to reduce rates of MIs and stent thromboses, but will be associated with a moderate increase in significant bleeds. In this group

there does not appear to be an increase in fatal, CABG-related or TIMI major bleeds. The favorable results in the PCI subset can be criticized on methodological grounds, but clinically appear to be useful.

- In ACS patients not considered for an invasive strategy, the standard-dose regimen of clopidogrel is appropriate.
- In all ACS patients, aspirin at a daily dose of 75–100 mg or 300–325 mg appears equally effective in preventing cardiovascular events and has similar safety profiles up to 30 days of follow-up.

The key findings of the CURRENT-OASIS trial will likely have an impact on medical treatment guidelines as they highlight the importance of high dosing $P2Y_{12}$ blockade in ACS patients undergoing PCI. However, the potential implication is that all ACS patients should be given the 600-mg loading dose "upstream" prior to planned PCI.

Conclusions

ACS is a major health problem associated with premature mortality and morbidity and a major economic burden. Improved diagnostic tools and algorithms, new medical therapies, and an early invasive strategy have led to a significant improvement of outcome in this disease. Recent clinical trials have informed us about the benefits and risks of intensified medical treatment and lead to changes in the management of ACS. These results enforce the need for large clinical trial programs, supported by private, industry, and public funding, to detect treatment effects in ACS to improve patient care in this high-risk population.

References

1. Widimsky P, Wijns W, Fajadet J, et al.; European Association for Percutaneous Cardiovascular Interventions. Reperfusion therapy for ST elevation acute myocardial infarction in Europe: description of the current situation in 30 countries. *Eur Heart J* 2010; 31:943–957
2. Pitts SR, Niska RW, Xu J, Burt CW. National Hospital Ambulatory Medical Care Survey: 2006 emergency department summary. National Health Statistics Reports, No. 7. Hyattsville, MD: National Center for Health Statistics, 2008
3. Ferguson JL, Beckett GJ, Stoddart M, Walker SW, Fox KAA. Myocardial 3 infarction redefined: the new ACC/ESC definition, based on cardiac troponin, increases the apparent incidence of infarction. *Heart* 2002;88:343–347.
4. Thygesen K, Alpert JS, White HD, on behalf of the Joint ESC/ACCF/AHA/WHF Task Force for the Redefinition of Myocardial Infarction. Universal definition of myocardial infarction. *Eur Heart J* 2007;28:2525–2538.
5. Canto JG, Goldberg RJ, Hand MM, et al. Symptom presentation of women with acute coronary syndromes: myth vs reality. *Arch Intern Med* 2007;167:2405–2413.
6. Braunwald E. Unstable angina. A classification. *Circulation* 1989;80:410–414.
7. Hamm CW, Braunwald E. A classification of unstable angina revisited. *Circulation* 2000;102:118–122.
8. Pope JH, Aufderheide TP, Ruthazer R, et al. Missed diagnoses of acute cardiac ischemia in the emergency department. *N Engl J Med* 2000;342:1163–1170.

9. Sabatine MS, Antman EM. The Thrombolysis in Myocardial Infarction risk score in unstable angina/non-ST-segment elevation myocardial infarction. *J Am Coll Cardiol* 2003;41 (Suppl S):89S–95S.

10. Eagle KA, Lim MJ, Dabbous OH, et al. A validated prediction model for all forms of acute coronary syndrome: estimating the risk of 6-month postdischarge death in an international registry. *JAMA* 2004;291:2727–2733.

11. Ryan TJ, Antman EM, Brooks NH, et al. 1999 update: ACC/AHA guidelines for the management of patients with acute myocardial infarction. *J Am Coll Cardiol* 1999; 36:890–911.

12. Kushner FG, Hand M, Smith SC Jr, et al. 2009 focused updates: ACC/AHA guidelines for the management of patients with ST-elevation myocardial infarction (updating the 2004 guideline and 2007 focused update) and ACC/AHA/SCAI guidelines on percutaneous coronary intervention (updating the 2005 guideline and 2007 focused update) a report of the American College of Cardiology Foundation/American Heart Association Task Force on Practice Guidelines. *J Am Coll Cardiol* 2009;54:2205–2241.

13. Shave R, Dawson E, Whyte G, et al. The cardiospecificity of the third-generation cTnT assay after exercise-induced muscle damage. *Med Sci Sports Exerc* 2002;34:651–654.

14. Harris BM, Nageh T, Marsden JT, Thomas MR, Sherwood RA. Comparison of cardiac troponin T and I and CK-MB for the detection of minor myocardial damage during interventional cardiac procedures. *Ann Clin Biochem* 2000;37:764–769.

15. Morrow DA, Cannon CP, Rifai N, et al. Ability of minor elevations of troponins I and T to predict benefit from an early invasive strategy in patients with unstable angina and non-ST elevation myocardial infarction: results from a randomized trial. *JAMA* 2001; 286:2405–2412.

16. Musso PCI, Vidano E, Zambon D, Panteghini M. Cardiac troponin elevations in chronic renal failure: prevalence and clinical significance. *Clin Biochem* 1999;32:125–130.

17. Kraemer BF, Seizer P, Geisler T, et al. Persistent troponin elevation in a patient with cardiac amyloidosis. *Clin Cardiol* 2009;32:E39–42.

18. Jeremias A, Gibson CM. Narrative review: alternative causes for elevated cardiac troponin levels when acute coronary syndromes are excluded. *Ann Intern Med* 2005;142: 786–791.

19. Reichlin T, Hochholzer W, Bassetti S, et al. Early diagnosis of myocardial infarction with sensitive cardiac troponin assays. *N Engl J Med* 2009;361:858–867.

20. Keller T, Zeller T, Peetz D, et al. Sensitive troponin I assays in early diagnosis of acute myocardial infarction. *N Engl J Med* 2009;361:868–877.

21. Morrow DA. Clinical application of sensitive troponin assays. *N Engl J Med* 2009; 361:913–915.

22. Adams JE, Schectman KB, Landt Y, Ladenson JH, Jaffe AS. Comparable detection of acute myocardial infarction by creatine kinase MB isoenzyme and cardiac troponin I. *Clin Chem* 1994;40:1291.

23. Wu AH, Apple FS, Gibler WB, Jesse RL, Warshaw MM, Valdes R Jr. National Academy of Clinical Biochemistry Standards of Laboratory Practice: recommendations for the use of cardiac markers in coronary artery diseases. *Clin Chem* 1999;45:1104–1121.

24. Dakik HA, Mahmarian JJ, Kimball KT, et al. Prognostic value of exercise 201Tl tomography in patients treated with thrombolytic therapy during acute myocardial infarction. *Circulation* 1996;94:2735–2742.

25. Mahmarian JJ, Dwivedi G, Lahiri T. Role of nuclear cardiac imaging in myocardial infarction: postinfarction risk stratification. *J Nucl Cardiol* 2004;11:186–209.

26. Brown KA, Heller GV, Landin RS, et al. Early dipyridamole (99m)Tc-sestamibi single photon emission computed tomographic imaging 2 to 4days after acute myocardial

infarction predicts in-hospital and post-discharge cardiac events: comparison with sub-maximal exercise imaging. *Circulation* 1999;100:2060–2066.

27. Mahmarian JJ, Shaw LJ, Olszewski GH, Pounds BK, Frias ME, Pratt CM; INSPIRE Investigators. Adenosine sestamibi SPECT post-infarction evaluation (INSPIRE) trial: A randomized, prospective multicenter trial evaluating the role of adenosine Tc-99m sestamibi SPECT for assessing risk and therapeutic outcomes in survivors of acute myocardial infarction. *J Nucl Cardiol* 2004;11:458–469.

28. Santana CA, Garcia EV, Faber TL, *et al.* Diagnostic performance of fusion of myocardial perfusion imaging (MPI) and computed tomography coronary angiography. *J Nucl Cardiol* 2009;16:201–211.

29. Hoffmann U, Bamberg F, Chae CU, *et al.* Coronary computed tomography angiography for early triage of patients with acute chest pain: the ROMICAT (Rule Out Myocardial Infarction using Computer Assisted Tomography) trial. *J Am Coll Cardiol* 2009;53: 1642–1650.

30. Flett AS, Westwood MA, Davies LC, Mathur A, Moon JC. The prognostic implications of cardiovascular magnetic resonance. *Circ Cardiovasc Imaging* 2009;2:243–250.

31. Kwong RY, Schussheim AE, Rekhraj S, *et al.* Detecting acute coronary syndrome in the emergency department with cardiac magnetic resonance imaging. *Circulation* 2003;107: 538–544.

32. Ingkanisorn WP, Kwong RY, Bohme NS, *et al.* Prognosis of negative adenosine stress magnetic resonance in patients presenting to an emergency department with chest pain. *J Am Coll Cardiol* 2006;47:1427–1432.

33. Farkouh ME, Smars PA, Reeder GS, *et al.* A clinical trial of a chest-pain observation unit for patients with unstable angina. Chest Pain Evaluation in the Emergency Room (CHEER) Investigators. *N Engl J Med* 1998;339:1882–1888.

34. Farkouh ME, Smars PA, Reeder GS, *et al.* A clinical trial of a chest-pain observation unit for patients with unstable angina. Chest Pain Evaluation in the Emergency Room (CHEER) Investigators. *N Engl J Med* 1998;339:1882–1888.

35. Smith SC Jr, Benjamin EJ, Bonow RO, *et al*; World Heart Federation and the Preventive Cardiovascular Nurses Association.AHA/ACCF Secondary Prevention and Risk Reduction Therapy for Patients with Coronary and other Atherosclerotic Vascular Disease: 2011 update: a guideline from the American Heart Association and American College of Cardiology Foundation. *Circulation* 2011;124:2458–2473.

36. Anderson JL, Adams CD, Antman EM, *et al.* ACC/AHA 2007 guidelines for the management of patients with unstable angina/non-ST-Elevation myocardial infarction: a report of the American College of Cardiology/American Heart Association Task Force on Practice Guidelines (Writing Committee to Revise the 2002 Guidelines for the Management of Patients With Unstable Angina/Non-ST-Elevation Myocardial Infarction) developed in collaboration with the American College of Emergency Physicians, the Society for Cardiovascular Angiography and Interventions, and the Society of Thoracic Surgeons endorsed by the American Association of Cardiovascular and Pulmonary Rehabilitation and the Society for Academic Emergency Medicine. *J Am Coll Cardiol* 2007;50:e1–e157.

37. James SK, Roe MT, Cannon CP, *et al.*; PLATO Study Group. Ticagrelor versus clopidogrel in patients with acute coronary syndromes intended for non-invasive management: substudy from prospective randomised PLATelet inhibition and patient Outcomes (PLATO) trial. *BMJ* 2011;342:d3527.

38. Tricoci P, Huang Z, Held C, *et al.*; TRACER Investigators.Thrombin-receptor antagonist vorapaxar in acute coronary syndromes. *N Engl J Med* 2012;366:20–33.

39. O'Donoghue ML, Bhatt DL, Wiviott SD, *et al.*; LANCELOT-ACS Investigators. Safety and tolerability of atopaxar in the treatment of patients with acute coronary syndromes:

the lessons from antagonizing the cellular effects of Thrombin–Acute Coronary Syndromes Trial. *Circulation* 2011;123:1843–1853.

40. Kastrati A, Mehilli J, Neumann FJ, *et al.*; Intracoronary Stenting and Antithrombotic: Regimen Rapid Early Action for Coronary Treatment 2 (ISAR-REACT 2) Trial Investigators. Abciximab in patients with acute coronary syndromes undergoing percutaneous coronary intervention after clopidogrel pretreatment: the ISAR-REACT 2 randomized trial. *JAMA* 2006;295:1531–1538.

41. Roffi M, Chew DP, Mukherjee D, *et al.* Platelet glycoprotein IIb/IIIa inhibition in acute coronary syndromes. Gradient of benefit related to the revascularization strategy. *Eur Heart J* 2002;23:1441–1448.

42. Effect of glycoprotein IIb/IIIa receptor blocker abciximab on outcome in patients with acute coronary syndromes without early coronary revascularisation: the GUSTO IV-ACS randomised trial. *Lancet* 2001;2001:1915–1924.

43. Stone GW, McLaurin BT, Cox DA, *et al.*; ACUITY Investigators. Bivalirudin for patients with acute coronary syndromes. *N Engl J Med* 2006;355:2203–2216.

44. Stone GW, Witzenbichler B, Guagliumi G, *et al.* Bivalirudin during primary PCI in acute myocardial infarction. *N Engl J Med* 2008;358:2218–2230.

45. Kastrati A, Neumann FJ, Schulz S, *et al.*; ISAR-REACT 4 Trial Investigators. Abciximab and heparin versus bivalirudin for non-ST-elevation myocardial infarction. *N Engl J Med* 2011;365:1980–1989.

46. Van't Hof AW, Ten Berg J, Heestermans T, *et al.*; Ongoing Tirofiban In Myocardial infarction Evaluation (On-TIME) 2 study group. Prehospital initiation of tirofiban in patients with ST-elevation myocardial infarction undergoing primary angioplasty (On-TIME 2): a multicentre, double-blind, randomised controlled trial. *Lancet* 2008;372:537–546.

47. Ellis SG. The Facilitated Intervention with Enhanced Reperfusion Speed to Stop Events (FINESSE) trial. Presented at the European Society of Cardiology Annual Congress, Vienna, September 1–5, 2007.

48. Guigliano RP, White Ja, Bode C, *et al.* Early versus delayed, provisional eptifibatide in acute coronary syndromes. *N Engl J Med* 2009;360:2176–2190.

49. Stone GW, Bertrand ME, Moses JW, *et al.* Routine upstream initiation vs deferred selective use of glycoprotein IIb/IIIa inhibitors in acute coronary syndromes: the ACUITY Timing trial. *JAMA* 2007;297:591–602.

50. Gödicke J, Flather M, Noc M, *et al.* Early versus periprocedural administration of abciximab for primary angioplasty: a pooled analysis of 6 studies. *Am Heart J* 2005;150:1015.

51. Thiele H, Wöhrle J, Hambrecht R, Rittger H, Birkemeyer R, Lauer B, Neuhaus P, Brosteanu O, Sick P, Wiemer M, Kerber S, Kleinertz K, Eitel I, Desch S, Schuler G. Intracoronary versus intravenous bolus abciximab during primary percutaneous coronary intervention in patients with acute ST-elevation myocardial infarction: a randomised trial. *Lancet.* 2012;379(9819):923–931.

52. Thiele H, Schindler K, Friedenberger J, *et al.* Circulation. Intracoronary compared with intravenous bolus abciximab application in patients with ST-elevation myocardial infarction undergoing primary percutaneous coronary intervention: the randomized Leipzig immediate percutaneous coronary intervention abciximab IV versus IC in ST-elevation myocardial infarction trial. *Circulation* 2008;118:49–57.

53. Gu YL, Kampinga MA, Wieringa WG, *et al.* Intracoronary versus intravenous administration of abciximab in patients with ST-segment elevation myocardial infarction undergoing primary percutaneous coronary intervention with thrombus aspiration: the comparison of intracoronary versus intravenous abciximab administration during emergency reperfusion of ST-segment elevation myocardial infarction (CICERO) trial. *Circulation* 2010;122:2709–2717.

54. Ferguson JJ, Califf RM, Antman EM, *et al*; SYNERGY Trial Investigators. Enoxaparin vs unfractionated heparin in high-risk patients with non-ST-segment elevation acute coronary syndromes managed with an intended early invasive strategy: primary results of the SYNERGY randomized trial. *JAMA* 2004;292:45–54.

55. Antman EM, Morrow DA, McCabe CH, *et al*. Enoxaparin versus unfractionated heparin with fibrinolysis for ST-elevation myocardial infarction. *N Engl J Med* 2006;354: 1477–1488.

56. Fifth Organization to Assess Strategies in Acute Ischemic Syndromes Investigators, Yusuf S, Mehta SR, Chrolavicius S, *et al*. Comparison of fondaparinux and enoxaparin in acute coronary syndromes. *N Engl J Med* 2006;354:1464–1476.

57. Mehta SR, Granger CB, Eikelboom JW, *et al*. Efficacy and safety of fondaparinux versus enoxaparin in patients with acute coronary syndromes undergoing percutaneous coronary intervention. Results from the OASIS-5 trial. *J Am Coll Cardiol* 2007;50:1742–1751.

58. Steg PG, Jolly SS, Mehta SR, *et al*. FUTURA/OASIS-8 Trial Group. Low-dose vs standard-dose unfractionated heparin for percutaneous coronary intervention in acute coronary syndromes treated with fondaparinux: the FUTURA/OASIS-8 randomized trial. *JAMA* 2010;304:1339–1349.

59. Yusuf S, Mehta SR, Chrolavicius S, *et al.*; OASIS-6 Trial Group. Effects of fondaparinux on mortality and reinfarction in patients with acute ST-segment elevation myocardial infarction: the OASIS-6 randomized trial. *JAMA* 2006;295:1519–1530.

60. Stone GW, McLaurin BT, Cox DA, *et al.*; ACUITY Investigators. Bivalirudin for patients with acute coronary syndromes. *N Engl J Med* 2006;355:2203–2216.

61. Stone GW, Witzenbichler B, Guagliumi G, *et al.*; HORIZONS-AMI Trial Investigators. Bivalirudin during primary PCI in acute myocardial infarction. *N Engl J Med* 2008; 358:2218–2230.

62. Oldgren J, Budaj A, Granger CB, Khder Y, Roberts J, Siegbahn A, Tijssen JG, Van de Werf F, Wallentin L; RE-DEEM Investigators. Dabigatran vs. placebo in patients with acute coronary syndromes on dual antiplatelet therapy: a randomized, double-blind, phase II trial. *Eur Heart J*. 2011;32(22):2781–2789.

63. Alexander JH, Lopes RD, James S, Kilaru R, He Y, Mohan P, Bhatt DL, Goodman S, Verheugt FW, Flather M, Huber K, *et al.*; APPRAISE-2 Investigators. Apixaban with antiplatelet therapy after acute coronary syndrome. *N Engl J Med* 2011;365:699–708.

64. Mega JL, Braunwald E, Mohanavelu S, *et al.*; ATLAS ACS-TIMI 46 study group. Rivaroxaban versus placebo in patients with acute coronary syndromes (ATLAS ACS-TIMI 46): a randomised, double-blind, phase II trial. *Lancet* 2009;374:29–38.

65. Mega JL, Braunwald E, Wiviott SD, *et al.*; ATLAS ACS 2–TIMI 51 Investigators. Rivaroxaban in patients with a recent acute coronary syndrome. *N Engl J Med* 2012;366: 9–19.

66. Ryden L, Ariniego R, Arnman K, *et al*. A double-blind trial of metoprolol in acute myocardial infarction. Effects on ventricular tachyarrhythmias. *N Engl J Med* 1983;308:614.

67. Friedman, LM, Byington, RP, Capone, RJ, Furberg, CD. Effect of propranolol in patients with myocardial infarction and ventricular arrhythmia. *J Am Coll Cardiol* 1986;7:1.

68. Doughty RN, Whalley GA, Walsh HA, *et al*. Effects of carvedilol on left ventricular remodeling after acute myocardial infarction: the CAPRICORN Echo Substudy. *Circulation* 2004;109:201.

69. Poulsen, SH, Jensen, SE, Egstrup, K. Effects of long-term adrenergic beta-blockade on left ventricular diastolic filling in patients with acute myocardial infarction. *Am Heart J* 1999;138:710.

70. Task Force for Diagnosis and Treatment of Non-ST-Segment Elevation Acute Coronary Syndromes of European Society of Cardiology, Bassand JP, Hamm CW, Ardissino D,

et al. Guidelines for the diagnosis and treatment of non-ST-segment elevation acute coronary syndromes. *Eur Heart J* 2007;28:1598–1660.

71. Canadian Cardiovascular Society; American Academy of Family Physicians; American College of Cardiology; American Heart Association, Antman EM, Hand M, Armstrong PW, *et al.* 2007 focused update of the ACC/AHA 2004 guidelines for the management of patients with ST-elevation myocardial infarction: a report of the American College of Cardiology/American Heart Association Task Force on Practice Guidelines. *J Am Coll Cardiol* 2008;51:210–247.

72. Chen ZM, Pan HC, Chen YP, *et al.* Early intravenous then oral metoprolol in 45,852 patients with acute myocardial infarction: randomised placebo-controlled trial *Lancet* 2005;366:1622–1632.

73. Briel M, Schwartz GG, Thompson PL, *et al.* Effects of early treatment with statins on short-term clinical outcomes in acute coronary syndromes: a meta-analysis of randomized controlled trials. *JAMA* 2006;295:2046–2056.

74. Hulten E, Jackson JL, Douglas K, George S, Villines TC. The effect of early, intensive statin therapy on acute coronary syndrome: a meta-analysis of randomized controlled trials. *Arch Intern Med* 2006;166:1814–1821.

75. Grines CL, Browne KF, Marco J, *et al.* A comparison of immediate angioplasty with thrombolytic therapy for acute myocardial infarction. The Primary Angioplasty in Myocardial Infarction Study Group. *N Engl J Med* 1993;328:673–679.

76. The Global Use of Strategies to Open Occluded Coronary Arteries in Acute Coronary Syndromes (GUSTO-IIb) Angioplasty Substudy Investigators. A clinical trial comparing primary coronary angioplasty with tissue plasminogen activator for acute myocardial infarction. *N Engl J Med* 1997;336:1621–1628.

77. Di Mario C, Dudek D, Piscione F, *et al.* Immediate angioplasty versus standard therapy with rescue angioplasty after thrombolysis in the Combined Abciximab REteplase Stent Study in Acute Myocardial Infarction (CARESS-in-AMI): an open, prospective, randomised, multicentre trial. *Lancet* 2008;371:559–568.

78. Cantor WJ, Fitchett D, Borgundvaag B, *et al.* Routine early angioplasty after fibrinolysis for acute myocardial infarction. *N Engl J Med* 2009;360:2705–2718.

79. Pinto DS, Kirtane AJ, Nallamothu BK, *et al.* Hospital delays in reperfusion for ST-elevation myocardial infarction: implications when selecting a reperfusion strategy *Circulation* 2006;114:2019–2025.

80. Mehta SR, Granger CB, Boden WE, *et al.*; TIMACS Investigators. Early versus delayed invasive intervention in acute coronary syndromes. *N Engl J Med* 2009;360:2165–2175.

81. Montalescot G, Cayla G, Collet JP, *et al.*; ABOARD Investigators. Immediate vs delayed intervention for acute coronary syndromes: a randomized clinical trial. *JAMA* 2009; 302:947–954.

82. Yusuf S, Zhao F, Mehta SR, Chrolavicius S, Tognoni G, Fox KK; Clopidogrel in Unstable Angina to Prevent Recurrent Events Trial Investigators. Effects of clopidogrel in addition to aspirin in patients with acute coronary syndromes without ST-segment elevation. *N Engl J Med* 2001;345:494–502.

83. Mehta SR, Yusuf S, Peters RG, *et al.* Effects of pre-treatment with clopidogrel and aspirin followed by long-term therapy in patients undergoing percutaneous coronary intervention: the PCI-CURE study. *Lancet* 2001;358:527–533.

84. Weintraub WS, Mahoney EM, Lamy A, *et al.*; CURE Study Investigators. Long-term cost-effectiveness of clopidogrel given for up to one year in patients with acute coronary syndromes without ST-segment elevation. Weintraub WS, Mahoney EM, Lamy A, Culler S, Yuan Y, Caro J, Gabriel S, Yusuf S; CURE Study Investigators. *J Am Coll Cardiol* 2005;45:838–845.

85. Wiviott SD, Braunwald E, McCabe CH, *et al.*; TRITON-TIMI 38 Investigators. Prasugrel versus clopidogrel in patients with acute coronary syndromes. *N Engl J Med* 2007; 357:2001–2015.

86. Anderson JR, Cain KC, Gelber RD. Analysis of survival by tumor response. *J Clin Oncol* 1983;1:710–719.

87. Unger EF. Weighing benefits and risks—the FDA's review of prasugrel. *N Engl J Med* 2009;361:942–945.

88. National Institute for Health and Clinical Excellence. Final appraisal determination—Prasugrel for the treatment of acute coronary syndromes with percutaneous coronary intervention. Issue date: August 2009.

89. Gurbel PA, Bliden KP, Butler K, *et al.* Randomized double-blind assessment of the ONSET and OFFSET of the antiplatelet effects of ticagrelor versus clopidogrel in patients with stable coronary artery disease: the ONSET/OFFSET study. *Circulation* 2009;120: 2577–2585.

90. Wallentin L, Becker RC, Budaj A, *et al.* Ticagrelor versus clopidogrel in patients with acute coronary syndromes. *N Engl J Med* 2009;361:1045–1057.

91. Cannon CP, Harrington RA, James S, *et al.*; PLATelet inhibition and patient Outcomes Investigators. Comparison of ticagrelor with clopidogrel in patients with a planned invasive strategy for acute coronary syndromes (PLATO): a randomised double-blind study. *Lancet* 2010;375:283–293.

92. Mehta SR, Bassand JP, Chrolavicius S, *et al.*; CURRENT-OASIS 7 Steering Committee. Design and rationale of CURRENT-OASIS 7: a randomized, 2 × 2 factorial trial evaluating optimal dosing strategies for clopidogrel and aspirin in patients with ST and non-ST-elevation acute coronary syndromes managed with an early invasive strategy. *Am Heart J* 2008;156:1080–1088.e1.

CHAPTER 5

Heart failure

Christopher M. O'Connor[1] and Wendy Gattis Stough[1,2]
[1]Duke University Medical Center, Durham, NC, USA
[2]Campbell University School of Pharmacy, Buies Creek, NC, USA

Epidemiology

Heart failure is a highly prevalent and burdensome cardiovascular disease throughout the world. In the US, an estimated 5.7 million people have heart failure and 670 000 new cases are diagnosed annually [1]. Among the US Medicare population, the estimated incidence of heart failure is 29.1%, and the prevalence is 121 persons per 1000 eligible Medicare beneficiaries [2]. The prevalence of heart failure in the Medicare population has steadily increased from 1994 to 2003 [2]. In 2004, the total mortality attributed to heart failure was 292 214, and heart failure contributed to an estimated 1 106 000 hospital discharges in 2006 [1]. The estimated 1- and 5-year risk adjusted mortality for heart failure among Medicare beneficiaries is 27.5% and 62.2%, respectively [2]. The estimated direct and indirect cost of heart failure for 2009 in the US is $37.2 billion [1]. Among European countries where data are available, the estimated prevalence of heart failure approaches 10–20% in patients aged 70–80 years. The mortality rate is 50% at 4 years, with a 40% annual rate of heart failure hospitalization or death [3].

Pathophysiology

The understanding of heart failure pathophysiology has changed substantially over the last 20 years. Historically, heart failure was viewed as primarily a hemodynamic disorder in which cardiac output declined with increasing preload and afterload. The neurohormonal hypothesis emerged in the 1980s and 1990s, recognizing that the sympathetic nervous and renin–angiotensin–aldosterone systems were activated in the setting of heart failure and associated with poor prognosis [4–8]. It is now understood that the pathophysiological progression of heart failure is multifactorial, involving cardiac injury, neurohormonal activation, altered hemodynamics, cardiac remodeling, inflammatory processes, and genetic factors [9,10].

Cardiovascular Clinical Trials: Putting the Evidence into Practice, First Edition.
Edited by Marcus D. Flather, Deepak L. Bhatt, and Tobias Geisler.
© 2013 Blackwell Publishing Ltd. Published 2013 by Blackwell Publishing Ltd.

Cardiac remodeling is now recognized as a major component of the pathophysiological process that leads to progressive heart failure. It results from a myriad of mechanical, neurohormonal, molecular, cellular, and genetic factors that alter the size, shape, and function of the left ventricle. It is characterized by hypertrophy, apoptosis, interstitial fibrosis, and thinning of the ventricular wall [10]. At the molecular level, neurohormones, including norepinephrine, angiotensin, and endothelin, are released in response to myocyte injury (myocardial infarction [MI]) and/or stretch. These hormones promote expression of altered proteins, resulting in myocyte hypertrophy. This process ultimately leads to progressive deterioration in cardiac performance and increased neurohormonal activation. The neurohormonal and cytokine activation may stimulate collagen release, which leads to fibrosis and extracellular matrix remodeling. Ultimately, remodeling leads to many cellular changes, including hypertrophy, necrosis, apoptosis, fibrosis, and fibroblast proliferation [11].

Identifying therapeutic agents with the ability to promote reverse remodeling has been an area of intense investigation in recent years, in an effort to interrupt the pathophysiological progression of heart failure. Angiotensin converting enzyme (ACE) inhibitors, angiotensin receptor blockers (ARBs), beta-blockers, and aldosterone receptor antagonists have all been shown to prevent or reverse the remodeling process. Concurrently, these agents have also been shown to improve survival and reduce morbidity [12–19]. In addition to pharmacological therapies, cardiac resynchronization therapy (CRT) has been shown to induce reverse remodeling while improving clinical outcomes [20,21]. These findings have stimulated many experts in the field to encourage the use of ventricular remodeling endpoints in clinical trials and to call on regulators to accept ventricular remodeling as a surrogate endpoint for clinical outcome [22,23].

Clinical presentation: registry data

Several registries conducted in the heart failure population have revealed important information about the clinical characteristics and presentation of heart failure patients. These include the Acute Decompensated Heart Failure National Registry (ADHERE) (n = 107362), Organized Program to Initiate Life Saving Treatment in Patients Hospitalized for Heart Failure (OPTIMIZE-HF) (n = 48612), and the The Registry to Improve the Use of Evidence-Based Heart Failure Therapies in the Outpatient Setting (IMPROVE HF) (n = 43000) in the US, and the Euro Heart Failure Survey (EHFS) (n = 14907) in Europe [24–29].

The high prevalence of heart failure in the elderly is reflected in the age of patients enrolled in these registries, which ranged from 68.7 to 73 years (Table 5.1 [24,30–36]). The distribution of men and women was relatively equal across all registries, except for the IMPROVE-HF outpatient heart failure registry, which included predominately men. In the registries where patients with preserved systolic function were included, 46–55% of patients had preserved ejection fraction.

Table 5.1 Heart failure demographics and clinical characteristics: registry data.

Characteristic	ADHERE (n = 105388) [24,30–32]	OPTIMIZE (n = 48612) [33,34]	IMPROVE-HF (n = 15381) [29]	EHFS I (n = 11327) [35,36]	EHFS II (n = 3580) [27]
Mean (SD) age (years)	72.4 (14)	73	68.7 (13.2)	71	69.9(12.5)
African–American (%)	20	22	9.1	N/A	N/A
Male (%)	48	48	71	53	61.3
Mean (SD) LVEF (%)	34.4 (16.1)	NR	25.5	<40% in 45%	38 ± 15
Preserved LVF (%)	46	49	N/A	55	34.3% in ≥45%
Mean (SD) systolic blood pressure (mmHg)	144 (32.6)	142	120 (18.9)	133	Median 135/80 IQR 110–160/70–90
Body mass index (kg/m²)	NR	NR	NR	<20 in 4% >30 in 24%	26.8
Length of stay (days)	4.3 (median)	4	N/A	11	9
Mortality	In-hospital: 4%	In-hospital: 4% 60–90 day post-discharge 9%	NR	In-hospital: 6.9%	In-hospital: 6.8%
CAD (%)	57	50	Ischemic etiology 65.2	68	53.6
Hypertension (%)	73	71	61.7	53	62.5
Diabetes (%)	44	42	34	27	32.8
Renal insufficiency (%)	30	30	NR	17	Renal failure 16.8
Mean SCr (mg/dL)	1.8	ND	1.42 (SD 2.21)	>1.7 in 16% >2.3 in 7%	NR
Atrial fibrillation (%)	31	31	30.8	42	38.7

CAD, coronary artery disease; IQR, interquartile range; N/A, not applicable; NR, not reported; SCr, serum creatinine; VEF, left ventricular ejection fraction.

The registry data also highlight the prevalence of comorbidities among heart failure patients. The majority of patients across all registries had coronary artery disease and hypertension. The mean systolic blood pressure indicated the presence of pre-hypertension or Stage I hypertension in the majority of patients. In addition, 27–44% had diabetes, approximately 30% had renal impairment, and 30% had atrial fibrillation (Table 5.1). For patients presenting acutely, acute dyspnea, rales, orthopnea, and peripheral edema are the most common signs and symptoms [24,32,33,37].

Data from the in-hospital registries revealed a consistently high in-hospital mortality across registries. In-hospital mortality was 4% in the ADHERE and OPTIMIZE registries, and slightly higher in the European registries (6.8–6.9%) [24–27]. An analysis of hospitalizations for heart failure among 2540838 Medicare beneficiaries from 2001 to 2005 found an in-hospital mortality rate of 4.2% [38]. OPTIMIZE-HF reported a post-discharge (60–90 days) mortality of 9%. Similar rates were observed by Curtis *et al*, in the US Medicare beneficiary study, with 30-day, 180-day, and 1-year mortality rates of 11%, 26%, and 37%, respectively [38].

Several factors were identified in ADHERE and OPTIMIZE-HF that predicted in-hospital and post-discharge mortality (Table 5.2) [39–41]. A predictive nomogram was generated from the OPTIMIZE-HF prognostic model that can be used to estimate expected mortality at 60 days [40] (Table 5.3). In addition to these factors, several other prognostic variables have been identified from other databases. An analysis of the Sudden Cardiac Death in Heart Failure Trial (SCD-HeFT) revealed that implantable cardioverter defibrillator (ICD) shocks were associated with an increased risk of all-cause mortality (HR 5.68; 95% CI, 3.97–8.12, p < 0.001) [42]. Progressive heart failure was the most common cause of death among these patients. In the US Medicare elderly population, additional variables found to predict mortality included male

Table 5.2 Predictors of in-hospital and post-discharge mortality in heart failure.

Increase mortality	Decrease mortality
Increased blood urea nitrogen	Increased systolic blood pressure (up to
Increased serum creatinine	160 mmHg)
Increased age	Heart failure as primary cause of admission
Increased heart rate	Increased diastolic blood pressure (up to
Decreased serum sodium	100 mmHg)
Liver disease	Hyperlipidemia/statin prescribed at discharge
Prior cerebrovascular accident or	Smoker within past year
transient ischemic attack	New-onset heart failure
Peripheral vascular disease	African-American
Left ventricular systolic dysfunction	ACE inhibitor at admission
Chronic obstructive pulmonary disease	Beta-blocker at admission
Depression	Beta-blocker at discharge
Lower extremity edema	Weight
Discharge serum creatinine	

Data from ADHERE and OPTIMIZE registries [39–41].

Table 5.3 Risk prediction nomogram for mortality to 60 days. (Reproduced from O'Connor et al. [40], with permission.)

Age (years)	Score	Weight (kg)	Score	SBP (mmHg)	Score	Sodium (mEq/L)	Score	Creatinine (mg/dL)	Score
25	0	60	9	80	24	110	12	0	0
35	2	80	7	100	20	115	10	1	5
45	5	100	5	120	17	120	8	2	9
55	7	120	3	140	13	125	6	3	14
65	10	140	2	160	11	130	4	4	19
75	12			180	9	135	2		
85	15			200	8	140	0		
95	17			220	6				
				240	4				
				260	2				
				280	0				
	+		+		+		+		+

Add the total number of points for clinical evaluation from the above table _____

Baseline risk factors	Score
History of liver disease	8
History of depression	4
History of reactive airway disease	4
Total from clinical evaluation	_____
Total score	_____

gender, acute MI, cardiogenic shock, dementia, functional disability, psychiatric disorders, cancer, peripheral vascular disease, pneumonia, malnutrition, arrhythmias, trauma, and valvular disease [38].

Standard management strategies

Pharmacological therapies

Several pharmacological therapies form the cornerstone of evidence-based heart failure therapy. Many of these agents have been established as standard heart failure care for an extended period of time and will only briefly be reviewed in this chapter.

ACE inhibitors

ACE inhibitors are recommended in all patients with symptomatic heart failure and systolic dysfunction, unless contraindications are present [3,43,44]. The Cooperative North Scandinavian Enalapril Survival Study (CONSENSUS) and Studies of Left Ventricular Dysfunction Treatment (SOLVD-T) demonstrated improved survival for patients treated with ACE inhibitors [45,46]. These agents have also been shown to reduce the need for hospitalization for heart failure, even among patients with asymptomatic systolic dysfunction [47].

The majority of patients with heart failure are candidates for ACE inhibitor therapy. Generally, ACE inhibitors should be avoided in patients with a history of angioedema, bilateral renal artery stenosis, or severe aortic stenosis, and in patients with unstable hypotension who are at risk of cardiogenic shock. Pregnancy is a contraindication to these drugs. ACE inhibitors may worsen hyperkalemia, and patients with a serum potassium of greater than 5.5 mmol/L should be prescribed an ACE inhibitor cautiously with close monitoring. Patients with elevated serum creatinine may receive an ACE inhibitor, but these patients should also be closely monitored. The dose may need to be reduced or the drug discontinued if serum creatinine increases [44].

Angiotensin receptor blockers

An ARB are recommended for patients with heart failure who are ACE inhibitor intolerant, primarily due to cough or angioedema, and also have a role as add-on therapies to existing ACE inhibitor treatment. Patients who do not tolerate ACE inhibitors from the standpoint of worsening renal function, hyperkalemia, or hypotension are likely to have the same response to ARBs, and these drugs should also be used cautiously with close monitoring in those patients [44]. In the Candesartan in Heart Failure Assessment of Reduction in Morbidity and Mortality (CHARM) Alternative study, candesartan was associated with a 23% reduction (HR 0.77; 95% CI, 0.67–0.89; $p = 0.0004$) in the primary endpoint of cardiovascular death or heart failure hospitalization among patients who were intolerant of ACE inhibitors [48].

An ARB is also recommended for patients who remain symptomatic despite optimal treatment with ACE inhibitors and beta-blockers [3,44]. Several studies have evaluated an ARB as add-on therapy to an ACE inhibitor. The Valsartan Heart Failure Trial (Val-HeFT) demonstrated a 13% reduction (RR 0.87; 97.5% CI, 0.77–0.97, p = 0.009) in the combined endpoint of mortality and morbidity for patients randomized to valsartan as compared to placebo. Mortality alone was similar between groups. Background ACE inhibitors were used in 93% of patients in this study [49]. In the CHARM-Added trial, candesartan was associated with a 15% reduction (HR 0.85; 95% CI, 0.75–0.96; p = 0.011) in the primary endpoint of cardiovascular death or heart failure hospitalization as compared to placebo, with 100% of patients receiving background ACE inhibitor therapy [50]. Notably, combination therapy is associated with a higher risk of hyperkalemia and increase in serum creatinine; thus, patients should be carefully chosen for and closely monitored with this treatment approach.

In patients with post-MI left ventricular (LV) systolic dysfunction and/or heart failure symptoms, the ARB valsartan was shown to be non-inferior to the ACE inhibitor captopril for the endpoints of mortality alone and fatal and non-fatal cardiovascular events in the Valsartan in Acute Myocardial Infarction (VALIANT) trial [51]. The combination of valsartan and captopril was not associated with improvements in clinical outcomes, but the rate of adverse events was higher in this group; thus, there is no advantage to using combination therapy in these patients. The use of an ARB in post-MI patients with a reduced ejection fraction or heart failure symptoms who are intolerant to an ACE inhibitor is recommended by the American College of Cardiology (ACC)/American Heart Association (AHA) guidelines (class I recommendation) [44].

In the Irbesartan in Heart Failure with Preserved Ejection Fraction (I-PRESERVE) study, irbesartan failed to demonstrate a clinical effect in this population [52]. The study enrolled 4128 patients with heart failure symptoms (New York Heart Association [NYHA] II–IV) and a left ventricular ejection fraction (LVEF) of 45% or greater. Patients were required to have been hospitalized at least once during the previous 6 months. Patients were randomized to irbesartan or placebo, and the primary endpoint was all -cause mortality or cardiovascular hospitalization. In the irbesartan group, 36% died or experienced a cardiovascular hospitalization compared to 37% in the placebo group (HR 0.95; 95% CI, 0.86–1.05; p = 0.35) [52]. No between-group differences were detected in any of the secondary endpoints. These findings emphasize the need to achieve a better understanding of the pathophysiology of heart failure with preserved systolic function and to identify effective treatments for this prevalent condition.

Beta-adrenergic blockers

Beta-blockers, in conjunction with ACE inhibitors, are the cornerstone of heart failure pharmacotherapy. Use of an evidence-based beta-blocker (bisoprolol, carvedilol, or metoprolol succinate CR/XL) is recommended for all patients

Table 5.4 Primary results from clinical trials of beta-blockers in heart failure.

Trial	Primary endpoint	HR (95% CI)	p-value
CIBIS-II [53]	All-cause mortality	0.66 (0.54–0.81)	<0.0001
COPERNICUS [55]	All-cause mortality	0.65 (0.52–0.81)	0.00013
MERIT-HF [54]	All-cause mortality	0.66 (0.53–0.81)	0.0062

with current or prior heart failure symptoms and reduced systolic dysfunction who are without contraindications [3,44]. These recommendations are based on the three major randomized, clinical trials evaluating beta-blockers in heart failure: the Cardiac Insufficiency Bisoprolol Study (CIBIS II), Carvedilol Prospective Randomized Cumulative Survival trial (COPERNICUS), and Metoprolol Randomized Intervention Trial in Congestive Heart Failure (MERIT-HF) [53–55]. Each of these trials demonstrated a remarkably consistent 34–35% reduction in the primary endpoint of all-cause mortality for patients randomized to beta-blockade compared to placebo (Table 5.4). The Study of the Effects of Nebivolol Intervention on Outcomes and Rehospitalization in Seniors with Heart Failure (SENIORS) trial randomized 2128 patients aged 70 years or older with a history of heart failure to nebivolol or placebo. The primary outcome (mortality or all-cause hospitalization) occurred in 332 patients (31.1%) on nebivolol compared with 375 (35.3%) on placebo (HR 0.86; 95% CI, 0.74–0.99; p = 0.039), indicating a benefit of nebivolol in this elderly population with heart failure, and nebivolol was well tolerated. Nebivolol is licensed for this indication in Europe and many other countries but not in the US [56]. All patients in these studies were receiving background ACE inhibitor therapy.

Beta-blockers inhibit the deleterious effects of the sympathetic nervous system on heart failure progression, prevent/reverse cardiac remodeling, and reduce the risk for sudden cardiac death. Beta-blockers are generally well tolerated, but patients should be clinically stable from a volume standpoint prior to beta-blocker initiation. They should be initiated at low doses and titrated at 1–2-week intervals to reduce the risk for short-term worsening of heart failure symptoms.

Aldosterone antagonists

An aldosterone antagonist is recommended for patients with systolic dysfunction and severe heart failure symptoms (NYHA class III or IV) despite optimal pharmacological therapy [3,44]. In the Randomized Aldactone Evaluation Study (RALES), spironolactone reduced the risk of all-cause mortality by 30% compared to standard therapy (RR 0.69; 95% CI, 0.58–0.82; p < 0.001) [57]. Hyperkalemia is a significant complication of spironolactone therapy, but had an incidence of only 2% in the RALES trial. However, outside of the rigorous follow-up of a clinical trial, much higher rates of hyperkalemia have been reported [58,59]. Careful patient selection and close laboratory monitoring help to minimize hyperkalemia-related complications in these patients.

Guidelines recommend that spironolactone only be initiated in patients with a serum creatinine of 2.5 mg/dL or less in men or 2.0 mg/dL or less in women, and a serum potassium of 5.0 mEq/L or less [44].

The aldosterone antagonist eplerenone has been shown to improve outcomes in post-MI patients with LV dysfunction and heart failure. Eplerenone reduced all-cause mortality by 15% (RR 0.85, 95% CI, 0.75–0.96; p = 0.008) and cardiovascular death or cardiovascular hospitalization by 13% (RR 0.87; 95% CI, 0.72–0.94; p = 0.005) in the Eplerenone Post-Acute Myocardial Infarction Heart Failure Efficacy and Survival Study (EPHESUS) [60].

In the Eplerenone in patients with systolic heart failure and mild symptoms (EMPHASIS HF) trial, 2737 patients with NYHA class II heart failure and an ejection fraction of less than 35% were randomized to eplerenone (up to 50 mg daily) or placebo. The trial was stopped prematurely after a median follow-up of 21 months. The primary outcome of cardiovascular death or hospitalization for heart failure occurred in 18.3% of patients in the eplerenone group compared to 25.9% in the placebo group (HR 0.63; 95% CI, 0.54–0.74; p < 0.001), and 12.5% of patients receiving eplerenone and 15.5% of those receiving placebo died (HR 0.76; 95% CI, 0.62–0.93; p = 0.008). This study confirms the role of eplerenone in patients with systolic heart failure and mild symptoms [61].

Combination renin–angiotensin–aldosterone system inhibitors

ARBs or aldosterone antagonists are recommended in patients who remain symptomatic despite optimal therapy with ACE inhibitors and beta-blockers. Triple therapy with an ACE inhibitor, ARB, and aldosterone antagonist is not recommended due to the substantial risk for hyperkalemia or worsening renal function [3,44]. The decision whether to initiate an ARB or aldosterone antagonist must be made on an individual patient basis. The available evidence indicates that aldosterone antagonists are associated with a significant survival benefit. In contrast, the addition of an ARB has not been associated with improved survival, although this has reduced the rate of composite mortality and morbidity endpoints. Although the use of the combination of ACE inhibitor and ARB transiently suppresses aldosterone levels, it does not achieve complete aldosterone blockade [56,62,63]. Finally, the ACC/AHA heart failure guidelines give a class I recommendation to the initiation of an aldosterone antagonist in appropriate patients and a class IIb recommendation for the addition of an ARB [44]. Thus, in many patients, it may be desirable to initiate aldosterone blockade rather than an ARB, unless this is contraindicated or not tolerated.

Hydralazine and isosorbide dinitrate

The combination of hydralazine and a nitrate may be used in patients with symptomatic systolic heart failure who do not tolerate an ACE inhibitor or ARB because of renal insufficiency or hyperkalemia, and in some cases, angioedema [44]. The combination of hydralazine and isosorbide dinitrate has a more specific role in the management of African-American patients with heart failure. The African American Heart Failure Trial (A-HeFT) randomized 1050 black patients with NYHA class III–IV heart failure to isosorbide dinitrate plus hydralazine or placebo in addition to standard therapy [64]. The primary endpoint was a composite score of weighted values for all-cause mortality, heart failure hospitalization, and quality of life. The trial was stopped early after a 43% reduction in all-cause mortality (HR 0.57; p = 0.01) was observed in the isosorbide dinitrate plus hydralazine group. A significant beneficial effect on the primary composite score was also observed (p = 0.01). In patients who remain symptomatic after ACE inhibitor and beta-blocker therapy, the addition of hydralazine and isosorbide dinitrate is reasonable [44]. The evidence supporting this approach is strongest for the African-American population.

Device therapies

Multiple clinical trials have demonstrated a survival benefit for patients with systolic dysfunction randomized to implantable cardioverter defibrillator (ICD) therapy as compared to optimal medical care [65,66]. Cardiac resynchronization therapy (CRT) has also been shown to improve symptoms and quality of life, and to reduce mortality in patients with chronic heart failure [21,67]. These devices are now part of recommended therapy as outlined by the ACC/AHA, Heart Failure Society of America (HFSA), and European Society of Cardiology (ESC) guidelines [3,43,44] (Table 5.5).

Implantable cardioverter defibrillator

Sudden cardiac death accounts for approximately half of all heart failure-related deaths, particularly in those patients with less severe symptoms [54]. SCD-HeFT randomized patients with stable, chronic NYHA class II or III heart failure due to ischemic or non-ischemic causes and LVEF of 35% or lower to an ICD, amiodarone, or placebo [65]. In this primary prevention study, the ICD reduced all-cause mortality by 23% (HR 0.77; 97.5% CI, 0.62–0.96; p = 0.007). Patients randomized to the ICD had improvements in several quality-of-life scales at 3 and 12 months, but the improvements did not persist to 30 months of follow-up [68]. In the Multicenter Automatic Defibrillator Implantation Trial II (MADIT II), an ICD reduced the risk of all-cause mortality by 31% (HR 0.69; 95% CI, 0.51–0.93; p = 0.016) as compared to conventional therapy among patients with a prior MI and LVEF of 30% or greater [66].

Despite the evidence supporting the use of ICDs, data indicate they are underused in eligible patients. In particular, usage differs according to both race and gender, with women and black patients receiving ICDs less often than white men [69]. Differences in ICD use according to hospital characteristics have also been reported from large national registries [70,71].

Cardiac resynchronization therapy

It is estimated that cardiac dyssynchrony affects 15–30% of patients with heart failure, resulting in decreased systolic function and increased systolic volumes [20]. By applying biventricular stimulation, CRT aims to restore appropriate activation of the intraventricular septum and LV free wall. Initial studies observed improvements in NYHA functional class, quality of life, 6-minute

Table 5.5 Guideline recommendations for device therapies.

	Implantable cardioverter defibrillator (ICD)	Cardiac resynchronization therapy (CRT)
ACC/ AHA [44]	An ICD is recommended as secondary prevention to prolong survival in patients with current or prior symptoms of heart failure and reduced LVEF who have a history of cardiac arrest, ventricular fibrillation, or hemodynamically destabilizing ventricular tachycardiac (class I, level of evidence A) ICD therapy is recommended for primary prevention to reduce total mortality by a reduction in SCD in patients with ischemic heart disease who are at least 40 days post-MI, have LVEF ≤30%, with NYHA functional class II or III symptoms while undergoing chronic optimal medical therapy, and have reasonable expectation of survival with a good functional status for >1 year (class I, level of evidence A) Recommended for primary prevention to reduce total mortality by a reduction in SCD in patients with non-ischemic cardiomyopathy who have LVEF ≤30%, with NYHA functional class II or III symptoms while undergoing chronic optimal medical therapy, and have reasonable expectation of survival with a good functional status for >1 year (class I, level of evidence B) Placement of an ICD is reasonable in patients with LVEF 30–35% of any origin with NYHA function class II or III symptoms who are taking chronic optimal medical therapy and who have reasonable expectation of survival with good functional status of >1 year (class II, level of evidence B)	Patients with LVEF ≤35%, sinus rhythm, and NYHA class III or ambulatory class IV symptoms despite recommended optimal medical therapy, and who have cardiac dyssynchrony, defined as a QRS duration >0.12 ms, should receive CRT unless contraindicated (class I, level of evidence A)

(continued)

Table 5.5 (continued)

	Implantable cardioverter defibrillator (ICD)	Cardiac resynchronization therapy (CRT)
ESC [3]	ICD therapy for secondary prevention is recommended for survivors of ventricular fibrillation and also for patients with documented hemodynamically unstable VT and/or VT with syncope, LVEF ≤40%, on optimal medical therapy, and with an expectation of survival with good function status for >1 year (class I, level of evidence A) ICD therapy for primary prevention is recommended to reduce mortality in patients with LV dysfunction due to prior MI or who are at least 40 days post-MI, have an LVEF ≤35%, in NYHA functional class II or III, receiving optimal medical therapy, and who have a reasonable expectation of survival with good functional status for >1 year (class I, level of evidence A) ICD therapy for primary prevention is recommended to reduce mortality in patients with non-ischemic cardiomyopathy with an LVEF ≤35%, in NYHA functional class II or III, receiving optimal medical therapy, and who have a reasonable expectation of survival with good functional status for >1 year (class I, level of evidence B)	CRT with pacemaker function (CRT-P) is recommended to reduce morbidity and mortality in patients in NYHA III–IV class who are symptomatic despite optimal medical therapy, and who have a reduced EF (LVEF ≤35%) and QRS prolongation (QRS ≥120 ms) (class I, level of evidence A) CRT with defibrillator function (CRT-D) is recommended to reduce morbidity and mortality in patients in NYHA III–IV class who are symptomatic despite optimal medical therapy, and who have a reduced EF (LVEF ≤35%) and QRS prolongation (QRS ≥120 ms) (class I, level of evidence A)
HFSA [43]	Prophylactic ICD placement should be considered (LVEF ≤30%) or may be considered (LVEF 31–35%) for those with mild-to-moderate heart failure symptoms (NYHA II–III) (level of evidence A) Concomitant ICD placement should be considered in patients undergoing implantation of a biventricular pacing device (level of evidence B) ICD placement is not recommended in chronic, severe, refractory heart failure when there is no reasonable expectation for improvement (level of evidence C) ICD implantation is recommended for survivors of cardiac arrest from ventricular fibrillation or hemodynamically unstable sustained VT without evidence of acute MI or if the event occurs >48 hours after the onset of infarction in the absence of a recurrent ischemic event (level of evidence A)	Biventricular pacing should be considered for patients with sinus rhythm, a widened QRS interval (≥120 ms) and severe LV systolic dysfunction (LVEF ≤35% with LV dilatation >5.5 cm) who have persistent, moderate-to-severe heart failure (NYHA III) despite optimal medical therapy (level of evidence A) Selected ambulatory NYHA IV patients may be considered for biventricular pacing therapy (level of evidence B) Biventricular pacing therapy is not recommended in patients who are asymptomatic or have mild heart failure symptoms (level of evidence C)

ACC, American College of Cardiology; AHA, American Heart Association; ESC, European Society of Cardiology; HFSA, Heart Failure Society of America; LVEF, left ventricular function; MI, myocardial infarction; NYHA, New York Heart Association; SCD, sudden cardiac death; VT, ventricular tachycardia.

walk distance, exercise test duration, and ejection fraction for patients randomized to CRT [67]. In the Comparison of Medical Therapy, Pacing, and Defibrillation in Heart Failure (COMPANION) trial, CRT was associated with a 19% reduction (HR 0.81; 95% CI, 0.69–0.96; p = 0.014) in the primary endpoint of all-cause death or all-cause hospitalization among patients with NYHA class III–IV heart failure, LVEF of 35% or less, and QRS duration of 120 ms or longer. The effect of CRT alone on all-cause mortality did not reach statistical significance (HR 0.76; 95% CI, 0.58–1.01; p = 0.059) [20]. Patients randomized to CRT plus ICD demonstrated a 20% reduction (HR 0.8; 95% CI. 0.68–0.95; p = 0.01) in all-cause death or hospitalization and a 36% reduction (HR 0.64; 95% CI; 0.48–0.86; p = 0.003) in all-cause mortality.

The Cardiac Resynchronization Heart Failure (CARE-HF) study evaluated CRT alone in 813 patients with NYHA class III–IV symptoms, LVEF of 35% or less, LV end-diastolic dimension (LVEDD) of at least 30 mm, and a QRS duration of 120 ms or longer [21]. CRT reduced the primary endpoint of all-cause mortality or cardiovascular hospitalization by 37% (HR 0.63; 95% CI, 0.51–0.77; p < 0.001). CRT was also associated with a 36% reduction in all-cause mortality (HR 0.64; 95% CI, 0.48–0.85; p < 0.002). Echocardiographic measurements also improved for the CRT group as compared to placebo, including higher ejection fraction, lower end-systolic volume index, smaller area of mitral regurgitation, and shorter interventricular mechanical delay, indicating that CRT exerted favorable effects on remodeling [21].

Additional data from MADIT-CRT suggest that patients with less symptomatic heart failure (ischemic cardiomyopathy in NYHA class I or II and non-ischemic cardiomyopathy class II), LVEF of 30% or less, and QRS duration of 130 ms or longer also benefit from CRT [72].

Left ventricular assist device

The applications of LV assist devices (LVADs) are largely limited to use as a bridge to transplantation and managing patients with acute, severe myocarditis [3]. Data from the International Society for Heart and Lung Transplantation (ISHLT) Mechanical Circulatory Support Device database indicate that 78% of devices were implanted as a bridge to transplant during 2002–2004 [73]. LVADs may also be used as permanent or destination therapy in selected patients with refractory heart failure and an estimated 1-year mortality exceeding 50% [44]. Destination therapy was the goal of implantation in 12% of cases in the ISHLT Mechanical Circulatory Support Device database [73]. Data supporting the approach of destination therapy were generated in the Randomized Evaluation of Mechanical Assistance for the Treatment of Congestive Heart Failure (REMATCH) trial. This study evaluated the long-term use of the HeartMate XVE (Thoratec, Pleasanton, CA, USA) in patients with chronic end-stage heart failure and contraindications to cardiac transplantation [74]. The primary endpoint of the study was all-cause mortality. A total of 129 patients with NYHA class IV symptoms, LVEF of 25% or less, and VO$_2$ max of 12 mL/kg/min or less, or a requirement for continuous infusion inotropes were randomized to LVAD or optimal medical therapy. Patients who received the LVAD had a 48% reduction in the risk of all-cause mortality as compared to the group receiving optimal therapy [74]. One-year survival was 52% in the device group and 25% in the medical therapy group (p = 0.002). At 2 years, the survival was 23% for the LVAD group and 8% in the optimal medical therapy group, a difference that was of borderline statistical significance (p = 0.09). Patients randomized to receive the LVAD had improvements in their SF-36 and Beck Depression Inventory scores and NYHA functional classification at 1 year. Serious adverse events related to the device were common with a probability of infection of 28%. The rate of device failure was 35% at 24 months [74].

Long *et al.* reported the results of 42 patients treated with LVAD therapy compared with optimal medical management [75]. The HeartMate XVE, approved by the FDA, was used in this study. The investigators compared the results for these 42 patients with those from the REMATCH trial. Patients treated with destination therapy in this study had a 40% lower rate of death as compared to the REMATCH population. The mortality rate due to sepsis was lower, and overall adverse events were 61% lower with destination therapy as compared to the REMATCH population. Specifically, the rate of sepsis was 63% lower, infection was 89% lower, and device failure was 73% lower as compared to REMATCH. Thus, this non-random comparison suggests that significant advances are being made in device therapy. In 2002, the HeartMate XVE was approved by the FDA for destination therapy in certain terminally ill patients who are not heart transplant candidates.

Ultrafiltration

Ultrafiltration carries a class IIa recommendation (level of evidence B) for the reduction of pulmonary or peripheral edema and correction of hyponatremia in symptomatic patients who are refractory to diuretics [3]. The Ultrafiltration versus Intravenous Diuretics for Patients Hospitalized for Acute Decompensated Heart Failure (UNLOAD) study (n = 200) demonstrated a greater degree of weight loss at 48 hours among patients randomized to ultrafiltration versus those treated with standard-care intravenous diuretics [76]. At 90 days, patients receiving ultrafiltration had fewer heart failure hospitalizations, rehospitalization days, and unscheduled visits as compared to patients receiving intravenous diuretics alone. No adverse safety signals were detected. More data are needed to guide patient selection and to evaluate clinical outcomes related to this therapy. Ultrafiltration is the focus of an ongoing study being conducted by the National Heart, Lung, and Blood Institute Heart Failure Network.

Surgical therapies

Revascularization

The majority of patients (~65%) with chronic heart failure have concomitant coronary artery disease [7]. Current practice regarding revascularization with percutaneous coronary intervention (PCI) or coronary artery bypass graft

(CABG) surgery is largely based on observational data. The majority of clinical trials evaluating CABG either excluded patients with heart failure, only included small numbers of heart failure patients, or only included patients with mild-to-moderate heart failure symptoms [77,78].

The National Institutes of Health sponsored a study to evaluate the role of surgical therapies in the management of patients with heart failure. The Surgical Treatment for Ischemic Heart Failure (STICH) trial was designed to determine whether CABG surgery was superior to guideline-based medical therapy in terms of survival. In addition, the study also addressed the issue of whether surgical ventricular reconstruction (SVR) in addition to CABG would improve hospitalization-free survival in patients with significant anterior wall dysfunction [78]. Overall, 2136 patients with coronary artery disease amenable to revascularization and an LVEF of 35% or less were enrolled in STICH. Of these, 1000 patients were included in the hypothesis 2 (SVR plus CABG vs CABG alone) component of the trial. These patients were randomized to SVR plus CABG (n = 501) or CABG alone (n = 499) [79]. After a median follow-up of 48 months, there was no statistical difference in the occurrence of all-cause mortality or cardiac hospitalization between groups (58% CABG plus SVR vs 59% CABG; HR 0.99; 95% CI, 0.84–1.17; p = 0.9). Symptoms of angina and heart failure improved for both groups, with no difference between groups detected. Patients randomized to CABG plus SVR had a significantly higher reduction in mean end-systolic volume index as compared to patients randomized to CABG alone (p < 0.001) [79]. For hypothesis 1, eligible patients with a mean ejection fraction of 28% were randomized to medical therapy alone (n = 602) or CABG plus medical therapy (n = 610) [80]. The primary outcome of all-cause mortality occurred in 244 patients (41%) in the medical therapy group and 218 (36%) in the CABG plus medical therapy group (HR 0.86; 95% CI, 0.72–1.04; p = 0.12). Death from any cause or hospitalization for cardiovascular causes occurred in 411 patients (68%) in the medical therapy group and 351 (58%) in the CABG group (HR with CABG, 0.74; 95% CI, 0.64–0.85; p < 0.001). In patients with coronary artery disease and heart failure, CABG plus medical therapy did not show a significant reduction in mortality compared with medical therapy alone, but there was a clear reduction in the secondary outcome of death or cardiovascular hospitalization. In a substudy published at the same time by Bonow *et al;*, there did not appear to be a link between the presence of myocardial viability and benefit of CABG [81]. Currently, the evidence from STICH suggests there is no clear indication for routine CABG in patients with mild-to-moderate angina and impaired LV function. This does not rule out the potential benefits of CABG in patients with heart failure or LV dysfunction in the presence of myocardial ischemia in the dysfunctional territories, but it is unclear if this question will be answered in a randomized trial. In the interim, the current heart failure guidelines recommend that patients with heart failure and angina are considered for revascularization therapy [3,44]. Patient and procedure selection should be according to the recommendations in the guidelines for chronic stable angina and for CABG surgery [82,83].

Valvular surgery

Valvular heart disease may be the underlying etiology for heart failure, or it may provoke worsening symptoms in patients with heart failure. Optimal medical management should be implemented prior to undergoing any valvular surgery.

As with revascularization procedures, few randomized studies have specifically evaluated clinical outcomes among patients with heart failure and valvular disease. Surgery is generally recommended among eligible patients with heart failure symptoms and severe aortic stenosis or aortic regurgitation, or in asymptomatic patients with severe aortic stenosis or aortic regurgitation who have systolic dysfunction [3]. Although symptoms, LV function, and possibly clinical outcomes may improve after surgery, surgical risk is highest as LV function declines. Mitral valve surgery (preferably repair) is recommended for patients with LVEF of greater than 30%. It may be considered in patients with lower LVEF (<30%), but only in patients who are refractory to pharmacological treatment and have a low risk profile [3]. In patients with functional mitral regurgitation, the use of CRT may decrease mitral regurgitation by improving LV geometry and papillary muscle dyssynchrony. Thus, it may be reasonable to optimize medical therapy and consider CRT therapy prior to surgery in CRT eligible patients [3].

Transplantation

Cardiac transplantation is the only established, long-term, treatment of advanced heart failure. Over 80 000 transplants have been performed globally [84]. The estimated annual number of transplants performed worldwide exceeds 5000. Clinical outcomes continue to improve in cardiac transplant patients. The median survival for patients surviving the first year post-transplantation is 13 years [84].

In the US, 2705 patients are on the national waiting list for a heart transplant. In comparison, there were 1668 total deceased donors from January to September 2008. It is not known whether all of these were suitable heart donors [85]. Because the number of ideal donor hearts is limited, consideration has been given to alternate heart transplants. Non-standard donor hearts are increasingly being used for higher risk recipients and critically ill patients. Recipients who would traditionally not be candidates for transplantation are being placed on alternate recipient lists. These patients include those of advanced age, or those with other comorbidities such as diabetes, or renal or pulmonary disease. Patients aged 60 years or older now account for 25% of all recipients [83]. The donor hearts used in these tranplants are those from older donors (≥50 years of age now accounts for >12% of donors [83]) with some degree of coronary artery disease, impaired LV function, or hypertrophy. Research is ongoing to determine the clinical outcomes of patients transplanted on the alternate heart list.

Exercise training

Exercise training or physical activity is recommended for stable patients with systolic dysfunction by the ACC, AHA, ECC, and Canadian Cardiovascular

Society heart failure guidelines [3,44,86]. However, these recommendations have largely been based on data from relatively small single-center trials that were often not well controlled or adequately powered to evaluate clinical outcomes such as mortality and morbidity.

The Heart Failure and A Controlled Trial Investigating Outcomes of Exercise Training (HF-ACTION) trial was designed to address this important question. HF-ACTION randomized 2331 patients with NYHA class II–IV heart failure symptoms and LVEF of 35% or less on optimal heart failure pharmacological and device therapy to exercise training or usual care [84]. Patients were exceptionally treated at baseline, with 93% receiving an ACE inhibitor or ARB, 95% a beta blocker, 45% an aldosterone antagonist, 40% an ICD, and 18% CRT. The exercise training arm consisted of supervised exercise training for approximately 3 months (36 sessions), followed by home-based training. The usual care group received standard care, which included the recommendation that patients participate in physical activity most days of the week. All patients were followed for 24 months. The primary endpoint was the composite of mortality or hospitalization from any cause [87]. Exercise training was associated with a 7% reduction in the risk of the primary endpoint as compared to usual care (HR 0.93; 95% CI, 0.84–1.02; $p = 0.13$). However, after adjustment for baseline characteristics that were highly predictive of death or hospitalization, exercise training was associated with a significant reduction in this composite endpoint (HR 0.89; 95% CI, 0.81–0.99; $p = 0.03$). Mortality alone was not significantly different between the groups (exercise training 16% vs usual care 17%). The secondary endpoint of cardiovascular mortality and heart failure hospitalizations was also favorably affected by exercise training (unadjusted HR 0.87; 95% CI, 0.75–1.00; $p = 0.06$; adjusted HR 0.85; 95% CI, 0.74–0.99; $p = 0.03$). These benefits were observed despite lower than expected adherence in the exercise training group and a higher rate of physical activity among usual care patients. Importantly, exercise training was found to be safe in this trial, with no differences in adverse events between groups. These data support the current guideline recommendation of exercise training for patients with heart failure symptoms and systolic dysfunction in addition to evidence-based pharmacological and device therapies [88].

Current challenges of heart failure: acute heart failure syndromes

In contrast to chronic heart failure, few significant advances in the management of patients with acute heart failure syndromes (AHFS) have been realized. None of the agents used in the treatment of AHFS has been shown to reduce mortality or improve long-term outcomes. Management is largely focused on improving symptoms and stabilizing the patient.

Pharmacological fluid management

Loop diuretics are recommended in patients with evidence of congestion and volume overload. The ECC recommends an initial furosemide dose of

20–40 mg intravenously that can then be increased according to renal function and history of chronic diuretic use [3]. The lowest diuretic dose should be prescribed that achieves symptomatic relief and volume goals. Data from the Evaluation Study of Congestive Heart Failure and Pulmonary Artery Catheterization Effectiveness (ESCAPE) study suggest that diuretic dose is a significant predictor of mortality even after adjusting for other important prognostic variables [89]. An analysis from the ADHERE registry revealed an association between furosemide doses of 160 mg/day or greater and a higher risk for in-hospital mortality, longer intensive care unit stay, longer overall length of stay, and adverse renal effects [90].

Alternatives to loop diuretics are currently under investigation. While these agents may not fully replace loop diuretics in the management of heart failure, they may allow for lower loop diuretic doses to be used, which in turn may be associated with improved outcomes. Oral vasopressin receptor antagonists and adenosine receptor antagonists are two drug classes that may offer some advantages over existing diuretic therapy. Oral vasopressin antagonists induce a free water aquaresis and have been associated with greater reductions in body weight and urine output as compared to diuretics alone [91,92]. These agents also improve serum sodium levels and are not associated with hypokalemia. However, their effect on clinical outcomes has been neutral in studies to date [93]. Adenosine receptor antagonists increase urine flow and induce natriuresis, and they have been shown to prevent reductions in renal function associated with loop diuretic use [94–96]. Phase 3 clinical trials are underway with several agents in these drug classes to determine their influence on clinical outcomes and potential role in the management of heart failure.

Vasodilators

Vasodilator therapy may also be appropriate in patients with congestion or edema with systolic blood pressure above 90 mmHg. These agents should not be used in patients with low systolic blood pressure or evidence of cardiogenic shock. Intravenous nitrates or sodium nitroprusside decreases filling pressures and improves dyspnea quickly in patients with AHFS. Although vasodilators are widely used in the management of AHFS, data are lacking that evaluate their effects on long-term outcomes.

Nesiritide is a recombinant form of human B-type natriuretic peptide. It has venous and arterial vasodilating properties. In the Vasodilation in the Management of Acute CHF (VMAC) study, nesiritide reduced pulmonary capillary wedge pressure to a greater extent than placebo (p < 0.001) and nitroglycerin (p = 0.03) at 3 hours [97]. There were no differences between the nesiritide and nitroglycerin group in dyspnea scores or global clinical status. However, some questions were raised regarding the safety of nesiritide in terms of worsening renal function [98] and mortality [99]. Nesiritide is currently being studied in a large, randomized trial to evaluate its effects on clinical outcomes [100]. Other natriuretic peptides are also under development. Ularitide is a synthetic analog of the renal natriuretic peptide urodilatin that has been shown to preserve renal function in patients with AHFS [101], and it is currently being studied in the Ularitide Global Evaluation in Acute Decompensated Heart Failure (URGENT) trial [102].

Inotropes

Inotropes have a role in the management of patients with AHFS who have evidence of cardiogenic shock, low systolic blood pressure, hypoperfusion, and/or low cardiac output [3]. They are not effective among patients with volume overload in the absence of low cardiac output or hypoperfusion. Although inotropic therapy improves cardiac output and other hemodynamic parameters over the short term, these drugs may have deleterious effects by increasing myocardial oxygen consumption and possibly contributing to myocardial injury, and they should be discontinued as soon as possible. In the Outcomes of a Prospective Trial of Intravenous Milrinone for Exacerbations of Chronic Heart Failure (OPTIME-CHF), milrinone did not reduce the number of days of cardiovascular hospitalization or death as compared to placebo in patients hospitalized for worsening heart failure [103]. Milrinone was associated with worse outcomes among patients with ischemic heart disease and arrhythmias in this study [104,105]. Retrospective analyses from several randomized trials and registry databases have demonstrated consistent associations between inotrope use and increased mortality [31,106–108].

Levosimendan is a novel inotropic agent that increases cardiac output by binding to cardiac troponin C and sensitizing cardiac myofilaments to calcium. It also has vasodilatory properties. Since its actions are independent of the beta-adrenergic receptor, it was hypothesized to be a safer and more effective inotropic agent as compared to existing inotropic therapies, particularly dobutamine. In comparison to dobutamine in the Survival of Patients With Acute Heart Failure in Need of Intravenous Inotropic Support (SURVIVE), levosimendan was associated with a greater reduction in B-type natriuretic peptide (BNP) levels at 24 hours ($p < 0.001$), but there were no differences between groups in all-cause mortality at 180 days (26% levosimendan vs 28% dobutamine; $p = 0.4$) [109]. In a meta-analysis of 5480 patients in 45 randomized clinical trials of levosimendan, the overall mortality rate was 17.4% (507 of 2915) among levosimendan-treated patients and 23.3% (598 of 2565) in the combined placebo or active control group (RR 0.80; 95% CI 0.72–0.89]; $p < 0.001$), with a significant effect in the subgroup of cardiac surgery trials [110]. Thus levosimendan may be a promising agent in selected acute heart failure patients and is licensed in Europe but not in the US.

Istaroxime is another novel agent for AHFS under development. It inhibits sodium–potassium adenosine triphosphatase (ATPase) and stimulates sarcoplasmic reticulum calcium ATPase isoform 2, which promotes both an inotropic and lusitropic response. Istaroxime has improved systolic and diastolic function without increasing myocardial oxygen consumption in animal models of heart failure. In the HORIZON-HF trial, istaroxime significantly lowered pulmonary capillary wedge pressure (PCWP), heart rate, and LV end-diastolic volume. Systolic blood pressure and cardiac index increased.

Neurohormones, renal function, or troponin I did not change in response to istaroxime therapy [111]. Future trials will determine the role of istaroxime in the management of AHFS.

Conclusion

Many successful and important advances have been made in the field of heart failure over the past 20–30 years. Although these advances have been associated with improvements in clinical outcomes, the mortality and morbidity rate among patients with heart failure remains high. In addition, identification of therapies that reduce mortality and morbidity for patients with AHFS is an unmet need and current challenge facing heart failure researchers and clinicians. The prevalence of heart failure will increase as the population ages, making it imperative to discover new and effective therapies to further improve outcomes for these patients.

References

1. Lloyd-Jones D, Adams R, Carnethon M, *et al*. Heart disease and stroke statistics–2009 update. A report From the American Heart Association Statistics Committee and Stroke Statistics Subcommittee. *Circulation* 2009;119:480–486.
2. Curtis LH, Whellan DJ, Hammill BG, *et al*. Incidence and prevalence of heart failure in elderly persons, 1994–2003. *Arch Intern Med* 2008;168:418–424.
3. Dickstein K, Cohen-Solal A, Filippatos G, *et al*. ESC Guidelines for the diagnosis and treatment of acute and chronic heart failure 2008: the Task Force for the Diagnosis and Treatment of Acute and Chronic Heart Failure 2008 of the European Society of Cardiology. Developed in collaboration with the Heart Failure Association of the ESC (HFA) and endorsed by the European Society of Intensive Care Medicine (ESICM). *Eur Heart J* 2008;29:2388–2442.
4. Cohn JN, Levine TB, Olivari MT, *et al*. Plasma norepinephrine as a guide to prognosis in patients with chronic congestive heart failure. *N Engl J Med* 1984;311:819–823.
5. Francis GS, Goldsmith SR, Levine TB, Olivari MT, Cohn JN. The neurohumoral axis in congestive heart failure. *Ann Intern Med* 1984;101:370–377.
6. Francis GS, Benedict C, Johnstone DE, *et al*. Comparison of neuroendocrine activation in patients with left ventricular dysfunction with and without congestive heart failure. A substudy of the Studies of Left Ventricular Dysfunction (SOLVD). *Circulation* 1990;82:1724–1729.
7. Levine TB, Francis GS, Goldsmith SR, Simon AB, Cohn JN. Activity of the sympathetic nervous system and renin-angiotensin system assessed by plasma hormone levels and their relation to hemodynamic abnormalities in congestive heart failure. *Am J Cardiol* 1982;49:1659–1666.
8. Mann DL, Kent RL, Parsons B, Cooper G. Adrenergic effects on the biology of the adult mammalian cardiocyte. *Circulation* 1992;85:790–804.
9. Schrier RW, Abraham WT. Hormones and hemodynamics in heart failure. *N Engl J Med* 1999;341:577–585.
10. Jessup M, Brozena S. Heart failure. *N Engl J Med* 2003;348:2007–2018.
11. Cohn JN, Ferrari R, Sharpe N. Cardiac remodeling–concepts and clinical implications: a consensus paper from an international forum on cardiac remodeling. Behalf of an International Forum on Cardiac Remodeling. *J Am Coll Cardiol* 2000;35:569–582.

12. Greenberg B, Quinones MA, Koilpillai C, *et al.* Effects of long-term enalapril therapy on cardiac structure and function in patients with left ventricular dysfunction. Results of the SOLVD echocardiography substudy. *Circulation* 1995;91:2573–2581.

13. Hall SA, Cigarroa CG, Marcoux L, *et al.* Time course of improvement in left ventricular function, mass and geometry in patients with congestive heart failure treated with beta-adrenergic blockade. *J Am Coll Cardiol* 1995;25:1154–1161.

14. Lowes BD, Gill EA, Abraham WT, *et al.* Effects of carvedilol on left ventricular mass, chamber geometry, and mitral regurgitation in chronic heart failure. *Am J Cardiol* 1999;83:1201–1205.

15. Quinones MA, Greenberg BH, Kopelen HA, *et al.* Echocardiographic predictors of clinical outcome in patients with left ventricular dysfunction enrolled in the SOLVD registry and trials: significance of left ventricular hypertrophy. Studies of left ventricular dysfunction. *J Am Coll Cardiol* 2000;35:1237–1244.

16. Remme WJ, Riegger G, Hildebrandt P, *et al.* The benefits of early combination treatment of carvedilol and an ACE-inhibitor in mild heart failure and left ventricular systolic dysfunction. The carvedilol and ACE-inhibitor remodelling mild heart failure evaluation trial (CARMEN). *Cardiovasc Drugs Ther* 2004;18:57–66.

17. Waagstein F, Stromblad O, Andersson B, *et al.* Increased exercise ejection fraction and reversed remodeling after long-term treatment with metoprolol in congestive heart failure: a randomized, stratified, double-blind, placebo-controlled trial in mild to moderate heart failure due to ischemic or idiopathic dilated cardiomyopathy. *Eur J Heart Fail* 2003;5:679–691.

18. Wong M, Staszewsky L, Latini R, *et al.* Valsartan benefits left ventricular structure and function in heart failure: Val-HeFT echocardiographic study. *J Am Coll Cardiol* 2002;40:970–975.

19. Zannad F, Alla F, Dousset B, Perez A, Pitt B. Limitation of excessive extracellular matrix turnover may contribute to survival benefit of spironolactone therapy in patients with congestive heart failure: insights from the randomized aldactone evaluation study (RALES). Rales Investigators. *Circulation* 2000;102:2700–2706.

20. Bristow MR, Saxon LA, Boehmer J, *et al.* Cardiac-resynchronization therapy with or without an implantable defibrillator in advanced chronic heart failure. *N Engl J Med* 2004;350:2140–2150.

21. Cleland JG, Daubert JC, Erdmann E, *et al.* The effect of cardiac resynchronization on morbidity and mortality in heart failure. *N Engl J Med* 2005;352:1539–1549.

22. Cohn JN. Remodeling as an end-point in heart failure therapy. *Cardiovasc Drugs Ther* 2004;18:7–8.

23. Konstam MA, Udelson JE, Anand IS, Cohn JN. Ventricular remodeling in heart failure: a credible surrogate endpoint. *J Card Fail* 2003;9:350–353.

24. Adams KF, Jr., Fonarow GC, Emerman CL, *et al.* Characteristics and outcomes of patients hospitalized for heart failure in the United States: rationale, design, and preliminary observations from the first 100,000 cases in the Acute Decompensated Heart Failure National Registry (ADHERE). *Am Heart J* 2005;149:209–216.

25. Fonarow GC, Abraham WT, Albert NM, *et al.* Organized Program to Initiate Lifesaving Treatment in Hospitalized Patients with Heart Failure (OPTIMIZE-HF): rationale and design. *Am Heart J* 2004;148:43–51.

26. Cleland JG, Swedberg K, Cohen-Solal A, *et al.* The Euro Heart Failure Survey of the EUROHEART survey programme. A survey on the quality of care among patients with heart failure in Europe. The Study Group on Diagnosis of the Working Group on Heart Failure of the European Society of Cardiology. The Medicines Evaluation Group Centre for Health Economics University of York. *Eur J Heart Fail* 2000;2:123–132.

27. Nieminen MS, Brutsaert D, Dickstein K, *et al.* Euro Heart Failure Survey II (EHFS II): A survey on hospitalized acute heart failure patients. Description of population. *Eur Heart J* 2006;27:2725–2736.

28. Fonarow GC, Yancy CW, Albert NM, *et al.* Improving the use of evidence-based heart failure therapies in the outpatient setting: the IMPROVE HF performance improvement registry. *Am Heart J* 2007;154:12–38.

29. Fonarow GC, Yancy CW, Albert NM, *et al.* Heart failure care in the outpatient cardiology practice setting: findings from IMPROVE-HF. *Circ Heart Fail* 2008;1:98–106.

30. Fonarow GC. Overview of Acutely Decompensated Congestive Heart Failure (ADHF): A Report from the ADHERE Registry. *Heart Fail Rev* 2004;9:179–185.

31. Abraham WT, Adams KF, Fonarow GC, *et al.* In-hospital mortality in patients with acute decompensated heart failure requiring intravenous vasoactive medications: an analysis from the Acute Decompensated Heart Failure National Registry (ADHERE). *J Am Coll Cardiol* 2005;46:57–64.

32. ADHERE Q3 2004 National Benchmark Report, 2005. www.adhereregistry.com

33. Gheorghiade M, Zannad F, Sopko G, *et al.* Acute heart failure syndromes: current state and framework for future research. *Circulation* 2005;112:3958–3968.

34. Yancy CW, Stough WG, Abraham WT, *et al.* Defining the natural history and improving quality of care for African Americans hospitalized with heart failure: A report from OPTIMIZE-HF [abstract]. *J Card Fail* 2005;11:S190.

35. Cleland JG, Swedberg K, Follath F, *et al.* The EuroHeart Failure survey programme– a survey on the quality of care among patients with heart failure in Europe. Part 1: patient characteristics and diagnosis. *Eur Heart J* 2003;24:442–463.

36. Komajda M, Follath F, Swedberg K, *et al.* The EuroHeart Failure Survey programme–a survey on the quality of care among patients with heart failure in Europe. Part 2: treatment. *Eur Heart J* 2003;24:464–474.

37. Rudiger A, Harjola VP, Muller A, *et al.* Acute heart failure: clinical presentation, one-year mortality and prognostic factors. *Eur J Heart Fail* 2005;7:662–670.

38. Curtis LH, Greiner MA, Hammill BG, *et al.* Early and Long-term Outcomes of Heart Failure in Elderly Persons, 2001–2005. *Arch Intern Med* 2008;168:2481–2488.

39. Fonarow GC, Adams KF, Jr., Abraham WT, Yancy CW, Boscardin WJ. Risk stratification for in-hospital mortality in acutely decompensated heart failure: classification and regression tree analysis. *JAMA* 2005;293:572–580.

40. O'Connor CM, Abraham WT, Albert NM, *et al.* Predictors of mortality after discharge in patients hospitalized with heart failure: an analysis from the Organized Program to Initiate Lifesaving Treatment in Hospitalized Patients with Heart Failure (OPTIMIZE-HF). *Am Heart J* 2008;156:662–673.

41. Abraham WT, Fonarow GC, Albert NM, *et al.* Predictors of in-hospital mortality in patients hospitalized for heart failure: insights from the Organized Program to Initiate Lifesaving Treatment in Hospitalized Patients with Heart Failure (OPTIMIZE-HF). *J Am Coll Cardiol* 2008;52:347–356.

42. Poole JE, Johnson GW, Hellkamp AS, *et al.* Prognostic importance of defibrillator shocks in patients with heart failure. *N Engl J Med* 2008;359:1009–1017.

43. Adams KF, Lindenfeld J, Arnold J, *et al.* Executive summary: HFSA 2006 Comprehensive Heart Failure Practice Guideline. *J Card Fail* 2006;12:10–38.

44. Hunt SA, Abraham WT, Chin MH, *et al.* ACC/AHA 2005 Guideline Update for the Diagnosis and Management of Chronic Heart Failure in the Adult: a report of the American College of Cardiology/American Heart Association Task Force on Practice Guidelines (Writing Committee to Update the 2001 Guidelines for the Evaluation and Management of Heart Failure): developed in collaboration with the American College

of Chest Physicians and the International Society for Heart and Lung Transplantation: endorsed by the Heart Rhythm Society. *Circulation* 2005;112:e154–e235.

45. The CONSENSUS Trial Study Group. Effects of enalapril on mortality in severe congestive heart failure. Results of the Cooperative North Scandinavian Enalapril Survival Study (CONSENSUS). *N Engl J Med* 1987;316:1429–1435.

46. The SOLVD Investigators. Effect of enalapril on survival in patients with reduced left ventricular ejection fractions and congestive heart failure. *N Engl J Med* 1991;325:293–302.

47. The SOLVD Investigators. Effect of enalapril on mortality and the development of heart failure in asymptomatic patients with reduced left ventricular ejection fractions. *N Engl J Med* 1992;327:685–691.

48. Granger CB, Ertl G, Kuch J, *et al.* Randomized trial of candesartan cilexetil in the treatment of patients with congestive heart failure and a history of intolerance to angiotensin-converting enzyme inhibitors. *Am Heart J* 2000;139:609–617.

49. Cohn JN, Tognoni G, Valsartan Heart Failure Trial Investigators. A randomized trial of the angiotensin-receptor blocker valsartan in chronic heart failure. *N Engl J Med* 2001; 345:1667–1675.

50. McMurray JJ, Ostergren J, Swedberg K, *et al.* Effects of candesartan in patients with chronic heart failure and reduced left-ventricular systolic function taking angiotensin-converting-enzyme inhibitors: the CHARM-Added trial. *Lancet* 2003;362:767–771.

51. Pfeffer MA, McMurray JJ, Velazquez EJ, *et al.* Valsartan, captopril, or both in myocardial infarction complicated by heart failure, left ventricular dysfunction, or both. *N Engl J Med* 2003;349:1893–1906.

52. Massie BM, Carson PE, McMurray JJ, *et al.* Irbesartan in patients with heart failure and preserved ejection fraction. *N Engl J Med* 2008;359:2456–2467.

53. CIBIS II Investigators. The Cardiac Insufficiency Bisoprolol Study II (CIBIS-II): a randomised trial. *Lancet* 1999;353:9–13.

54. MERIT-HF Investigators. Effect of metoprolol CR/XL in chronic heart failure: Metoprolol CR/XL Randomised Intervention Trial in Congestive Heart Failure (MERIT-HF). *Lancet* 1999;353:2001–2007.

55. Packer M, Coats AJ, Fowler MB, *et al.* Effect of carvedilol on survival in severe chronic heart failure. *N Engl J Med* 2001;344:1651–1658.

56. Flather MD, Shibata MC, Coats AJ, *et al.*; SENIORS Investigators. Randomized trial to determine the effect of nebivolol on mortality and cardiovascular hospital admission in elderly patients with heart failure (SENIORS). *Eur Heart J* 2005;26:215–225.

57. Pitt B, Zannad F, Remme WJ, *et al.* The effect of spironolactone on morbidity and mortality in patients with severe heart failure. Randomized Aldactone Evaluation Study Investigators. *N Engl J Med* 1999;341:709–717.

58. Juurlink DN, Mamdani MM, Lee DS, *et al.* Rates of hyperkalemia after publication of the Randomized Aldactone Evaluation Study. *N Engl J Med* 2004;351:543–551.

59. Svensson M, Gustafsson F, Galatius S, Hildebrandt PR, Atar D. How prevalent is hyperkalemia and renal dysfunction during treatment with spironolactone in patients with congestive heart failure? *J Card Fail* 2004;10:297–303.

60. Pitt B, Remme W, Zannad F, *et al.* Eplerenone, a selective aldosterone blocker, in patients with left ventricular dysfunction after myocardial infarction. *N Engl J Med* 2003;348: 1309–1321.

61. Zannad F, McMurray JJ, Krum H, *et al.*; EMPHASIS-HF Study Group. Eplerenone in patients with systolic heart failure and mild symptoms. *N Engl J Med* 2011;364:11–21.

62. Biollaz J, Brunner HR, Gavras I, Waeber B, Gavras H. Antihypertensive therapy with MK 421: angiotensin II–renin relationships to evaluate efficacy of converting enzyme blockade. *J Cardiovasc Pharmacol* 1982;4:966–972.

63. Staessen J, Lijnen P, Fagard R, Verschueren LJ, Amery A. Rise in plasma concentration of aldosterone during long-term angiotensin II suppression. *J Endocrinol* 1981;91: 457–465.

64. Taylor AL, Ziesche S, Yancy C, *et al*. Combination of isosorbide dinitrate and hydralazine in blacks with heart failure. *N Engl J Med* 2004;351:2049–2057.

65. Bardy GH, Lee KL, Mark DB *et al*. Amiodarone or an implantable cardioverter-defibrillator for congestive heart failure. *N Engl J Med* 2005;352:225–237.

66. Moss AJ, Zareba W, Hall WJ, *et al*. Prophylactic implantation of a defibrillator in patients with myocardial infarction and reduced ejection fraction. *N Engl J Med* 2002;346: 877–883.

67. Abraham WT, Fisher WG, Smith AL, *et al*. Cardiac resynchronization in chronic heart failure. *N Engl J Med* 2002;346:1845–1853.

68. Mark DB, Anstrom KJ, Sun JL, *et al*. Quality of life with defibrillator therapy or amiodarone in heart failure. *N Engl J Med* 2008;359:999–1008.

69. Hernandez AF, Fonarow GC, Liang L, *et al*. Sex and racial differences in the use of implantable cardioverter-defibrillators among patients hospitalized with heart failure. *JAMA* 2007;298:1525–1532.

70. Mehra MR, Yancy CW, Albert NM, *et al*. Evidence of clinical practice heterogeneity in the use of implantable cardioverter-defibrillators in heart failure and post-myocardial infarction left ventricular dysfunction: Findings from IMPROVE HF. *Heart Rhythm* 2009;6:1727–1734.

71. Shah B, Hernandez AF, Liang L, *et al*. Hospital variation and characteristics of implantable cardioverter-defibrillator use in patients with heart failure: data from the GWTG-HF (Get With The Guidelines-Heart Failure) registry. *J Am Coll Cardiol* 2009;53: 416–422.

72. Moss AJ, Hall WJ, Cannom DS, *et al*. Cardiac-resynchronization therapy for the prevention of heart-failure events. *N Engl J Med* 2009;361:1329–1338.

73. Deng MC, Edwards LB, Hertz MI, *et al*. Mechanical circulatory support device database of the International Society for Heart and Lung Transplantation: third annual report–2005. *J Heart Lung Transplant* 2005;24:1182–1187.

74. Rose EA, Gelijns AC, Moskowitz AJ, *et al*. Long-term mechanical left ventricular assistance for end-stage heart failure. *N Engl J Med* 2001;345:1435–1443.

75. Long JW, Kfoury AG, Slaughter MS, *et al*. Long-term destination therapy with the HeartMate XVE left ventricular assist device: improved outcomes since the REMATCH study. *Congest Heart Fail* 2005;11:133–138.

76. Costanzo MR, Guglin ME, Saltzberg MT, *et al*. Ultrafiltration versus intravenous diuretics for patients hospitalized for acute decompensated heart failure. *J Am Coll Cardiol* 2007;49:675–683.

77. Gheorghiade M, Sopko G, De LL, *et al*. Navigating the crossroads of coronary artery disease and heart failure. *Circulation* 2006;114:1202–1213.

78. Velazquez EJ, Lee KL, O'Connor CM, *et al*. The rationale and design of the Surgical Treatment for Ischemic Heart Failure (STICH) trial. *J Thorac Cardiovasc Surg* 2007;134: 1540–1547.

79. Jones RH, Velazquez EJ, Michler RE, *et al*. Coronary bypass surgery with or without surgical ventricular reconstruction. *N Engl J Med* 2009;360:1705–1717.

80. Velazquez EJ, Lee KL, Deja MA, *et al*. Coronary-artery bypass surgery in patients with left ventricular dysfunction. *N Engl J Med* 2011;364:1607–1616.

81. Bonow RO, Maurer G, Lee KL, *et al.*; STICH Trial Investigators. Myocardial viability and survival in ischemic left ventricular dysfunction. *N Engl J Med* 2011;364: 1617–1625.

82. Eagle KA, Guyton RA, Davidoff R, *et al*. ACC/AHA 2004 guideline update for coronary artery bypass graft surgery: a report of the American College of Cardiology/American Heart Association Task Force on Practice Guidelines (Committee to Update the 1999 Guidelines for Coronary Artery Bypass Graft Surgery). *Circulation* 2004;110: e340–e437.

83. Gibbons RJ, Abrams J, Chatterjee K, *et al*. ACC/AHA 2002 guideline update for the management of patients with chronic stable angina–summary article: a report of the American College of Cardiology/American Heart Association Task Force on practice guidelines (Committee on the Management of Patients With Chronic Stable Angina). *J Am Coll Cardiol* 2003;41:159–168.

84. Taylor DO, Edwards LB, Aurora P, *et al*. Registry of the International Society for Heart and Lung Transplantation: twenty-fifth official adult heart transplant report–2008. *J Heart Lung Transplant* 2008;27:943–956.

85. Organ Procurement and Transplantation Network, 2008. http://www.optn.org/data/

86. Arnold JM, Liu P, Demers C, *et al*. Canadian Cardiovascular Society consensus conference recommendations on heart failure 2006: diagnosis and management. *Can J Cardiol* 2006;22:23–45.

87. Whellan DJ, O'Connor CM, Lee KL, *et al*. Heart failure and a controlled trial investigating outcomes of exercise training (HF-ACTION): design and rationale. *Am Heart J* 2007;153:201–211.

88. O'Connor CM, Whellan DJ, Lee KL, *et al*. Efficacy and safety of exercise training in patients with chronic heart failure: HF-ACTION randomized controlled trial. *JAMA* 2009;301:1439–1450.

89. Hasselblad V, Gattis SW, Shah MR, *et al*. Relation between dose of loop diuretics and outcomes in a heart failure population: results of the ESCAPE trial. *Eur J Heart Fail* 2007;9:1064–1069.

90. Peacock WF, Costanzo MR, De MT, *et al*. Impact of Intravenous Loop Diuretics on Outcomes of Patients Hospitalized with Acute Decompensated Heart Failure: Insights from the ADHERE Registry. *Cardiology* 2008;113:12–19.

91. Gheorghiade M, Gattis WA, O'Connor CM, *et al*. Effects of tolvaptan, a vasopressin antagonist, in patients hospitalized with worsening heart failure: a randomized controlled trial. *JAMA* 2004;291:1963–1971.

92. Goldsmith SR, Elkayam U, Haught WH, Barve A, He W. Efficacy and safety of the vasopressin V1A/V2-receptor antagonist conivaptan in acute decompensated heart failure: a dose-ranging pilot study. *J Card Fail* 2008;14:641–647.

93. Konstam MA, Gheorghiade M, Burnett JC, Jr., *et al*. Effects of oral tolvaptan in patients hospitalized for worsening heart failure: the EVEREST Outcome Trial. *JAMA* 2007; 297:1319–1331.

94. Gottlieb SS, Skettino SL, Wolff A, *et al*. Effects of BG9719 (CVT-124), an A1-adenosine receptor antagonist, and furosemide on glomerular filtration rate and natriuresis in patients with congestive heart failure. *J Am Coll Cardiol* 2000;35:56–59.

95. Gottlieb SS, Brater DC, Thomas I, *et al*. BG9719 (CVT-124), an A1 adenosine receptor antagonist, protects against the decline in renal function observed with diuretic therapy. *Circulation* 2002;105:1348–1353.

96. Greenberg B, Thomas I, Banish D, *et al*. Effects of multiple oral doses of an A1 adenosine antagonist, BG9928, in patients with heart failure: results of a placebo-controlled, dose-escalation study. *J Am Coll Cardiol* 2007;50:600–606.

97. VMAC Investigators. Intravenous nesiritide vs nitroglycerin for treatment of decompensated congestive heart failure: a randomized controlled trial. *JAMA* 2002;287: 1531–1540.

98. Sackner-Bernstein JD, Skopicki HA, Aaronson KD. Risk of worsening renal function with nesiritide in patients with acutely decompensated heart failure. *Circulation* 2005;111:1487–1491.
99. Sackner-Bernstein JD, Kowalski M, Fox M, Aaronson K. Short-term risk of death after treatment with nesiritide for decompensated heart failure: a pooled analysis of randomized controlled trials. *JAMA* 2005;293:1900–1905.
100. Mohammed SF, Korinek J, Chen HH, Burnett JC, Redfield MM. Nesiritide in acute decompensated heart failure: current status and future perspectives. *Rev Cardiovasc Med* 2008;9:151–158.
101. Luss H, Mitrovic V, Seferovic PM, *et al*. Renal effects of ularitide in patients with decompensated heart failure. *Am Heart J* 2008;155:1012–1018.
102. Pang PS, Tavares M, Collins SP, *et al*. Design and rationale of the URGENT Dyspnea study: an international, multicenter, prospective study. *Am J Ther* 2008;15:299–303.
103. Cuffe MS, Califf RM, Adams KF, Jr., *et al*. Short-term intravenous milrinone for acute exacerbation of chronic heart failure: a randomized controlled trial. *JAMA* 2002;287:1541–1547.
104. Benza RL, Tallaj JA, Felker GM, *et al*. The impact of arrhythmias in acute heart failure. *J Card Fail* 2004;10:279–284.
105. Felker GM, Benza RL, Chandler AB, *et al*. Heart failure etiology and response to milrinone in decompensated heart failure: results from the OPTIME-CHF study. *J Am Coll Cardiol* 2003;41:997–1003.
106. O'Connor CM, Gattis WA, Uretsky BF, *et al*. Continuous intravenous dobutamine is associated with an increased risk of death in patients with advanced heart failure: insights from the Flolan International Randomized Survival Trial (FIRST). *Am Heart J* 1999;138:78–86.
107. Elkayam U, Tasissa G, Binanay C, *et al*. Use and impact of inotropes and vasodilator therapy in hospitalized patients with severe heart failure. *Am Heart J* 2007;153:98–104.
108. Costanzo MR, Johannes RS, Pine M, *et al*. The safety of intravenous diuretics alone versus diuretics plus parenteral vasoactive therapies in hospitalized patients with acutely decompensated heart failure: a propensity score and instrumental variable analysis using the Acutely Decompensated Heart Failure National Registry (ADHERE) database. *Am Heart J* 2007;154:267–277.
109. Mebazaa A, Nieminen MS, Packer M, *et al*. Levosimendan vs dobutamine for patients with acute decompensated heart failure: the SURVIVE Randomized Trial. *JAMA* 2007;297:1883–1891.
110. Landoni G, Biondi-Zoccai G, Greco M, *et al*. Effects of levosimendan on mortality and hospitalization. A meta-analysis of randomized controlled studies. *Crit Care Med* 2012;40:634–646.
111. Gheorghiade M, Blair JE, Filippatos GS, *et al*. Hemodynamic, echocardiographic, and neurohormonal effects of istaroxime, a novel intravenous inotropic and lusitropic agent: a randomized controlled trial in patients hospitalized with heart failure. *J Am Coll Cardiol* 2008;51:2276–2285.

CHAPTER 6

Atrial fibrillation

Chee W. Khoo and Gregory Y.H. Lip
University of Birmingham Centre for Cardiovascular Sciences, City Hospital, Birmingham, UK

Introduction

Atrial fibrillation (AF) is the most common sustained cardiac rhythm disorder encountered in clinical practice. AF is characterized by uncoordinated atrial activation which subsequently gives rise to atrial contraction failure. The ventricle rate is fast and irregular due to the chaotic atrial activation.

With an aging population, AF has become a major condition that requires extra resources for its management as well as the complications associated with it. AF is often associated with an increase in mortality and morbidity from thromboembolic events, including stroke, heart failure, and impaired quality of life. Only a third of patients with AF present to hospital [1]. Indeed, many patients with AF are asymptomatic and are not hospitalized until they develop complications. Hence, much of the management of AF is community based.

This chapter concentrates on clinical practice related to AF management. There are extensive reviews on the electrophysiology and pathophysiology of AF, which are beyond the scope of this chapter. As shown in Figure 6.1, many of the pathophysiological abnormalities of AF can be related to the symptoms associated with this arrhythmia.

Epidemiology

The prevalence and incidence of AF increase with advancing age. Much of the information on the epidemiology of AF comes from observation of predominantly white populations. The overall prevalence of AF was 6% in the Framingham and Rotterdam studies [2,3]. The Framingham study found a 1 in 4 lifetime risk of developing AF, for both men and women aged 40 and older [2]. Similar estimates have also been reported from the Rotterdam study [3]. The increase in the aging population in developed countries has led to a rise in the prevalence of AF. Another population study [4] reported a 13% rise in AF by 13% over the past two decades and estimated that 15.9 million people

Cardiovascular Clinical Trials: Putting the Evidence into Practice, First Edition.
Edited by Marcus D. Flather, Deepak L. Bhatt, and Tobias Geisler.
© 2013 Blackwell Publishing Ltd. Published 2013 by Blackwell Publishing Ltd.

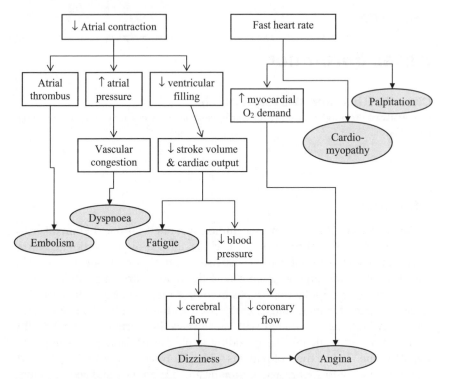

Figure 6.1 Pathophysiology and clinical symptoms in atrial fibrillation.

in the US will have AF by 2050. In another population-based study in West Scotland, the Renfrew-Paisley study [5], the prevalence of AF amongst patients aged 45–64 years was 6.5%. The prevalence increased with age and was higher in males. The incidence of AF was 0.54 cases per 1000 person years. The largest screening study for AF is the Screening for Atrial Fibrillation in the Elderly (SAFE) study [6] which showed a baseline prevalence of 7%, increasing to 10% for patients aged 75 years and older. This study also showed that an opportunistic screening strategy was more cost-effective than a systematic screening strategy.

AF often occurs in association with other cardiovascular diseases or risk factors (Table 6.1). Patients with hypertension and diabetes have shown an increased risk of developing AF [7,8]. Other known risk factors include coronary artery disease, valvular heart disease, hyperthyroidism, and high alcohol intake. There is also a strong family history associated with AF, with a risk as high as 30% [9].

Some patients do not have any obvious etiological factor predisposing to AF. In young subjects, usually aged younger than 65 years, a diagnosis of "lone AF" is made. This is essentially a diagnosis of exclusion, and is only made if the subject has no history of cardiovascular disease or hypertension; no abnormal cardiac signs on physical examination; a normal check X-ray and

Table 6.1 Etiological risk factors for atrial fibrillation.

- Increasing age
- Hypertension
- Diabetes
- Congestive heart failure
- Valvular heart disease
- Cardiac surgery
- Hyperthyroidism
- High alcohol intake
- Lung diseases

Table 6.2 Temporal patterns of atrial fibrillation.

Type of pattern	Onset duration	Comment
New onset	Within 48 hours	Acute
Paroxysmal	<7 days	Acute, often self-limiting, can be recurrent episodes
Persistent	7 days or more	Recurrent episodes, need DC or drug cardioversion
Long-standing persistent	≥1 year when it is decided to adopt a rhythm control state	
Permanent	>1 year	Chronic, non-cardioverted with DC or drug

DC, direct current.

electrocardiogram (apart from AF, with no evidence of prior myocardial infarction [MI] or left ventricular hypertrophy [LVH]); and normal atria, valves, and left ventricular size (and function) on echocardiography. There are implications of labeling someone as "lone AF" as this group is often considered as being "at low risk", although recent data have been inconclusive.

Clinical classification

The clinical presentation of AF is generally classified according to the temporal pattern of presentation [10] (Tables 6.2 and 6.3). This type of classification is based on duration of onset of the rhythm disorder. The main purpose of this classification is to help guide the approach to management and treatment objectives (Table 6.3).

The overall non-surgical management strategies for AF are based on rhythm control, rate control, and antithrombotic therapy. Patients with AF have to be assessed thoroughly, and their management guided by symptoms, whether there is any hemodynamic compromise, and other associated co-morbidities [11].

• Clinical presentations
• Hemodynamics
• Degrees of congestive cardiac failure
• Rates of thromboembolic complications
• Modes of treatment

Table 6.3 Differences between subsets of atrial fibrillation.

Table 6.4 Treatment modalities for atrial fibrillation.

Treatment	Indications
Antiarrhythmic drug (AAD)	Cardioversion; maintenance of sinus rhythm
Direct current cardioversion (DCCV)	Cardioversion
Rate control drug (RCD)	Ventricular rate control
Non-pharmacological treatment: • Surgical ablation • Electrophysiology-guided treatment • Devices	See Table 6.14
Antithrombotic treatment (ATT)	Thromboprophylaxis
Treatment of heart failure	

Management

The treatment objectives in AF are mainly symptom relief, reduction of thromboembolic events, and avoidance of concomitant heart failure. Management of associated comorbidities is essential. There are numerous ways to achieve these objectives. Table 6.4 summarizes the main treatment modalities for AF. As discussed previously, the temporal pattern of AF can help guide the approach to management and treatment objectives. All patients with AF have to be assessed for thromboembolic risk and then appropriate antithrombotic treatment can be initiated.

The main objective in the management of paroxysmal AF is to reduce paroxysmal events and maintain sinus rhythm, hence antiarrhythmic drugs are used. Heart rate control is the main objective of management in patients with permanent AF, and thus, rate control drugs are used.

For patient with persistent AF, both a rhythm and a rate control strategy can be used as first-line management, and many patients will need both [12,13]. Table 6.5 summarizes the management of AF according to the temporal pattern of classification.

New-onset atrial fibrillation

The first presentation of AF is usually termed new-onset AF or acute AF. At least 25% of all admissions for AF are of recent onset [12,13]. The treatment

Table 6.5 Treatment of atrial fibrillation according to temporal classification.

Type of atrial fibrillation (AF)	Treatment option
Paroxysmal AF	No therapy, AAD for cardioversion DCCV ATT
Recurrent paroxysmal AF	No symptoms: RCD, ATT Symptoms: RCD, ATT, maintenance AAD, EP
Persistent AF	RCD, ATT, AAD cardioversion, DCCV
Recurrent persistent AF	No symptoms: RCD, ATT Symptoms: RCD, ATT, DCCV, maintenance AAD, EP
Permanent AF	RCD Long-term AAT EP
New onset	Refer to Figure 6.2

AAD, antiarrhythmic drug; ATT, antithrombotic therapy; DCCV, direct current cardioversion; EP, electrophysiology; RCD, rate control drugs.

Table 6.6 Principles of acute atrial fibrillation management.

- Control of rapid ventricular rate
- Treat concomitant heart failure
- Acute cardioversion to sinus rhythm
- Thromboembolic prevention
- Treat underlying/precipitating cause
- Prevention of relapse

options differ widely, depending upon the clinical and hemodynamic condition of the individual patient. The principles of acute AF management are listed in Table 6.6.

Recommendations from the UK National Institute for Health and Clinical Excellence (NICE) [10] for the management of acute onset AF state that:
- In AF patients with life threatening-hemodynamic instability, electrical cardioversion should be performed, irrespective of the duration of AF.
- In AF patients with non–life-threatening hemodynamic instability, electrical cardioversion should be performed. If there is delay in arranging electrical cardioversion, amiodarone can be used.
- In patients with known Wolff–Parkinson–White syndrome, flecainide may be used as alternative pharmacological cardioversion. Other atrioventricular nodal blocking agents, such as diltiazem, verapramil, and digoxin, should not be used.

• In patients with known permanent AF and hemodynamic instability that is mainly caused by poor ventricular rate control, a pharmacological rate control strategy should be used.

• If urgent rate control is indicated, intravenous beta-blockers or rate-limiting calcium-channel blockers should be employed. Amiodarone can be used if these two agents are contraindicated or ineffective.

Cardioversion

Patients who are hemodynamically compromised due to a rapid ventricular rate should be cardioverted. If life-threatening, emergency electrical cardioversion can be used with heparin as antithrombotic cover. Both electrical and pharmacological cardioversion can safely be performed in patients who do not have valvular heart disease and present with recent onset (<48 hours) of AF using heparin (unfractionated or low molecular weight) as antithrombotic cover.

In patients who have longer duration of AF (>48 hours), a formal anticoagulation with international normalized ratio (INR) of 2.0 or more is recommended for a minimum of 3 weeks before attempted cardioversion. Immediate cardioversion can be performed if a transesophageal echocardiogram can be arranged to rule out thrombus formation.

The success rate of pharmacological agents (class I and III) in cardioversion varies widely and is dependent on the duration of AF. For patients who have AF for longer periods of time, the success rate is only 15–30% [10]. If pharmacological cardioversion fails, electrical cardioversion can still be attempted. Trial evidence for urgent cardioversion in acute AF is sparse.

The systematic review as part of the NICE guidelines identified two studies [14,15] that showed no difference in the success rate of cardioversion between electrical and pharmacological cardioversion. Patients who failed pharmacological cardioversion as the initial treatment option and then went on to have electrical cardioversion were more likely to have successful cardioversion as compared to the reverse strategy (96% vs 84%, respectively) [14].

The NICE guidelines therefore recommend that in patients with AF without hemodynamic instability for whom cardioversion is indicated:

• The advantages and disadvantages of both pharmacological and electrical cardioversion should be discussed with patients before initiating treatment.

• Where AF onset was within 48 hours previously, either pharmacological or electrical cardioversion should be performed.

• For those with more prolonged AF (onset >48 hours previously), electrical cardioversion should be the preferred initial treatment option.

Note that pretreatment with class I and III drugs helps facilitate electrical cardioversion and prevent recurrent AF [16]. However, many of the trials were not performed in acute-onset AF.

Table 6.7 summarizes the common pharmacological agents used for cardioversion of AF.

Table 6.7 Common pharmacological agents cardioversion of atrial fibrillation.

Drug	Dose for cardioversion	Dose for maintenance	Comments
Flecainide	200 mg orally	50–150 mg b.i.d.	Not for patient with structural heart disease
Propafenone	600 mg orally; 1.5–2.0 mg/kg IV over 10–20 min	150–300 mg b.i.d.	As above
Amiodarone	6 mg/kg bolus over 30–60 min, then 1200 mg IV over 24 hours	600 mg daily for 1 week, then 400 mg daily for second week, followed by 200 mg o.d.	Good heart rate control Proven effectiveness Beware of hypotension Prolong QT interval and Torsades de pointes
Sotalol	5–10 mg slowly IV, may be repeated	120–160 mg b.i.d.	Conversion rate is slow Proarrhythmia risk is high.

IV, intravenously; b.i.d., twice daily; o.d., once daily.

Rate control

A patient who is hemodynamically stable, relatively asymptomatic or presents with longer duration of AF (>48 hours) should be treated with a rate control strategy with appropriate antithrombotic therapy. This strategy will allow sufficient time to determine the cause and precipitating factors for the rhythm disorder.

The pooled analysis from the Atrial Fibrillation Follow-up Investigation of Rhythm Management (AFFIRM) and Rate Control vs Electrical cardioversion (RACE) [17] suggested that the aim should be a resting heart rate of <100 beats/min. A well-controlled heart rate would relieve symptoms and improve the patient's hemodynamic status.

The rate-limiting calcium-channel blockers (verapamil and diltiazem) and beta-blockers are very effective in controlling heart rate during AF, and current management guidelines recommend these drug classes as first-line therapy for rate control. Both groups of drug have to be used with caution in patients with heart failure or hypotension.

Digoxin, which has a slow onset, is often used in patient with fast AF and acute heart failure due to its negative chronotropic and positive inotropic effects [18]. The combination of digoxin with rate-limiting calcium channel blockers and beta-blockers might be needed to control ventricular rate, but a combination of verapamil and beta-blockers should be avoided due to the risk of ventricular asystole.

Amiodarone is a safe alternative if other drugs are ineffective or contraindicated in controlling ventricular rate, especially in patient with severe heart failure or hypotension. Intravenous amiodarone should be given via a central venous line due to the risk of thrombophlebitis.

Trial evidence for urgent rate control in acute AF is sparse. The systematic review as part of the NICE guideline identified three studies [19–21]. One study [19] found that the use of rate-limiting agents such as beta-blockers, rate-limiting calcium-calcium blockers or digoxin to be an effective strategy in reducing ventricular rate in 75% of AF patients with a fast ventricular rate. Another study [22] with the rate-limiting calcium channel blocker diltiazem, showed similar results. For patients who were hemodynamically unstable, two studies [20,21] found the intravenous administration of amiodarone to be an effective strategy to control ventricular rate.

Table 6.8 summarizes the common drugs used for rate control in AF.

The management of patient with new-onset AF is summarized in Figure 6.2.

Table 6.8 Drugs for rate control in atrial fibrillation.

Drug	Dose for rate control	Dose for maintenance	Comments
Esmolol	0.5 mg/kg IV bolus	0.05–0.2 mg/kg/min IV	Hypotension, asthma/COPD
Propranolol	1 mg over 1 min, repeat if necessary to max of 10 mg	10–40 mg q.d.s.	Non-selective, asthma/COPD
Metoprolol	5 mg IV bolus, repeated twice at 2-min intervals	50–200 mg daily in divided dose	Useful in concomitant ischemic heart disease
Amiodarone	6 mg/kg bolus over 30–60 min, then 1200 mg IV over 24 hours	600 mg daily for 1 week, then 400 mg daily for second week, followed by 200 mg o.d.	Cardioversion may occur; proven effectiveness Beware of prolonged QT interval, Torsades de pointes
Diltiazem	120–360 mg orally, daily in divided dose	120–360 mg orally, daily in divided dose	Hypotension, promotes heart failure Improves rate control with digoxin
Verapamil	5–10 mg IV over 2 min	40–120 mg t.d.s.	Negative inotropic, not to be used with beta-blockers, increase digoxin level
Digoxin	0.25 mg IV over 2 hours, up to 1.5 mg	62.5–250 μg orally o.d.	Slow onset Beware of digitalis toxicity

COPD, chronic obstructive pulmonary disease; IV, intravenously; o.d., once daily; q.d.s., four times a day; t.d.s., three times a day.

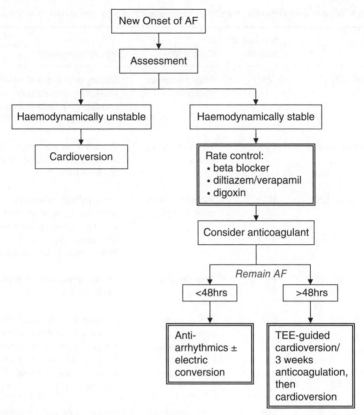

Figure 6.2 Management of new-onset atrial fibrillation (AF). TEE, transesophageal echocardiography.

Paroxysmal atrial fibrillation

Patients who have infrequent paroxysmal attacks or few symptoms, a "no drug treatment" strategy or "pill-in-the-pocket" strategy can be considered [10,23]. Patients best suited for this strategy are those without a history of left ventricular dysfunction or valvular or ischemic heart disease,; have a resting heart rate of greater than 70 beats/min and systolic blood pressure of greater than 100 mmHg; and are able to follow instruction and know when and how to take the medication when needed.

In one trial by Alboni *et al.* [23], the "pill-in-the-pocket" approach with class Ic agents (flecainide and propafenone) for the treatment of paroxysmal AF was studied in a highly selected population of 210 patients. The average number of admissions per month for emergency treatment was significantly lower with the "pill-in-the-pocket" strategy as compared with conventional treatment.

There is a large trial evidence-base for antiarrhythmic drug therapy in paroxysmal AF. The systematic review as part of the NICE guidelines

Table 6.9 Randomized controlled trials of propafenone compared with sotalol or amiodarone.

Study	Number of patients	Comparison	Results/comments
Lee *et al*. [24]	73	Propafenone vs sotalol	Equally effective and safe in preventing attacks and alleviating symptoms over a minimum of 3 months
Kochiadakis *et al*. [25]	–	Propafenone vs sotalol	Propafenone was more effective in maintaining sinus rhythm in the long term
Bellandi *et al*. [26]	300	Propafenone vs sotalol vs placebo	No significant difference between propafenone and sotalol; both drugs were superior to placebo. 63% vs 73% vs 35% remain in sinus rhythm
Reimold *et al*. [27]	100	Propafenone vs sotalol	Equally effective in maintaining sinus rhythm
Roy *et al*. [28]	403	Amiodarone vs sotalol or propafenone	Amiodarone was more effective than sotalol or propafenone in the prevention of AF recurrence. 65% vs 37% remain in sinus rhythm, mean follow-up of 16 months
Kochiadakis *et al*. [29]	146	Propafenone vs amiodarone	Recurrent AF at 24 months: 83% vs 40%

AF, atrial fibrillation.

identified nine studies comparing class I, II, and III agents. The results of these trials are summarized in Tables 6.9 [24–29] and 6.10 [30–32]. Class Ic, II, and III agents were effective in maintaining sinus rhythm. The class III agent, amiodarone, was more effective but had more side effects. The trials do not suggest a benefit for digoxin in reducing paroxysms of AF; in fact, a paradoxical worsening of paroxysmal AF may occur. The NICE guidelines [10] therefore recommend that the best drugs for the management of paroxysmal AF are class 1c (flecainide, propafenone) and beta-blockers.

For patients who have frequent symptomatic paroxysmal AF and in whom prophylaxis is needed, a beta-blocker should be the first-line therapy. In patients who do not respond to beta-blockers and have no structural heart disease, a class Ic agent or sotalol can be tried.

A new class III agent, dronedarone, has been useful as an antiarrhythmic in paroxysmal AF and for facilitating cardioversion in patients with persistent AF. In the ATHENA trial, dronedarone significantly reduced the risk of car-

Table 6.10 Randomized controlled trials of sotalol compared with amiodarone or beta-blockers.

Study	Number of patients	Comparison	Results/comments
Kochiadakis et al. [30]	186	Amiodarone vs sotalol vs placebo	Both amiodarone and sotalol were more effective than placebo in maintaining sinus rhythm Amiodarone was more effective than sotalol but caused more side effects
Kochiadakis et al. [31]	214	Amiodarone vs sotalol vs propafenone	Amiodarone and propafenone were superior to sotalol in maintaining long-term normal sinus rhythm in patients with atrial fibrillation Amiodarone was associated with more side effects, although it tended to be superior to propafenone
Steeds et al. [32]	41	Sotalol vs atenolol	No significant difference in the frequency of recurrence of AF

AF, atrial fibrillation.

diovascular hospitalizations in patients with associated risk factors [33]. However, this drug should not be used in patients with permanent AF or associated heart failure [34,35].

If this approach still fails to provide adequate reduction in symptoms and paroxysms, either amiodarone or referral for non-pharmacological intervention (see later) should be considered. Digoxin does not reduce paroxysmal events. Patients who are on long-term medications for paroxysmal AF should be kept under review to assess the need for continued treatment and the development of any side effects.

Persistent atrial fibrillation

Both rate-control and rhythm-control strategies can be used in patients with persistent AF. Clinical trials [36–40] comparing rhythm control and rate control for persistent AF have consistently shown there is no significant difference between the two strategies (Table 6.11).

The NICE guidelines [10] give recommendations for an initial rate/rhythm control strategy in persistent AF (Table 6.12). Since the publication of these guidelines, results from the AF-CHF trial have reported that rate control was not an inferior strategy to rhythm control in subjects with heart failure due to left ventricular systolic dysfunction [40].

For a patient who is successfully cardioverted under the rhythm control strategy, beta-blockers can be used to help maintain sinus rhythm. Where beta-blockers are ineffective, not tolerated or contraindicated, class Ic agents can be tried provided the patient has no structural heart disease. As discussed above, dronedarone is useful to facilitate cardioversion [41], although less

Table 6.11 Clinical trials comparing rate-control and rhythm-control strategies in persistent atrial fibrillation (AF).

Study	Number of patients	Comparison	Results/comments
Hohnloser et al. [36] (PIAF)	252	Rate control (diltiazem) vs rhythm control (amiodarone)	Over 1 year, both arms yielded similar result in symptomatic improvement. Exercise tolerance was better but hospital admission more frequent with the rhythm-control strategy
Van Gelder et al. [37] (RACE)	522	Rate limiting agents vs serial cardioversion and antiarrhythmic drugs; both groups received anticoagulant drugs	Mean follow-up of 2.3 years, rate control was not inferior to rhythm control for the prevention of death and morbidity from cardiovascular causes
Wyse et al. [38] (AFFIRM)	4060	Rate control vs rhythm control; anticoagulant was mandatory for rate control arm but not rhythm control	Mortality at 5 years: 21.3% vs 23.8%. Hospitalization and side effects rates were higher for the rhythm control group. Rhythm control offered no survival advantage over rate control
Carlsson et al. [39] (STAF)	200	Rate control (with anticoagulant) vs rhythm control	After a mean of 19.6 months, no difference in primary endpoint between rate control (10/100) and rhythm control (9/100)
Roy et al. [40] (AF-CHF)	1376	Rate control vs rhythm control in patients with AF and congestive heart failure	Mean follow-up of 37 months, primary and secondary outcomes were similar in the two groups; the composite of death from cardiovascular causes, stroke, or worsening heart failure was 43% vs 46%

Table 6.12 NICE recommendations for initial rate/rhythm control strategy in persistent atrial fibrillation (AF).

Rate control strategy	Rhythm control strategy
Age > 65	Younger patient
Contraindications to antiarrhythmic drugs	"Lone" AF
Coronary artery disease	Congestive heart failure
No congestive heart failure	AF secondary to treated/corrected precipitant
Unsuitable for cardioversion	

efficacious in maintaining sinus rhythm (but better tolerated) compared to amiodarone [42].

If dronedarone fails or the patient has structural heart disease, amiodarone is the next option. If the patient fails to remain in sinus rhythm despite antiarrhythmic drugs (or non-pharmacological measures, where relevant), then a rate control strategy should be adopted to prevent relapse.

Permanent atrial fibrillation

Patients who have AF for a long period of time, as well as those who have failed or are unsuitable for cardioversion, should be treated with a rate control strategy. A heart rate of 60–80 beats/min at rest and 90–115 beats/min at moderate exercise is generally considered adequate controlled [43]. In order to maintain an equivalent cardiac output, it has been suggested that AF patients should probably have a faster heart rate than patients in sinus rhythm [44].

There is a large trial evidence-base for drug therapy in permanent AF. The systematic review as part of the NICE guidelines [10] identified eight studies of beta-blockers, calcium channel blockers, and digoxin (Table 6.13) [45–52]. These showed that both calcium-channel blockers and beta-blockers were more effective as monotherapy than digoxin in controlling heart rate during exercise. However, there was no difference during normal daily activities.

Another systematic review of drugs for permanent AF by Segal *et al.* [53] identified 45 articles that evaluated 17 drugs. The conclusion was that calcium-channel blockers (verapamil or diltiazem) or select beta-blockers were more effective in controlling heart rate at rest and during exercise for patients with AF, without a clinically important decrease in exercise tolerance. Digoxin was useful when rate control during exercise was unimportant. The NICE guidelines [10] recommend that the best drugs for management of permanent AF are the beta-blockers and rate-limiting calcium-channel blockers. These are effective as monotherapy for rate control.

Some patients will need a combination of drugs to control ventricular rate. When monotherapy is inadequate, beta-blockers or rate-limiting calcium-channel blockers should be given in combination with digoxin to control heart rate only during normal activities. Rate-limiting calcium-channel blockers should be given with digoxin to control heart rate during both normal activities and exercise. Amiodarone or non-pharmacological methods can be used if further rate control is needed or with failure of the initial drugs.

Non-pharmacological treatments

Antiarrhythmic drugs have limited efficacy and proarrhythmic risks. This has prompted the exploration of alternative non-pharmacological therapies to treat AF. Most of the non-pharmacological approaches are directed at eliminating the triggers and modifying the electrophysiological substrate for the prevention and treatment of AF.

Table 6.13 Randomized controlled trials of ventricular rate control in permanent atrial fibrillation (AF).

Study	Number of patients	Comparison	Results/comments
Khand et al. [45]	47	First phase: carvedilol and digoxin vs digoxin Second phase: carvedilol vs digoxin	Combination of carvedilol and digoxin was superior to either carvedilol or digoxin alone in the management of AF in patients with heart failure
Farshi et al. [46]	12	Digoxin vs diltiazem vs atenolol vs digoxin + diltiazem vs digoxin + atenolol	Digoxin and diltiazem, as single agents, are least effective for controlling ventricular rate in atrial fibrillation during daily activity Digoxin + atenolol produced the most effective rate control
Wong et al. [47]	10	Four phases (placebo, digoxin, digoxin with half-dose labetalol, and full-dose labetalol)	No difference in average heart rate between digoxin and labetalol at rest During exercise, labetalol was more effective in controlling heart rate
Maragno et al. [48]	19	Diltiazem + digoxin vs digoxin alone	Diltiazem was more effective in controlling heart rate during exercise than digoxin
Lewis et al. [49]	10	Diltiazem vs Digoxin vs Combination treatment	Diltiazem resulted in lower heart rate during exercise compared with digoxin Combination treatment was more effective in controlling heart rate over 24 hours compared with monotherapy
Pomfret et al. [50]	8	Verapamil vs digoxin vs combination treatment	Verapamil alone and combination therapy were shown to give greater control of heart rate at work than digoxin alone
Roth et al. [51]	12	240 mg diltiazem vs 360 mg diltiazem vs digoxin vs combination therapies	240 mg diltiazem with digoxin was more effective than monotherapy in controlling heart rate at rest and during exercise
Lang et al. [52]	52	Different phases: no therapy; digoxin 0.25 mg and 0.5 mg daily; digoxin 0.25 mg and verapamil; and verapamil alone	Heart rate at rest and during all levels of exercise was better controlled with combination therapy or with verapamil alone

Table 6.14 summarizes the indications for and adverse effects of non-pharmacological treatments for AF.

There is increasing trial evidence for the role of catheter ablation in AF (Table 6.15). These studies [54–56] show that the success rate of catheter ablation is clearly dependent upon the duration of AF. Patients with paroxysmal AF are more likely to remain in sinus rhythm after catheter ablation as compared to persistent or permanent AF patients.

Table 6.14 Non-pharmacological (but non-surgical) treatments for atrial fibrillation (AF).

	Current indications	Adverse effects
Device therapies:		
Atrial pacing	Patients with conventional indications for a pacemaker	
Defibrillator	Patients with conventional indications for an implantable cardioverter defibrillator	Shock discomfort Early reinitiation of AF
AV nodal ablation and permanent pacing	Symptomatic patients refractory to other rate-control and rhythm-control treatments Patients who already have an implanted pacemaker or defibrillator	Pacemaker dependence Sudden death early after ablation (<0.1%)
Catheter ablation	Symptomatic patients refractory to AADs Young patients with lone AF Patients unable or unwilling to take long-term AADs	Vascular access complications (1%) Stroke and transient ischemic attack (1%) Pronounced pulmonary vein stenosis (<1%) Proarrhythmia (10–20%) Rare: valvular, phrenic nerve and esophagus injury

AADs, antiarrhythmic drugs; AV, atrioventricular.

Table 6.15 Studies on catheter ablation in atrial fibrillation (AF).

Study	Number of patients	Results/outcomes
Pappone et al. [54]	179 paroxysmal AF 72 permanent AF	At mean follow-up of 10 months, 85% of paroxysmal AF patients and 68% of permanent AF patients remained AF-free
Vasamreddy et al. [55]	21 paroxysmal AF 22 persistent AF 27 permanent AF	At mean follow-up of 6 months, 76% (53 patients) were AF-free, including 14 patients taking antiarrhythmic drugs
Oral et al. [56]	58 paroxysmal AF 12 persistent AF	At 5 month follow-up, 70% of paroxysmal and 22% of persistent AF patients were free from recurrence AF

Thromboembolism prevention

AF is associated with increased risk of thromboembolic events. The risk of stroke or thromboembolism is four- to five-fold across all age groups, and is similar in patients with either paroxysmal or permanent AF [57]. Antithrombotic therapy becomes an essential part of AF management. Individual patients should be assessed for thromboembolic risk, contraindications, and comorbidities prior to commencing antithrombotic therapy.

There are numerous randomized controlled clinical trials of thromboprophylaxis in AF patients, some of which are summarized below.

Warfarin versus placebo

Table 6.16 summarizes the clinical trials comparing warfarin with either a control or placebo. The results of these trials and the meta-analysis of adjusted-dose warfarin [58–65] in AF patients when compared with placebo showed a two-thirds reduction in the relative risk of ischemic stroke or systemic embolism.

Aspirin versus placebo

Table 6.17 summarizes the clinical trials comparing antiplatelet therapy either with placebo or a control. These studies had marked differences in the dosage of aspirin (50–1200 mg/day) and follow-up period (1.2–4.0 years). The relative risk reductions were similar in all trials with the exception of the SPAF-1 trial [54], which showed a relative risk reduction of 42% versus placebo/control The SPAF-1 trial was the only trial that showed a significant benefit of aspirin for stroke prevention in patients with AF, but there were internal inconsistencies within the trial for the aspirin effect, which was less apparent in the elderly and also, aspirin did not prevent severe strokes [70].

A recent meta-analysis [58] showed that antiplatelet drugs, when compared with controls, reduced stroke risk by 22%. When the meta-analysis was confined to aspirin-only trials compared with placebo or no treatment, aspirin was associated with a non-significant reduction in the incidence of stroke of 19%, with no impact on mortality. The evidence for aspirin for stroke prevention in AF is rather weak, and increasing data show that the risk of major bleeding (including intracranial hemorrhage) with aspirin is not significantly different from warfarin, especially in the elderly [71].

Warfarin versus antiplatelet therapy

A meta-analysis of large randomized trials [58] involving 12 963 participants in 12 trials demonstrated a 64% reduction in stroke risk with adjusted-dose warfarin as compared to a 22% reduction risk with aspirin. The Clopidogrel plus aspirin versus oral anticoagulation for atrial fibrillation in the Atrial fibrillation Clopidogrel Trial with Irbesartan for prevention of Vascular Events (ACTIVE-W) [72], the largest of these trials, showed that the combined use of aspirin and clopidogrel did not offer protection against stroke above that from

Table 6.16 Trials comparing warfarin with placebo/control for stroke prevention in atrial fibrillation.

Study	Number of patients (warfarin)	Target INR	Comparison	Thromboembolic events/patients RRR (%) Comments
AFASAK [60]	671 (335)	2.8–4.2	Warfarin (335) vs placebo (336)	5/335 vs 21/336 54
BAATAF [61]	420 (212)	1.5–2.7	Warfarin (212) vs placebo (208)	3/212 vs 13/208 78
CAFA [62]	378 (187)	2.0–3.0	Warfarin (187) vs placebo (191)	6/187 vs 9/191 33
EAFT [63] (secondary prevention study)	439 (225)	2.5–4.0	Warfarin (225) vs placebo (214)	20/225 vs 50/214; 68; mean follow up of 2.3 years, annual rate of outcome event was 8% vs 17%
SPAF-I [64]	421 (210)	2.0–4.5	Warfarin (210) vs placebo (211)	8/210 vs 19/211 60
SPINAF [65]	571 (281)	1.4–2.8	Warfarin (281) vs placebo (290)	7/281 vs 23/290 70 Over a mean follow-up of 1.8 years, the annual event rate among of patients aged over 70 years of age was 4.8% in the placebo group and 0.9% in the warfarin group (risk reduction, 0.79)

AFASAK, Atrial Fibrillation, Aspirin, Anticoagulation trial; BAATAF, Boston Area Anticoagulation Trial for Atrial Fibrillation; CAFA, Canadian Atrial Fibrillation Anticoagulation trial; EAFT, European Atrial Fibrillation Trial; INR, international normalized ratio; RRR, relative risk reduction; SPAF, Stroke Prevention in Atrial Fibrillation trial; SPINAF, Stroke Prevention in Non-rheumatic Atrial Fibrillation trial.

aspirin alone, and the combination therapy was inferior to adjusted-dose warfarin. The trial was stopped early because of the clear evidence of superiority of adjusted-dose warfarin.

The Birmingham Atrial Fibrillation Treatment of the Aged (BAFTA) study [73] was conducted in 973 patients with AF aged 75 years or older in the primary care setting. It was a randomized trial comparing warfarin (INR 2–3) and aspirin (75 mg/day), with an average follow-up of 2.7 years. The result showed that warfarin was significantly more effective than aspirin in preventing stroke (by >50%, with a nearly 2% annual absolute risk reduction), without any excess in the risk of major bleeding.

Table 6.17 Trials comparing aspirin with placebo/control for stroke prevention in atrial fibrillation.

Study	Number of patients (aspirin)	Doses	Comparison	Thromboembolic event/patients RRR (%) Comments
AFASAK [60]	672 (336)	75 mg/day	Aspirin vs placebo	16/336 vs 19/336 17
EAFT [63]	782 (404)	300 mg/day	Aspirin vs placebo	88/404 vs 90/378 11
ESPS II [66]	211 (104)	50 mg/day	Aspirin vs placebo	17/104 vs 23/107 At mean follow-up of 2 years, stroke risk was reduced by 18% with aspirin when compared with placebo
SPAF-I [64]	1120 (552)	325 mg/day	Aspirin vs placebo	25/552 vs 44/568; 44
UK-TIA [67]	28 (13) 36 (21)	300 mg/day 1200 mg/day	Aspirin vs placebo	3/13 vs 4/15 17 5/21 vs 4/15 14 Aspirin reduces stroke risk by about 20%
JAST [68]	871 (426)	150 mg/day	Aspirin vs no treatment	20/426 vs 19/445 −10
LASAF [69]	195 (104) 181 (90)	125 mg/day 125 mg/alt day	Aspirin vs no treatment	4/104 vs 3/91 −17 1/90 vs 3/91 67

AFASAK, Atrial Fibrillation, Aspirin, Anticoagulation trial; EAFT, European Atrial Fibrillation Trial; ESPS, European Stroke Prevention Study; JAST, Japan Atrial Fibrillation Stroke Trial; LASAF, Low-dose Aspirin, Stroke, Atrial Fibrillation; RRR, relative risk reduction; SPAF, Stroke Prevention in Atrial Fibrillation trial; UK-TIA, United Kingdom Transient Ischaemic Attack.

Combined warfarin and antiplatelet therapy

A meta-analysis by Dentali *et al.* [74] compared oral anticoagulation with combined aspirin–oral anticoagulation in 10 randomized controlled trials of patients with different indications for anticoagulation therapy. The benefits of combined therapy were confined to patients with mechanical heart valves. There was no significant difference in the risk of arterial thromboembolism in patients with AF. The risk of bleeding was increased with combined therapy.

Other trials [75–77] have investigated the effectiveness of oral anticoagulant in combination with antiplatelet therapy for the prevention of stroke in AF patients. Combined therapy did not show a beneficial effect when compared with anticoagulant therapy alone.

Combined aspirin and clopidogrel therapy versus placebo

The benefit of dual antiplatelet therapy (aspirin and clopidogrel) in AF patients at increased risk for stroke who are unsuitable for oral anticoagulation therapy were evaluated in a study arm of the Atrial fibrillation Clopidogrel Trial with Irbesartan for prevention of Vascular Events (ACTIVE) – ACTIVE-A [78]. Patients unsuitable for warfarin (i.e., poor INR control, increased bleeding risk, drug interactions, or patient preference) were randomized to aspirin with placebo versus aspirin with clopidogrel. The primary outcome was a composite of major vascular events, including stroke, myocardial ischemia, non-central nervous system (CNS) systemic embolism, or cardiovascular death. A total of 7554 patients were enrolled from 580 centers in 33 countries, with a median follow-up of 3.6 years. Patients randomized to dual antiplatelet therapy showed a significant reduction in the primary endpoint (6.6 vs 7.6, relative risk reduction 11%; $p < 0.01$), which was substantially due to the relative risk reduction of stroke (28%; $p < 0.001$). However, the additional prevention of thrombotic events was at the expense of significantly higher rates of major bleedings (2.0 vs 1.3; $p < 0.001$).

Antithrombotic treatment with direct thrombin inhibitors

The direct thrombin inhibitors (DTIs) allow thrombin activity to be blocked as well as preventing fibrin formation from fibrinogen. This inhibits both free and fibrin-bound thrombin.

In the Randomized Evaluation of Long-Term Anticoagulant Therapy (RE-LY) study, the reversible oral DTI dabigatran etexilate, a prodrug of dabigatran, was compared to warfarin in AF patients [79]. The trial randomized 18 113 patients with AF (mean age 71 years) and at least one additional risk factor for stroke to blinded treatment with dabigatran at either 110 mg or 150 mg b.i.d. or unblinded prophylaxis with warfarin adjusted to an INR of 2.0–3.0. Over a median 2-year follow-up, the annualized rates of the primary endpoint of stroke and systemic embolism were 1.53% for the low-dose dabigatran group, 1.11% for the high-dose group, and 1.69% for the warfarin group. The relative risks versus warfarin were 0.91 (95% CI, 0.74–1.11) for the low-dose group ($p < 0.001$ for non-inferiority) and 0.66 (95% CI, 0.53–0.82) for the high-dose group ($p < 0.001$ for superiority). The rate of major bleeding was 3.36% per year in the warfarin group, as compared with 2.71% per year in the low-dose dabigatran group (RR with dabigatran, 0.80; 95% CI, 0.69–0.93; $p = 0.003$) and 3.11% per year in the high-dose group (RR 0.93; 95% CI, 0.81–1.07; $p = 0.31$). The main side effect of dabigatran is severe dyspepsia and this was a major reason for the increased premature break off of study drug treatment with dabigatran in this trial. In summary, the results showed the superiority of higher doses of dabigatran to warfarin, with a comparable bleeding risk to warfarin, and the non-inferiority of lower doses of dabigatran compared to warfarin, but with lower bleeding rates. Impressive phase 3 clinical trial data are also available for the oral factor Xa inhibitors, rivaroxaban and apixaban. Rivaroxaban was compared to warfarin in the ROCKET-AF trial [80], which showed that it was non-inferior to warfarin for the primary endpoint of stroke and systemic embolism, with a similar rate of major bleeding. As with the other new oral anticoagulants, rivaroxaban was associated with significantly less hemorrhagic stroke and intracranial hemorrhage.

Apixaban was compared to warfarin in the ARISTOTLE trial [81], which showed that it was superior to warfarin by 21% in reducing the primary endpoint of stroke and systemic embolism, largely by reducing hemorrhagic stroke; there was no significant difference in ischemic stroke with apixaban compared to warfarin. Apixaban was also compared to aspirin in patients who had refused or failed warfarin therapy in the AVERROES trial. Apixaban was superior to aspirin in reducing the primary endpoint of stroke and systemic embolism, with a similar rate of major bleeding (and intracranial hemorrhage) and better tolerability [82].

Triple antithrombotic therapy

AF patients need antithrombotic therapy for thromboembolic prevention. Patients with coronary artery disease (CAD) need antiplatelet therapy. About 20–30% of the AF population has coexisting CAD [83]. The management of these patients who present with an acute coronary syndrome (ACS) remains a complex issue. A recent consensus document from the European Society of Cardiology Working Group on Thrombosis provided detailed guidance on antithrombotic therapy following coronary artery stenting in this subgroup of AF patients [84].

Stroke risk stratification

From the above meta-analysis and clinical trials, oral anticoagulation (warfarin) has been proven to reduce stroke risk. The relative risk reduction with warfarin in preventing stroke is about 60% as compared to 20% with aspirin. However, not all AF patients are suitable for oral anticoagulation. Individual patients have to be assessed accordingly and their thromboembolic risk reviewed on a regular basis.

Appropriate risk stratification and choice of thromboprophylaxis in AF is not an easy task. The risk of stroke is not homogeneous amongst all AF patients and treatment has to balance stroke risk, contraindications, and comorbidities. In a recent meta-analysis [85], only prior stroke or transient ischemic attack, older age, hypertension, and diabetes were identified as consistent independent risk factors for stroke and thromboembolism.

Another systematic review [86] identified 12 different published schemes to aid assessment of thromboembolic risk, and concluded that there are substantial differences among the schemes designed to stratify stroke risk in patients with AF. Using the difference schemes on same cohort of patients would yield different results. The proportion classified as "high risk" would vary from 11% to 77% and proportion classified as "low risk" from 9% to 49% depending on which stroke risk stratification scheme was used. Table 6.18

Table 6.18 Main stroke risk stratification schemes.

Scheme	Risk strata		
	Low	Intermediate	High
AFI [87]	Age <65 years; no high risk factors	Age >65 years; no other risk factors	Previous stroke/TIA; history of hypertension, CAD or diabetes
SPAF [64]	No high-risk factors	History of hypertension or diabetes	Women aged >75 years; systolic blood pressure >160 mmHg; LV dysfunction (echocardiography or clinical)
CHADS$_2$ [88]	Score 0	Score 1–2	Score 3–6
Framingham [89]	Point scoring system based on age, sex, raised blood pressure, and diabetes Total score of 31 points: score 0–7 = low risk; 8–15 = intermediate risk; 16–31 = high risk		
ACCP [90]	≤75 years without other risk factors	One of the following risk factors: age >75 years, hypertension, diabetes, at least moderately impaired LV function or heart failure	Previous TIA/stroke/ systemic embolism; or two or more of the following risk factors: >75 years, at least moderately impaired LV function, hypertension, diabetes
NICE [10]	Age <65 years, without high-risk factors	Age ≥65 years without high risk factors; age <75 years with hypertension, diabetes or vascular disease	Previous stroke or TIA; age ≥75 years with hypertension, diabetes or vascular disease; impaired LV function on echocardiography; clinical evidence of valve disease or heart failure
ACC/AHA/ESC guidelines [43]	No risk factors	Age ≥75 years; hypertension; heart failure; impaired LV systolic function; or diabetes	Previous stroke/TIA/ systemic embolism; valve disease; more than one of: age ≥75 years, hypertension, heart failure, impaired LV systolic function, or diabetes
CHA$_2$DS$_2$-VASc [92]	No risk factors	Score = 1 (see Table 6.19)	Score = 2–9 (see Table 6.19)

ACC, American College of Cardiology; ACCP, American College of Chest Physicians; AFI, Atrial Fibrillation Investigators; CAD, coronary artery disease; AESC, European Society of Cardiology; LV, left ventricular; SPAF, Stroke Prevention in Atrial Fibrillation; TIA, transient ischemic attack.

Table 6.19 2009 Birmingham schema: CHA_2DS_2-VASc.

Risk factor	Score
Congestive heart failure/LV dysfunction	1
Hypertension	1
Age ≥75 years	2
Diabetes mellitus	1
Stroke/TIA/TE	2
Vascular disease (previous MI, PVD or aortic plaque)	1
Age 65–74	1
Sex category (female)	1

LV, left ventricular; MI, myocardial ischemia; PVD, peripheral vascular disease; TE, thromboembolism; TIA, transient ischemic attack.

summarizes the main stroke risk stratification schemes for patients with AF [10,43,64,86–92].

The $CHADS_2$ (score 1 point each on congestive heart failure, hypertension, age >75 years, diabetes; score 2 points for previous stroke or transient ischemic attack) is the most popular and well-validated scheme. It is simple to use, but it does not include echocardiographic left ventricular impairment or association with other vascular disease as high-risk factors. The $CHADS_2$ scheme has various limitations which have been the subject of debate [93,94], particularly its non-inclusion of many common stroke risk factors and its poor predictive value for high-risk patients as well as its inadequate identification of "truly low-risk" subjects who do not need any antithrombotic therapy [95].

The 2009 Birmingham Schema [92] refined the NICE stroke risk stratification schema into a risk factor-based approach by incorporating additional risk factors. The proposed scoring system, CHA_2DS_2-VASc score, is summarized in Table 6.19,: scores of 0 = low, 1 = intermediate, and ≥2 = high risk. This new scoring system has a marginally better C-statistic of 0.606 when compared with the classic $CHADS_2$ (0.561). This new schema also showed a low thromboembolic event rate in low-risk subjects and classified a small proportion of subjects into the intermediate-risk category. This new point-based schema could improve the clinical approach to stroke risk stratification in AF.

The 2010 ESC guidelines are based on this risk factor-based approach to stroke risk assessment, with use of the CHA_2DS_2-VASc score to complement the $CHADS_2$ score [96] (Table 6.20 and Figure 6.3). The CHA_2DS_2-VASc score has been validated in various independent cohorts and outperforms the $CHADS_2$ score in identifying "truly low-risk" patients; it is as good as, and possibly better, than the $CHADS_2$ score in identifying high-risk subjects [97,98].

Bleeding risk

The assessment of bleeding risk becomes part of the clinical assessment of patients with AF before starting anticoagulation therapy [99]. Patients who have risk factors for stroke also have increasing bleeding risk [99].

Table 6.20 Approach to thromboprophylaxis in patients with atrial fibrillation (Reproduced from Camm *et al.* [96] by permission of Oxford University Press).

Risk category	CHA_2DS_2-VASc score	Recommended antithrombotic therapy
One "major" risk factor or ≥2 "clinically relevant non-major" risk factors	≥2	OAC*
One "clinically relevant non-major" risk factor	1	Either OAC* or aspirin 75–325 mg daily Preferred: OAC rather than aspirin
No risk factors	0	Either aspirin 75–325 mg daily or no antithrombotic therapy Preferred: No antithrombotic therapy rather than aspirin

*Oral anticoagulation (OAC) such as a vitamin K antagonist (VKA), adjusted to an intensity range of INR 2.0–3.0 (target 2.5). New OAC drugs, which may be viable alternatives to a VKA, may ultimately be considered. CHA_2DS_2-VASc = cardiac failure, hypertension, age ≥75 years (doubled), diabetes, stroke (doubled), vascular disease, age 65–74 years, and sex category (female).

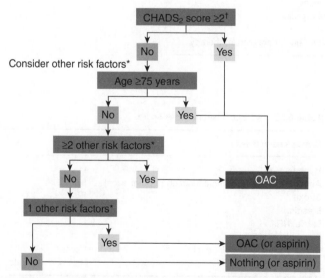

Figure 6.3 Stroke risk stratification algorithm from the ESC guidelines. †Congestive heart failure, hypertension, age ≥75 years, diabetes, stroke, transient ischemic attack, thromboembolism (doubled). *Other clinically relevant non-major risk factors: age 65–74 years, female sex, vascular disease. OAC, oral anticoagulation. (Reproduced from Camm *et al.* [96] by permission of Oxford University Press.)

A systematic review on nine studies by Hughes *et al.* [100] identified a total of eight possible risk factors: increasing age, polypharmacy, history of MI, cerebrovascular disease or previous bleeding events, gender, diabetes, and blood pressure. Conventional risk factors associated with bleeding are summarized in Table 6.21.

A recent study proposed a novel bleeding risk score as a practical tool to assess individual bleeding risk [101]. HAS-BLED (Table 6.22) has demonstrated a good predictive accuracy (C-statistic 0.72) within the study cohort. This accuracy improved in subgroups taking antiplatelet therapy alone (C-statistic 0.91) or no antithrombotic therapy (C-statistics 0.85). The HAS-BLED score has been validated in several independent cohorts [102–104]. This easy-to-use tool could support clinician in decision making regarding thromboprophylaxis therapy in AF patients.

Stroke risk has been balanced against bleeding risk in several net clinical benefit analyses. For the majority of AF patients, the absolute gain in stroke reduction with oral anticoagulation would outweigh the small absolute increase in serious bleeds [105].

Table 6.21 Risk factors associated with bleeding complications.

- Elderly age (>75 years)
- Uncontrolled hypertension
- Polypharmacy
- History of bleeding
- Anemia
- Concomitant use of antiplatelet therapy

Table 6.22 HAS-BLED bleeding risk score.

Clinical characteristic	Score
Hypertension	1
Abnormal liver and/or renal function (1 point each)	1 or 2
Stroke	1
Bleeding	1
Labile INRs	1
Elderly (age >65 years)	1
Drugs or alcohol (1 point each)	1 or 2
	Maximum 9 points

Hypertension: systolic blood pressure >160 mmHg. Abnormal renal function: dialysis, renal transplant or serum creatinine ≥ 200 μmol/L. Abnormal liver function: chronic hepatic disease or biochemical evidence of significant hepatic derangement (bilirubin >2x upper limit of normal, in association with AST/ALT/ALP >3x upper limit of normal). Bleeding: previous episodes, history of anemia, bleeding diathesis. Labile INR: unstable/high INRs or <60% time in therapeutic range. Drugs/alcohol: concomitant use of drugs (antiplatelet agents, non-steroidal anti-inflammatory drugs).

Conclusion

Patient who present with AF should be assessed carefully and thoroughly. All precipitating causes should be treated. The choice of treatment for the irregular rhythm itself is individually based. Both rhythm-control and rate-control therapy can be employed as first-line treatment, depending on the duration of the irregular rhythm. All patients who present with AF should also be assessed for their stroke and thromboembolic risk, and appropriate antithrombotic therapy should be started.

References

1. Lip GY, Golding DJ, Nazir M, Beevers DG, Child DL, Fletcher RI. A survey of atrial fibrillation in general practice: the West Birmingham Atrial Fibrillation project. *Br J Gen Pract* 1997;47:28.
2. Lloyd-Jones DM, Wang TJ, Leip EP, *et al.* Lifetime risk for development of atrial fibrillation: the Framingham heart study. *Circulation* 2004;110:1042–1046.
3. Heeringa J, van der Kuip DA, Hofman A, *et al.* Prevalence, incidence and lifetime risk of atrial fibrillation: the Roterdam study. *Eur Heart J* 2006;27:949–953.
4. Miyasaka Y, Barnes ME, Gersh BJ, *et al.* Secular trends in incidence of atrial fibrillation in Olmsted County, Minnesota, 1980 to 2000, and implications on the projections for future prevalence. *Circulation* 2006;114:119–125.
5. Stewart S, Hart CL, Hole DJ, McMurray JJ. Population prevalence, incidence, and predictors of atrial fibrillation in the Renfrew/Paisley study. *Heart* 2001;86:516–521.
6. Hobbs FD, Fitzmaurice DA, Mant J, *et al.* A randomized controlled trial and cost-effectiveness study of systematic screening (targeted and total population screening) versus routine practice for the detection of atrial fibrillation in people aged 65 and over. The SAFE study. *Health Technol Assess* 2005;9:1–74.
7. Psaty BM, Manolio TA, Kuller LH, *et al.* Incidence of and risk factors for atrial fibrillation in older adults. *Circulation* 1997;96:2455–2461.
8. Benjamin EJ, Levy D, Vaziri SM, D'Agostino RB, Belanger AJ, Wolf PA. Independent risk factors for atrial fibrillation in a population-based cohort: The Framingham Heart Study. *JAMA* 1994;271:840–844.
9. Fox CS, Parise H, D'Agostino RB Sr, *et al.* Parental atrial fibrillation as a risk factor for atrial fibrillation in offspring. *JAMA* 2004;291:2851–2855.
10. National Collaborating Centre for Chronic Conditions. *Atrial Fibrillation: national clinical guideline for management in primary and secondary care.* London: Royal College of Physicians, 2006 (http://rcplondon.ac.uk/pubs/books/af/index.asp).
11. Lip GY, Tse HF. Management of atrial fibrillation. *Lancet* 2007;370:604–618.
12. Lévy S, Maarek M, Coumel P, *et al.* Characterization of different subsets of atrial fibrillation in general practice in France. The ALFA study. *Circulation* 1999;99:3028–3035.
13. Davidson E, Weinberger I, Rotenberg Z, Fuchs J, Agmon J. Atrial fibrillation. Cause and time of onset. *Arch Intern Med* 1989;149:457–459.
14. de Paola AA, Figueiredo E, Sesso R, *et al.* Effectiveness and costs of chemical versus electrical cardioversion of atrial fibrillation. *Int J Cardiol* 2003;88:157–153.
15. Valencia MJ, Climent P, Marin O, *et al.* The efficacy of scheduled cardioversion in atrial fibrillation: comparison of two schemes of treatment: electrical versus pharmacological cardioversion. *Revista Espanola de Cardiologia* 2002;55:113–120.

16. Singh BN, Singh SN, Reda DJ, *et al.*; Sotalol Amiodarone Atrial Fibrillation Efficacy Trial (SAFE-T) Investigators. Amiodarone versus sotalol for atrial fibrillation. *N Engl J Med* 2005;352:1861–1872.

17. Van Gelder IC, Wyse DG, Chandler ML, *et al.*; RACE and AFFIRM Investigators. Does intensity of rate-control influence outcome in artial fribrillation An analysis of pooled date from the RACE and AFFIRM studies. *Europace* 2006;8:935–942.

18. Li Saw Hee FL, Lip GYH. Digoxin revisited. *Q J Med* 1998;91:259–264.

19. Michael JA, Stiell IG, Agarwal S, Mandavia DP. Cardioversion of paroxysmal atrial fibrillation in the emergency department. *Ann Emerg Med* 1999;33:379–387.

20. Kumar A. Intravenous amiodarone for therapy of atrial fibrillation and flutter in critically ill patients with severely depressed left ventricular function. *South Med J* 1996;89: 779–785.

21. Strasberg B, Arditti A, Sclarovsky S. Efficacy of intravenous amiodarone in the management of paroxysmal or new atrial fibrillation with fast ventricular response. *Int J Cardiol* 1985;7:47–55.

22. Wang HE, O'connor RE, Megargel RE, *et al.* The use of diltiazem for treating rapid atrial fibrillation in the out-of-hospital setting. *Ann Emerg Med* 2001;37:38–45.

23. Alboni P, Botto GL, Baldi N, *et al.* Outpatient treatment of recent-onset atrial fibrillation with the "pill-in-the-pocket" approach. *N Engl J Med* 2004;351:2384–2391.

24. Lee SH, Chen SA, Tai CT, *et al.* Comparisons of oral propafenone and sotalol as an initial treatment in patients with symptomatic paroxysmal atrial fibrillation. *Am J Cardiol* 1997;79:905–908.

25. Kochiadakis GE, Igoumenidis NE, Hamilos ME, *et al.* Sotalol versus propafenone for long-term maintenance of normal sinus rhythm in patients with recurrent symptomatic atrial fibrillation. *Am J Cardiol* 2004;94:1563–1566.

26. Bellandi F,Simonetti I, Leoncini M, *et al.* Long-term efficacy and safety of propafenone and sotalol for the maintenance of sinus rhythm after conversion of recurrent symptomatic atrial fibrillation. *Am J Cardiol* 2001;88:640–645.

27. Reimold SC, Cantillon CO, Friedman PL, Antman EM. Propafenone versus sotalol for suppression of recurrent symptomatic atrial fibrillation. *Am J Cardiol* 1993;71:558–563.

28. Roy D, Talajic M, Dorian P, *et al.* Amiodarone to prevent recurrence of atrial fibrillation. Canadian Trial of Atrial Fibrillation Investigators. *N Engl J Med* 2000;342:913–920.

29. Kochiadakis GE, Igoumenidis NE, Hamilos MI, *et al.* Long-term maintenance of normal sinus rhythm in patients with current symptomatic atrial fibrillation: amiodarone versus propafenone, both in low doses. *Chest* 2004;125:377–383.

30. Kochiadakis GE, Igoumenidis NE, Marketou ME, Kateboubos MD, Simantirakis EN, Vardas PE. Low dose amiodarone and sotalol in the treatment of recurrent, symptomatic atrial fibrillation: a comparative, placebo controlle study. *Heart* 2000;84:251–257.

31. Kochiadakis GE, Marketou ME, Igoumenidis NE, *et al.* Amiodarone, sotalol, or propafenone in atrial fibrillation: which is preferred to maintain normal sinus rhythm? *Pacing Clin Electrophysiol* 2000;23:1883–1887.

32. Steeds RD, Birchall AS, Smith M, Channer KS. An open label, randomised crossover study comparing sotalol and atenolol in the treatment of symptomatic paroxysmal atrial fibrillation. *Heart* 1999;82:170–173.

33. Hohnloser SH, Crijns HJ, van Eickels M, *et al.*; ATHENA Investigators. Effect of dronedarone on cardiovascular events in atrial fibrillation. *N Engl J Med.* 2009;360):668–678. Erratum in: *N Engl J Med* 2011;364:1481; *N Engl J Med* 2009;360:2487.

34. Connolly SJ, Camm AJ, Halperin JL, *et al.*; PALLAS Investigators. Dronedarone in high-risk permanent atrial fibrillation. *N Engl J Med* 2011;365:2268–2276. Erratum in: *N Engl J Med* 2012;366:672.

35. Køber L, Torp-Pedersen C, McMurray JJ, *et al.*; Dronedarone Study Group. Increased mortality after dronedarone therapy for severe heart failure. *N Engl J Med* 2008;358:2678–2687.

36. Hohnloser SH, Kuck KH, Lilienthal J. Rhythm or rate control in atrial fibrillation— Pharmacological Intervention in Atrial Fibrillation (PIAF): a randomised trial. *Lancet* 2000;356:1789–1794.

37. Van Gelder IC, Hagens VE, Bosker HA, *et al.*; Rate Control versus Electrical Cardioversion for Persistent Atrial Fibrillation Study Group. A comparison of rate control and rhythm control in patients with recurrent persistent atrial fi brillation. *N Engl J Med* 2002;347:1834–1840.

38. Wyse DG, Waldo AL, DiMarco JP, *et al.*; Atrial Fibrillation Follow-up Investigation of Rhythm Management (AFFIRM) Investigators. A comparison of rate control and rhythm control in patients with atrial fibrillation. *N Engl J Med* 2002;347:1825– 1833.

39. Carlsson J, Miketic S, Windeler J, *et al.*; STAF Investigators. Randomized trial of rate-control versus rhythm-control in persistent atrial fi brillation: the Strategies of Treatment of Atrial Fibrillation (STAF) study. *J Am Coll Cardiol* 2003;41:1690–1696.

40. Roy D, Talajic M, Nattel S, *et al.*; Atrial Fibrillation and Congestive Heart Failure Investigators. Rhythm control versus rate control for atrial fibrillation and heart failure. *N Engl J Med* 2008;358:2667–2677.

41. Singh BN, Connolly SJ, Crijns HJ, *et al*; EURIDIS and ADONIS Investigators. Dronedarone for maintenance of sinus rhythm in atrial fibrillation or flutter. *N Engl J Med* 2007;357:987–999.

42. Le Heuzey JY, De Ferrari GM, Radzik D, Santini M, Zhu J, Davy JM. A short-term, randomized, double-blind, parallel-group study to evaluate the efficacy and safety of dronedarone versus amiodarone in patients with persistent atrial fibrillation: the DIONYSOS study. *J Cardiovasc Electrophysiol* 2010;21:597–605.

43. Fuster V, Ryden LE, Cannom DS, *et al.* ACC/AHA/ESC 2006 guidelines for the management of patients with atrial fibrillation: full text: a report of the American College of Cardiology/American Heart Association Task Force on practice guidelines and the European Society of Cardiology Committee for Practice Guidelines (Writing Committee to Revise the 2001 guidelines for the management of patients with atrial fibrillation) developed in collaboration with the European Heart Rhythm Association and the Heart Rhythm Society. *Europace* 2006;8:651–745.

44. Rawles JM. What is meant by a 'controlled' ventricular rate in atrial fibrillation? *Br Heart J* 1990;63:157–161.

45. Khand AU, Rankin AC, Martin W, Taylor J, Gemmell I, Cleland JG. Carverdilol alone or in combination with digoxin for the management of atrial fibrillation in patients with heart failure? *J Am Coll Cardiol* 2003;42:1944–1951.

46. Farshi R, Kistner D, Sarma JS, Longmate JA, Singh BN. Ventricular rate control in chronic atrial fibrillation during daily activity and programmed exercise: a crossover open label study of five drug regimens. *J Am Coll Cardiol* 1999;33:304–310.

47. Wong CK, Lau CP, Leung WH, Cheng CH. Usefulness of labetalol in chronic atrial fibrillation. *Am J Cardiol* 1990;66:1212–1215.

48. Maragno I, Santostasi G, Gaion RM, *et al.* Low- and medium-dose diltiazem in chronic atrial fibrillation: comparison with digoxin and correlation with drug plasma levels. *Am Heart J* 1988;116:385–392.

49. Lewis RV, Laing E, Moreland TA, Service E, McDevitt DG. A comparison of digoxin, diltiazem and their combination in the treatment of atrial fibrillation. *Eur Heart J* 1988;9:279–283.

50. Pomfret SM, Beasley CR, Challenor V, Holgate ST. Relative efficacy of oral verapamil and digoxin alone and in combination for the treatment of patients with chronic atrial fibrillation. *Clin Sci (Lond)* 1988;74:351–357.

51. Roth A, Harrison E, Mitani G, Cohen J, Rahimtoola SH, Elkayam U. Efficacy and safety of medium-and high-dose diltiazem alone and in combination with digoxin for control of heart rate at rest and during exercise in patients with chronic atrial fibrillation. *Circulation* 1986;73:316–324.

52. Lang R, Klein HO, Weiss E, *et al*. Superiority of oral verapamil therapy to digoxin in treatment of chronic atrial fibrillation. *Chest* 1983;83:491–499.

53. Segal JB, McNamara RL, Miller MR, *et al*. The evidence regarding the drugs used for ventricular rate control. *J Fam Pract* 2000;49:47–59.

54. Pappone C, Oreto G, Rosanio S, *et al*. Atrial electroanatomic remodeling after circumferential radiofrequency pulmonary vein ablation: efficacy of an anatomic approach in a large cohort of patients with atrial fibrillation. *Circulation* 2001;104:2539–2544.

55. Vasamreddy CR, Dalal D, Eldadah Z, *et al*. Safety and efficacy of circumferential pulmonary vein catheter ablation of atrial fibrillation. *Heart Rhythm* 2005;2:42–48.

56. Oral H, Knight BP, Tada H, *et al*. Pulmonary vein isolation for paroxysmal and persistent atrial fibrillation. *Circulation* 2002;105:1077–1081.

57. Lip GY, Boss CJ. Antithrombotic treatment in atrial fibrillation. *Heart* 2006;92:155–161.

58. Hart RG, Pearce LA, Agullar MI. Antithrombotic therapy to prevent stroke in patients who have nonvalvular atrial fibrillation: a meta-analysis. *Ann Intern Med* 2007;146: 857–867.

59. Lip GY, Edwards SJ. Stroke prevention with aspirin, warfarin and ximelagatran in patients with non-valvular atrial fibrillation: a systemic review and meta-analysis. *Thromb Res* 2006;118:321–333.

60. Petersen P, Boysen G, Godtfredsen J, Andersen ED, Andersen B. Placebo-controlled, randomised trial of warfarin and aspirin for prevention of thromboembolic complications in chronic atrial fibrillation. The Copenhagen AFASAK study. *Lancet* 1989;1: 175–179.

61. The Boston Area Anticoagulation Trial for Atrial Fibrillation Investigators. The effect of low-dose warfarin on the risk of stroke in patients with nonrheumatic atrial fibrillation. *N Engl J Med* 1990;323:1505–1511.

62. Connolly SJ, Laupacis A, Gent M, Roberts RS, Cairns JA, Joyner C. Canadian Atrial Fibrillation Anticoagulation (CAFA) Study. *J Am Coll Cardiol* 1991;18:349–355.

63. Secondary prevention in non-rheumatic atrial fibrillation after transient ischaemic attack or minor stroke. EAFT (European Atrial Fibrillation Trial) Study Group. *Lancet* 1993;342:1255–1262.

64. Stroke Prevention in Atrial Fibrillation Study. Final results. *Circulation* 1991;84:527–539.

65. Ezekowitz MD, Bridgers SL, James KE, *et al*. Warfarin in the prevention of stroke associated with nonrheumatic atrial fibrillation. Veterans Affairs Stroke Prevention in Nonrheumatic Atrial Fibrillation Investigators. *N Engl J Med* 1992;327:1406–1412.

66. Diener HC, Cunha L, Forbes C, Sivenius J, Smets P, Lowenthal A. European Stroke Prevention Study. 2. Dipyridamole and acetylsalicylic acid in the secondary prevention of stroke. *J Neurol Sci* 1996;143:1–13.

67. Benavente O, Hart R, Koudstaal P, Laupacis A, McBride R. Antiplatelet therapy for preventing stroke in patients with non-valvular atrial fibrillation and no previous history of stroke or transient ischemic attacks. *Cochrane Database Syst Rev* 2000;(2):CD001925.

68. Japan Atrial Fibrillation Stroke Trial Group. Low-dose aspirin for prevention of stroke in low-risk patients with atrial fibrillation: Japan Atrial Fibrillation Stroke Trial. *Stroke* 2006;37:447–451.

69. Posada IS, Barriales V. Alternate-day dosing of aspirin in atrial fibrillation. LASAF Pilot Study Group. *Am Heart J* 1999;138:137–143.

70. Stroke Prevention in Atrial Fibrillation investigators. A differential effect of aspirin in prevention of stroke on atrial fibrillation. *J Stroke Cerebrovasc Dis* 1993;3:181–188.

71. Lip GY. The role of aspirin for stroke prevention in atrial fibrillation. *Nat Rev Cardiol* 2011;8:602–606.

72. ACTIVE Writing Group on behalf of the ACTIVE Investigators. Clopidogrel plus aspirin versus oral anticoagulation for atrial fibrillation in the atrial fibrillation clopidogrel trial with irbesartan for prevention of vascular events (ACTIVE W). *Lancet* 2006;367:1903–1912.

73. Mant J, Hobbs FD, Fletcher K, *et al.*; BAFTA investigators; Midland Research Practices Network (MidReC). Warfarin versus aspirin for stroke prevention in an elderly community population with atrial fibrillation (the Birmingham Atrial Fibrillation Treatment of the Aged Study, BAFTA): a randomised controlled trial. *Lancet* 2007;370:493–503.

74. Dentali F, Douketis JD, Lim W, Crowther M. Combined aspirin-oral anticoagulant therapy compared with oral anticoagulant therapy alone among patients at risk for cardiovascular disease. A meta-analysis of randomised trials. *Arch Intern Med* 2007;167: 117–124.

75. Gulløv AL, Koefoed BG, Petersen P, *et al.* Fixed minidose warfarin and aspirin alone and in combination vs adjusted-dose warfarin for stroke prevention in atrial fibrillation: Second Copenhagen Atrial Fibrillation, Aspirin, and Anticoagulation Study. *Arch Intern Med* 1998;158:1513–1521.

76. Hellemons BS, Langenberg M, Lodder J, *et al.* Primary prevention of arterial thromboembolism in non-rheumatic atrial fibrillation in primary care: randomised controlled trial comparing two intensities of coumarin with aspirin. *BMJ* 1999;319:958–964.

77. Adjusted-dose warfarin versus low-intensity, fixed-dose warfarin plus aspirin for high-risk patients with atrial fibrillation: Stroke Prevention in Atrial Fibrillation ? randomised clinical trial. *Lancet* 1996;348:633–638.

78. ACTIVE Investigators, Connolly SJ, Pogue J, Hart RG, *et al.* Effect of clopidogrel added to aspirin in patients with atrial fibrillation. *N Engl J Med* 2009;360:2066–2078.

79. Connolly SJ, Ezekowitz MD, Yusuf S, *et al.*; RE-LY Steering Committee and Investigators. Dabigatran versus warfarin in patients with atrial fibrillation. *N Engl J Med* 2009;361:1139–1151.

80. Patel MR, Mahaffey KW, Garg J, *et al.*; ROCKET AF Investigators. Rivaroxaban versus warfarin in nonvalvular atrial fibrillation. *N Engl J Med* 2011;365:883–891.

81. Granger CB, Alexander JH, McMurray JJ, *et al.*; ARISTOTLE Committees and Investigators. Apixaban versus warfarin in patients with atrial fibrillation. *N Engl J Med* 2011; 365:981–992.

82. Connolly SJ, Eikelboom J, Joyner C, *et al.*; AVERROES Steering Committee and Investigators. Apixaban in patients with atrial fibrillation. *N Engl J Med* 2011;364: 806–817.

83. Nieuwlaat R, Capucci A, Camm AJ, *et al.*; European Heart Survey Investigators. Atrial fibrillation management: a prospective survey in ESC member countries: the Euro Heart Survey on Atrial Fibrillation. *Eur Heart J* 2005;26:2422–2434.

84. Lip GY, Huber K, Andreotti F, *et al.*; European Society of Cardiology Working Group on Thrombosis. Management of antithrombotic therapy in atrial fibrillation patients presenting with acute coronary syndrome and/or undergoing percutaneous coronary intervention/ stenting. *Thromb Haemost* 2010;103:13–28.

85. Stroke Risk in Atrial Fibrillation Working Group. Independent predictors of stroke in patients with atrial fibrillation: a systematic review. *Neurology* 2007;69:546–554.

86. Stroke Risk in Atrial Fibrillation Working Group. Comparison of 12 risk stratification schemes to predict stroke in patients with nonvalvular atrial fibrillation. *Stroke* 2008;39:1902–1910.

87. Atrial Fibrillation Investigators. Risk factors for stroke and efficacy of antithrombotic therapy in atrial fibrillation: analysis of pooled data from five randomized controlled trials. *Arch Intern Med* 1994;154:1449–1457.

88. Gage BF, van Walraven C, Pearce L, *et al*. Selecting patients with atrial fibrillation for anticoagulation: stroke risk stratification in patients taking aspirin. *Circulation* 2004;110: 2287–2292.

89. Wang TJ, Massaro JM, Levy D, *et al*. A risk score for predicting stroke or death in indicviduals with new-onset atrial fibrillation in the community: the Framingham Heart Study. *JAMA* 2003;290:1049–1056.

90. Singer DE, Albers GW, Dalen JE, *et al*. Antithrombotic Therapy in Atrial Fibrillation: American College of Chest Physicians Evidence-Based Clinical Practice Guidelines (8TH Edition). *Chest* 2008;133:546–592.

91. Nieuwlaat R, Capucci A, Lip GY, *et al*. Antithrombotic treatment in real-life atrial fibrillation patients: a report from the Euro Heart Survey on Atrial Fibrillation. *Eur Heart J* 2006;27:3018–3026.

92. Lip GY, Nieuwlaat R, Pisters R, Lane DA, Crijns HJ. Refining clinical risk stratification for prediction stroke and thromboembolism in atrial fibrillation using a novel risk factor-based approach. *Chest* 2010;137:263–272.

93. Karthikeyan G, Eikelboom JW. The CHADS2 score for stroke risk stratification in atrial fibrillation–friend or foe? *Thromb Haemost* 2010;104:45–48.

94. Keogh C, Wallace E, Dillon C, Dimitrov BD, Fahey T. Validation of the CHADS2 clinical prediction rule to predict ischaemic stroke. A systematic review and meta-analysis. *Thromb Haemost* 2011;106:528–538.

95. Olesen J, Torp-Petersen C, Hansen ML, Lip GY. The value of the CHA$_2$DS$_2$-VASc score for refining stroke risk stratification in patients with atrial fibrillation with a CHADS$_2$ score 0–1: a nationwide cohort study. *Thromb Haemostat* 2012 [Epub ahead of print].

96. Camm AJ, Kirchhof P, Lip GY, *et al*. Guidelines for the management of atrial fibrillation: the Task Force for the Management of Atrial Fibrillation of the European Society of Cardiology (ESC). *Eur Heart J* 2010;31:2369–2429. Erratum in: *Eur Heart J* 2011;32:1172.

97. Olesen JB, Lip GY, Hansen ML, *et al*. Validation of risk stratification schemes for predicting stroke and thromboembolism in patients with atrial fibrillation: nationwide cohort study. *BMJ* 2011;342:d124.

98. Friberg L, Rosenqvist M, Lip GY. Evaluation of risk stratification schemes for ischaemic stroke and bleeding in 182 678 patients with atrial fibrillation: the Swedish Atrial Fibrillation cohort study. *Eur Heart J* 2012 [Epub ahead of print].

99. Lip GY, Andreotti F, Fauchier L, *et al*.; European Heart Rhythm Association. Bleeding risk assessment and management in atrial fibrillation patients. Executive Summary of a Position Document from the European Heart Rhythm Association [EHRA], endorsed by the European Society of Cardiology [ESC] Working Group on Thrombosis. *Thromb Haemost* 2011;106:997–1011.

100. Hughes M, Lip GY; on behalf of the Guideline Development Group for the NICE national clinical guideline for management of atrial fibrillation in primary and secondary care. Risk factors for anticoagulation-related bleeding complications in patients with atrial fibrillation: a systematic review. *Q J Med* 2007;100:599–607.

101. Pisters R, Lane DA, Nieuwlaat R, de Vos CB, Crijns HJ, Lip GY. A novel user-friendly score (HAS-BLED) to assess one-year risk of major bleeding in atrial fibrillation patients: The Euro Heart Survey. *Chest* 2010;138:1093–1100.

102. Friberg L, Rosenqvist M, Lip GY. Evaluation of risk stratification schemes for ischaemic stroke and bleeding in 182 678 patients with atrial fibrillation: the Swedish Atrial Fibrillation cohort study. *Eur Heart J* 2012 Jan 13 [Epub ahead of print].

103. Olesen JB, Lip GY, Hansen PR, *et al.* Bleeding risk in 'real world' patients with atrial fibrillation: comparison of two established bleeding prediction schemes in a nationwide cohort. *J Thromb Haemost* 2011;9:1460–1467.

104. Gallego P, Roldán V, Torregrosa JM, *et al.* Relation of the HAS-BLED bleeding risk score to major bleeding, cardiovascular events and mortality in anticoagulated patients with atrial fibrillation. *Circ Arrhythm Electrophysiol* 2012 Feb 7 [Epub ahead of print].

105. Olesen JB, Lip GY, Lindhardsen J, *et al.* Risks of thromboembolism and bleeding with thromboprophylaxis in patients with atrial fibrillation: A net clinical benefit analysis using a 'real world' nationwide cohort study. *Thromb Haemost* 2011;106:739–749.

CHAPTER 7

Electrophysiology and pacing

Irina Suman-Horduna and Sabine Ernst
National Heart and Lung Institute, Imperial College; Royal Brompton and Harefield Hospital, London, UK

Arrhythmias

Sinus rhythm

Under normal circumstances, the sinus node drives the normal rhythm with electrical activation spreading through atrial conduction fibers towards the atrioventricular node (AVN). The electrical impulse leaving the AVN reaches the ventricular myocardium through the His bundle, right and left bundle branches, and Purkinje network. The Purkinje system fans out throughout the ventricular endocardium, allowing the impulse to proceed from the specialized conduction system to the myocardial muscle.

The polarity of the sinus P wave is consistent with the sinus node location, thus positive in leads I, II, III, and aVF, and isoelectric in lead V1.

Mechanisms

Focal tachycardias

Automaticity is the property of a cell to undergo spontaneous depolarization. Enhanced normal automaticity refers to the acceleration of the discharge rate of normal pacemaker tissue, either the primary pacemaker of the heart, the sinus node, or the other latent pacemakers identified in the atrial myocardium, AVN or His–Purkinje system.

Re-entrant tachycardias

Re-entry is the most common mechanism of arrhythmias; it requires two anatomically and functionally separated pathways, a unidirectional block in one pathway, and an excitable gap (the time interval between the tail of the circuit and the leading edge of the next impulse). In the electrophysiology laboratory, re-entrant arrhythmias can be reproduced by introducing a premature stimulus that penetrates the excitable gap, blocks one pathway, and

Cardiovascular Clinical Trials: Putting the Evidence into Practice, First Edition.
Edited by Marcus D. Flather, Deepak L. Bhatt, and Tobias Geisler.
© 2013 Blackwell Publishing Ltd. Published 2013 by Blackwell Publishing Ltd.

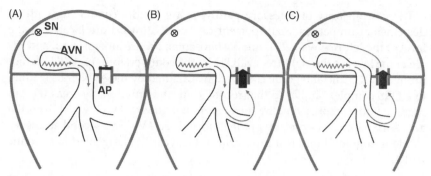

Figure 7.1 Concept of re-entrant tachycardia induction: example of orthodromic atrioventricular re-entrant tachycardia (AVRT). (A) During sinus rhythm the activation travels from the sinus node (SN) antegradely across the atrioventricular node (AVN). The accessory pathway (AP) is concealed and therefore there is no evidence of ventricular pre-excitation. (B) The electric impulse enters the AP retrogradely and thereby returns the activation back to the atria. (C) The impulse returns to the AVN antegradely and the loop is closed and an orthodromic AV re-entrant tachycardia is established.

slowly conducts antegradely over the other pathway. If the wave travels slowly enough to allow the blocked pathway to recover, the electrical activation can be retrogradely conducted to close the loop, resulting in a single beat of re-entry called an echo beat. If these echo beats are perpetuated, tachycardia results (Figure 7.1).

Supraventricular tachycardia (SVT) refers to regular, narrow QRS complex tachycardias, usually faster than 100 beats/min. These tachycardias are divided into three main categories: atrioventricular nodal re-entrant tachycardia (AVNRT), atrioventricular re-entrant tachycardia (AVRT) due to an accessory pathway, and atrial tachycardia (AT).

AVNRT is a re-entrant tachycardia involving two functionally different pathways within the AVN with different conduction properties. The most commonly encountered form of AVNRT (typical slow/fast AVNRT) requires a "dual nodal pathway physiology": one slow pathway (SP) with low-velocity conduction and a shorter refractory period, and one fast pathway (FP) that conducts faster and with a longer refractory period. The atrial activation (up the FP) occurs almost simultaneously with the ventricular activation (down the SP); therefore, on the surface electrocardiogram (EKG), the retrograde negative P wave is buried in the QRS complex and is thus invisible, or recorded as a small indentation at the end of the QRS complex (pseudo r' in the V1 and pseudo s' wave in the inferior leads).

AVRT is a re-entrant tachycardia that utilizes at least one accessory pathway as one limb. The association between manifest pre-excitation in sinus rhythm and episodes of paroxysmal tachycardia defines the Wolff–Parkinson–White (WPW) syndrome. If the accessory pathway is only capable of conducting retrogradely, the terminology used is "concealed accessory pathway."

The vast majority of accessory pathways are rapidly conducting with no decremental properties. Sixty percent of these pathways are located at the level of the left free wall, 27% are posteroseptal, 5% are anteroseptal, and 8% are at the level of the right free wall [1]. In the common form of AVRT (orthodromic AVRT), the antegrade conduction is assured by the AVN, thus leading to a QRS complex similar to that recorded in sinus rhythm, whereas the retrograde limb is represented by the accessory pathway. AVRT, which uses the accessory pathway as the antegrade limb and the AVN or a second accessory as the retrograde limb, is a rare form of tachycardia designated antidromic AVRT.

Atrial tachycardia
The mechanism of this tachycardia, which is confined to the atrial myocardium, may be focal or re-entrant (often related to atrial scaring). Focal ATs have preferential anatomical locations, like the crista terminalis, coronary sinus ostium, AV annulus, atrial appendages, and pulmonary veins.

Atrial flutter
Atrial flutter is a macrore-entrant arrhythmia with either an isthmus-dependent (typical or common) or a non–isthmus-dependent (uncommon) re-entrant circuit. The typical atrial flutter circuit has an obligatory critical component in the cavo-tricuspid isthmus (between the tricuspid annulus and inferior vena cava) and can turn in the clockwise (positive P waves in the inferior leads) or counterclockwise (negative P waves in the inferior leads) direction.

Atrial fibrillation (Table 7.1)
AF is the most common sustained arrhythmia encountered in clinical practice. Its prevalence increases with age, affecting less than 1% of those aged 50–59 years in the Framingham study but 9% of those aged 80–89 years [2].

On the EKG, P waves are replaced by rapid oscillations or fibrillatory waves that vary in amplitude, shape, and timing, and are associated with an irregular, frequently rapid ventricular response when atrioventricular (AV) conduction is intact. The ventricular response to AF depends on the electrophysiological properties of the AV node and other conducting tissues, the level of vagal and sympathetic tone, the presence or absence of accessory conduction pathways, and the action of drugs.

Table 7.1 Definitions of atrial fibrillation (AF).

Type	Duration	Termination
Paroxysmal AF	<7 days	Spontaneously
Persistent AF	>7 days	Requires medication or electrical cardioversion
Permanent AF	>1 year	No more attempts at cardioversion made
Longstanding persistent AF	>1 year	Only by catheter ablation

The current understanding of the pathogenesis of AF involves an arrhythmia trigger and substrate that allows for tachycardia perpetuation. The trigger for AF is usually located in the left atrium at the junction with one or more pulmonary veins [3]. The atrial tissue represents the substrate and this is prone to mechanical and electrical remodeling when additional factors like hypertension, aging, congestive heart failure or AF recurrence itself concur.

Ventricular arrhythmias

Ventricular tachycardias (VT) are classified according to the presence of an underlying cardiomyopathy, duration, morphology, hamodynamic consequences, and mechanism. Monomorphic VT exhibits a single QRS morphology, whereas during polymorphic VT the QRS morphology becomes multiform. Ventricular arrhythmias may be well tolerated and hemodynamically stable, or can have severe hemodynamic consequences leading to presyncope/syncope/sudden cardiac death (SCD)/sudden cardiac arrest.

Most often, ventricular arrhythmias are associated with various types of cardiomyopathy. The most common causes are coronary heart disease, heart failure, congenital heart disease, cardiomyopathies (dilated cardiomyopathy, hypertrophic cardiomyopathy, arrhythmogenic right ventricular cardiomyopathy). The underlying mechanism of a VT can be focal or re-entrant.

Torsade de pointes refers to a ventricular arrhythmia usually occurring in the setting of a long QT and characterized by the peculiar EKG feature of twisting of the peaks of the QRS complexes around the isoelectric line.

Ventricular fibrillation is characterized by a fast (>300bpm/200-ms cycle length) irregular ventricular rhythm with marked variability in QRS morphology and amplitude.

Pacing and pacing technologies

The first pacemakers were designed only to provide fixed-rate ventricular support in bradycardic patients. Nowadays, pacemakers are equipped with more complex algorithms to provide the patient with the best support for his/her medical condition.

A pacemaker system consists of the pulse generator and lead(s). The pulse generator contains the device circuitry and the battery, and the lead consists of the electrode, insulation, connector pin, and a fixation mechanism. The leads conduct the cardiac signals to the pulse generator (can) in either a bipolar (two electrodes at the tip of the lead) or unipolar (a single electrode at the tip of the lead with the can functioning as the second electrode) configuration. Most modern systems are bipolar to minimize the risks of sensing non-cardiac electrical signals.

Implantation procedure

The vast majority of pacemakers are implanted transvenously under local anesthetic, although epicardial leads can occasionally be implanted, especially in patients with congenital heart disease, pediatric patients or in postoperative

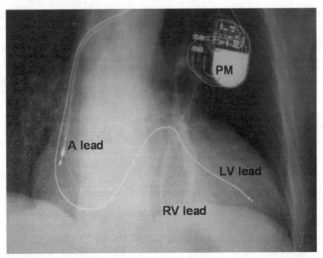

Figure 7.2 Pacemaker implantation and electrode positions. Typical positions of atrial (A) lead, right ventricular (RV) lead, and left ventricular (LV) lead as well as the pacemaker (PM) itself.

circumstances. For transvenous access, the cephalic, axillary or subclavian veins are commonly used. Cephalic vein leads are less prone to fracture and their insertion carries a lower risk of pneumothorax compared to subclavian access. Leads are usually placed in the right atrial appendage and right ventricular apex (Figure 7.2).

After lead placement, the electrical parameters (threshold, sensing, and impedance) of the leads are assessed. The pacing threshold is the minimum energy required to capture the myocardium. The initial programming of the output should be at least three times the threshold to ensure an adequate safety margin.

Sensing refers to the ability of the device to detect intracardiac electrical signals. In the acute settings, the intrinsic amplitude of the atrial and ventricular electrogram should be at least 1.5–1.8 mV and 4.5 mV, respectively. Sensitivity is a programmed value below which the device will ignore electrical signals. With the bipolar leads, sensitivity values can now be programmed to as low as 0.3 mV (i.e., very high sensitivity) and there is minimal risk of oversensing.

Lead impedance is assessed at implantation and routinely during follow-up. The lead impedance is a combination of the result of the intrinsic properties of the lead and the resistance at the interface of the electrode and the cardiac chamber.

Pacing modes are described using a three- to five-letter code, initially developed in 1970 and periodically updated (Table 7.2).

Complications after pacemaker implantation are rare (about 5–7%) and include infection, bleeding, pneumothorax, hemothorax, venous thrombosis, lead dislodgement, or cardiac tamponade.

Table 7.2 Pacing modes.

First letter	Second letter	Third I	Fourth letter	Fifth letter
Stimulation	Sensing	Response	Rate adaptation	Multisite pacing
A = Atrium	A = Atrium	I = Inhibition	R = Rate modulation	A = Atrium
V = Ventricle	V = Ventricle	T = Triggered	0 = None	V = Ventricle
D = A + V	D = A + V	D = I + T		D = A + V
0 = none	0 = none	0 = none		0 = none

Indications and differential pacing modes

Sinus node dysfunction and AV block are the most common indications for pacemaker implantation [4].

In single-chamber devices (AAI or VVI), after an intrinsic or paced event, the low rate timer is started, and at the end, if there is no event is sensed in the intervening period, a pacing output is delivered and the timer restarted. VVI pacing is most often used in patients with AF; the AAI mode is the preferred pacing mode in isolated sinus node dysfunction patients with normal AVN function.

In the DDD mode, pacing and sensing occur in both chambers. In addition, a sensed or paced beat in the atrium triggers a ventricular paced event unless an intrinsic QRS occurs spontaneously before the programmed AV delay. The AV delay is a programmable interval activated by a sensed or paced atrial event.

In the DDI mode, sensing and pacing occur in both the atria and ventricles, but a sensed atrial event does not start an AV interval and thus the ventricular pacing is not triggered by the sensed atrial events. Sequential dual chamber pacing at the low rate will only occur when no intrinsic atrial or ventricular activity is detected.

In the VDD mode, detection occurs both in the atrium and ventricle, but there is only pacing in the ventricle. Atrial-sensed events trigger ventricular pacing after a programmed AV delay, as in the DDD mode.

In the AOO, VOO, and DOO pacing modes, pacing occurs at a fixed programmed rate without sensing of the underlying rhythm. This pacing mode is sometimes used in pacemaker-dependent patients to avoid oversensing problems.

Electrophysiological assessment

Conventional mapping techniques

Diagnostic and ablation catheters are usually inserted using a Seldinger technique under local anesthesia. Most procedures can be undertaken only under conscious sedation, although approaches may differ between centers. General anesthesia is universally used in young adults or children or when external cardioversion is required. Some centers use the femoral vein exclusively, but access via the subclavian or jugular approach can be used, especially for coronary sinus cannulation.

A standard diagnostic electrophysiological study for investigation of SVT uses intracardiac recordings from standardized sites with characteristic intracardiac electrograms (Figure 7.3).

Baseline electrophysiological study

The usual techniques for stimulation are described below.

Atrial extrastimulus testing

The protocol for atrial stimulation uses a drive train of eight paced beats (S1) at a fixed cycle length followed by an extrastimulus (S2) delivered sequentially; the coupling interval of the extrastimulus is progressively shortened until the atrial refractoriness is reached. This protocol allows for characterization of the AVN dynamic properties (mostly its decremental properties manifested as progressive lengthening of the atrial to His bundle (AH) interval with shortening of the coupling interval of the extrastimulus), the presence of a dual AVN physiology or of an antegradely conducting alternative pathway. It can also be used for arrhythmia induction, sometimes with a second extrastimulus (S3) added.

Ventricular extrastimulus testing

A similar protocol is used for ventricular testing in order to assess the presence and pattern of the retrograde conduction. If the retrograde atrial activation is concentric (i.e., first atrial electrogram recorded in the septal area) and decremental (i.e., progressive lengthening of the ventriculoatrial interval with shorter S2 coupling interval), the ventriculoatrial retrograde conduction is likely to involve the AVN. If either of the above conditions is not fulfilled, the presence of a concealed alternative pathway should be suspected.

This protocol can also be used for arrhythmia induction; up to three extrastimuli (S2–S4), two different cycle lengths (typically 600 ms and 400 ms), and two pacing sites (right ventricle [RV] apex and RV outflow tract) are commonly used.

Other pacing protocols

Incremental (atrial or ventricular) pacing starts at a cycle length slightly shorter than the sinus rate; the pacing rate is then accelerated in small steps until the 1:1 conduction (antegrade if atrial pacing and retrograde if ventricular pacing) ceases; this point defines the antegrade/retrograde Wenckebach cycle length.

Burst pacing is at a fixed rate (atrial or ventricular) and is usually used for arrhythmia induction.

Myocardial mapping for arrhythmias

AVNRT, AVRT, some .ATs, and some forms of idiopathic VT.s can be successfully mapped and ablated using conventional mapping techniques under

(A)

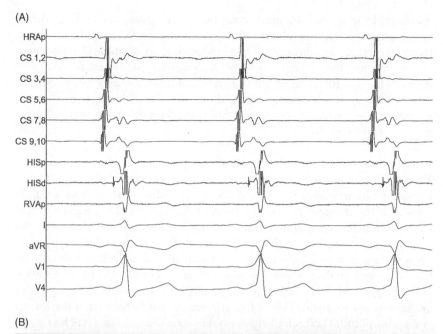

(B)

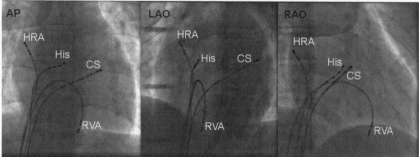

Figure 7.3 Endocavitary signals (upper panel) and corresponding electrode positions in anteroposterior (AP), left anterior oblique (LAO), and right anterior oblique (RAO) fluoroscopic views (lower panel) during electrophysiological study in a patient with a manifest left-sided accessory pathway. High right atrium (HRA): a quadripolar catheter is placed in contact with the right atrial wall, ideally on the high lateral wall near the superior vena cava–right atrium (RA) junction. Coronary sinus (CS): the coronary sinus is situated along the posterior mitral annulus allowing recording of the left atrial electrogram without need for direct left atrial access. A multipolar catheter is positioned via the RA through the CS ostium located at the inferoposterior aspect of the interatrial septum. His bundle (His): this catheter is used to record electrograms in the region of the AVN; at the correct location, it straddles the tricuspid annulus in its superoanterior part. It records the His bundle electrogram between the atrial and ventricular electrogram and allows assessment of the conduction time in the AVN (AH interval). Right ventricular apex (RVA): a quadripolar catheter is placed as close as possible to the right ventricular apex. His and RVA may be recorded via a single catheter; "p" denotes proximal bipole and "d" denotes distal bipole; I, aVR, V1, V4 represent surface EKG leads.

fluoroscopic guidance. In more complex arrhythmias, such as re-entrant tachycardias associated with underlying cardiomyopathy, procedural success requires correct identification of the underlying substrate and subsequent elimination of the critical part for tachycardia continuation. Mapping refers to the identification of the substrate and often requires more sophisticated techniques, including three-dimensional (3D) electroanatomical mapping, non-contact mapping, remote magnetic navigation, and intracardiac echocardiography.

Biosense CARTO® mapping system
The CARTO mapping system (Biosense, Diamond Bar, CA, USA) utilizes a low-level magnetic field (5×10^{-6} to 5×10^{-5} T) delivered from three separate coils in a locationpad positioned beneath the patient. The magnetic field strength from each coil is detected by a location sensor embedded in the tip of a specialized mapping catheter. This catheter can be moved along a chamber's surface to record local endocardial activation times relative to an arbitrarily chosen timing reference, while simultaneously recording location points to generate 3D chamber geometry (Figure 7.4). A voltage map can also be constructed to distinguish between areas of scar (which have the lowest voltage amplitude) and relatively normal tissue. Ablation sites will be tagged and this allows deployment of complex ablation strategies, such as long linear lesions (see below).

NavX® mapping system
The NavX® system (Endocardial Solutions, St Jude Medical, Inc, St Paul, MN, USA) is capable of displaying the 3D positions of multiple catheters. This is achieved by applying a low-level 5.6-kHz current through six orthogonally-located skin patches. The recorded voltage and impedance generated at each catheter's electrodes allows 3D appreciation of their location in space.

Non-contact mapping
The non-contact mapping system uses a multielectrode array catheter with 64 electrodes on its surface (Ensite; Endocardial Solutions Inc) to simultaneously record multiple areas of endocardial activation. Chamber geometry can be reconstructed by manipulating this mapping catheter within the chamber of interest. This simultaneous mapping system is particularly useful in mapping non-sustained arrhythmias and rhythm disturbances that are poorly tolerated hemodynamically.

Remote magnetic navigation
The magnetic navigation system (Niobe; Stereotaxis, Inc, St Louis, MO, USA) [5] consists of two permanent magnets capable of creating a relatively uniform magnetic field (0.08 T) on a distance of approximately 15 cm inside the chest of the patient. The mapping and ablation catheter is equipped with small permanent magnets positioned at the tip that align with the direction of the externally controlled magnetic field to enable the tip to be steered effectively.

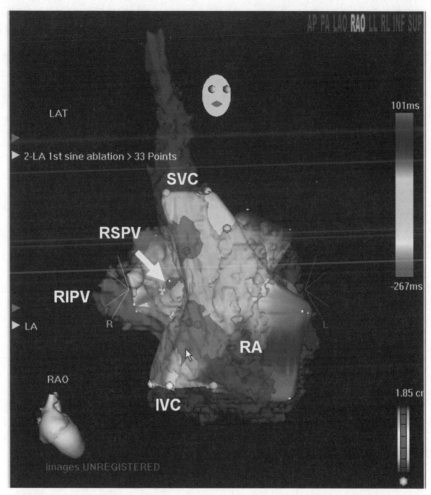

Figure 7.4 Example of three-dimensional electroanatomical mapping using CARTO (Biosense Webster). In a focal tachycardia, the activation wavefront spreads radially from the site of origin. Sequential mapping of the local activation time depicts the earliest site (arrow) just anterior to the septal pulmonary veins (right superior [RSPV] and inferior pulmonary veins [RIPV]). The right atrium (RA) is shown as well to demonstrate the spatial relationship of the superior (SVC) and inferior caval vein in relationship to the left atrium.

By changing the orientation of the outer magnets relative to each other, the orientation of the magnetic field changes and thereby leads to deflection of the catheter. In addition, a computer-controlled catheter advancer system (Cardiodrive unit; Stereotaxis Inc) is used to allow truly remote catheter navigation without the need for manual manipulation. The video workstation in conjunction with the Cardiodrive unit allows precise orientation of the catheter and is controlled by a mouse from inside the control room (Figure 7.5).

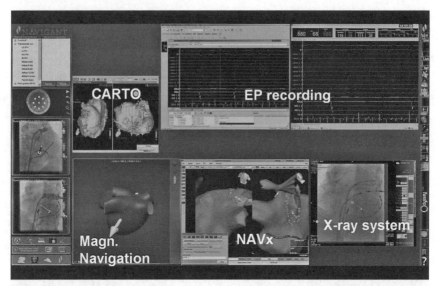

Figure 7.5 Example of a screen capture during a remote controlled atrial fibrillation procedure of the Odyssey system (Stereotaxis, Inc). All involved systems such as the fluoroscopy pictures, three-dimensional reconstructions on CARTO (Biosense Webster), three-dimensional mapping systems using NAVx technology (St Jude Medical), and the intracardiac signals (on a Bard recording system) are displayed simultaneously and are accessible using a single mouse and keyboard.

Ablation procedures

Most atrial and ventricular arrhythmias are amenable to catheter ablation. Nowadays, even complex scar-related arrhythmias can be treated with ablation with a reasonable chance of success.

"Simple" electrophysiological substrates

Catheter ablation is now first-line therapy for common re-entrant supraventricular arrhythmias (AVNRT, AVRT) and some forms of AT. The success rate is high (95%) with a relatively low risk (<3%) of major complications (AV block requiring permanent pacemaker, tamponade, stroke, myocardial infarction [MI] or patient death) and a low likelihood of recurrence (6%) [6].

Ablation for AVNRT

Targeting the slow pathway along the posteroseptal region of the tricuspid annulus is the common approach to ablate this type of arrhythmia. The endpoint for successful ablation is arrhythmia non-inducibility along with criteria for complete slow pathway ablation or slow pathway modification. In some circumstances, when arrhythmia is not inducible during the electrophysiological study, the surrogate endpoint of an accelerated junctional rhythm during ablation is a good indication of slow pathway ablation.

Ablation of an accessory pathway

For right-sided and septal accessory pathways, the tricuspid annulus is mapped using a catheter introduced most commonly from the right femoral vein. Two approaches can be considered to map the mitral annulus and ablate left-sided accessory pathways: the retrograde approach via the femoral artery and across the aortic valve to the left ventricle (LV), and trans-septal puncture with direct access to the left atrium. If the accessory pathway conducts ante-gradely, mapping along the annulus can be performed during sinus rhythm or during atrial pacing at a rate that can cause delay in the AVN and thus maximize pre-excitation. Mapping and ablation of an accessory pathway can also be performed by mapping the retrograde conduction. The aim is to locate the atrial insertion of the accessory pathway by seeking the earliest atrial electrogram during constant ventricular stimulation.

Right isthmus ablation for atrial flutter

In typical atrial flutter, the circuit passes through an anatomically well-defined channel—the isthmus between the inferior vena cava and the tricuspid annulus. To interrupt conduction across the isthmus, a series of lesions is created as the ablation catheter is gradually withdrawn from the ventricular aspect of the isthmus towards its caval end.

"Complex" electrophysiological substrates

Catheter ablation of atrial fibrillation

Catheter ablation of AF has been increasingly performed over the last decade with long-term arrhythmia control/cure rates of ~70% [7]. Catheter ablation of AF requires the introduction of multiple catheters into the heart, trans-septal catheterization, high levels of anticoagulation, and delivery of multiple lesions around the pulmonary vein ostia with or without additional atrial lines [8,9]. Major complications may occur, most significantly tamponade (1.2%), transient ischemic attack (0.53%), stroke (0.23%), and periprocedural death (0.05%) [10].

Mapping and ablation of focal tachycardias (atrial or ventricular)

Pace mapping

The origin of focal (atrial or ventricular) arrhythmias can be appreciated by comparing the 12-lead EKG morphology obtained by pacing from the mapping catheter with that during tachycardia or spontaneous ectopic beats. If the match is perfect in all 12 leads, a close proximity to the tachycardia focus is assumed and the site can be targeted for ablation. This technique is particularly useful when arrhythmia is non-sustained or poorly tolerated.

Activation mapping

During tachycardia the mapping catheter explores the earliest endocardial electrogram recorded relative to a fixed reference, which is usually the onset of the P wave or QRS complex on the surface EKG. Simultaneously, the suitable site for ablation should display a sharp initial negative deflection on the unipolar recording (QS morphology).

Mapping and ablation for macrore-entrant tachycardias (atrial or ventricular)

The purpose of mapping macrore-entrant tachycardias is to identify the circuit as well as the critical isthmus of the slow conducting zone to target the ablation. The main purpose of activation mapping during such tachycardias is to identify "mid-diastolic" potentials, which represent the slow conducting zone within the narrow isthmus of the circuit. Pace mapping is useful for identifying the exit region of the circuit.

Implantable defibrillators

Current indications for implantable cardioverter defibrillators (ICDs) derive from the inclusion criteria of several pivotal clinical trials and are included in the 2006 American College of Cardiology/American Heart Association/ European guidelines for the management of ventricular arrhythmias and the prevention of SCD [11], and are discussed below.

Technical basics

The ICD has several components: the pulse generator consisting of the battery, charging capacitor, and controlling circuitry, and specially designed leads with both rate-sensing electrodes and arrhythmia-sensing plus defibrillation coils.

Lead technology has evolved and modern ICDs now have integrated coils for defibrillation; one coil is in the distal part of the lead and lies along the diaphragmatic wall of the RV; the vector of the delivered shock is established between the can and this coil. Some leads are designed with a second coil placed within the superior vena cava, allowing a larger amount of the myocardium to be encompassed within the defibrillation field and usually resulting in less energy being required for defibrillation (lower defibrillation thresholds [DFTs]). In cases where the DFT is unacceptably high (i.e., <10-J safety margin between the DFT and the maximum output of the device), a subcutaneous array or coil can be tunneled from the pocket towards the posterolateral left chest wall. Additionally, an atrial and a LV pacemaker lead can be implanted for dual-chamber or biventricular ICDs, respectively.

The pulse generator consists of the metal housing which is the active part of the shock vector, internal circuitry, the battery (generally lasting for 5–7 years), and a high voltage capacitor for delivering the charge.

Lead integrity

Decreased values for pacing impedances might suggest lead insulation failure, whereas increased values may signify lead fracture. Shock impedance is another parameter routinely measured in ICD patients; it is an indicator of lead and circuitry integrity and its values vary between manufactures and ICD models.

Specific functions: tachyarrhythmia detection and therapy

In order to avoid inadequate device intervention, several detection algorithms have been developed to increase the ability to correctly discriminate between SVT and VT. They analyze the onset of the arrhythmia (sudden or gradual), assess stability or variability of the RR interval, or apply a morphology criterion which compares the baseline ventricular morphology to the electrogram during the arrhythmia. Dual-chamber ICDs have another important feature to help discriminate SVT from VT, which is based on analyzing atrial and ventricular rates, and the P and R relationship [12].

Apart from performing a pacing function similar to a pacemaker for treatment of bradyarrhythmias, ICDs are also able to treat tachyarrhythmias by different means: antitachycardia pacing (ATP), cardioversion, and defibrillation.

The ICD is usually programmed to deliver ATP as initial therapy in a tachycardia zone where VT is expected to be readily discriminated from an SVT, but not so fast as to lead to syncope. ATP can terminate VT in 70–75% of cases [13]. ATP works by delivering multiple extrastimuli at a rate faster than the tachycardia cycle length (TCL) and is usually only effective in terminating VT due to re-entry. Although ATP may terminate the VT, it also carries a risk of accelerating the tachycardia or converting it into polymorphic VT or VF.

The ICD can deliver shocks with a programmable amount of energy. Lower energy cardioverting shocks (5–20J) can be delivered quicker because the time required to charge the capacitor is shorter. High output devices are nowadays able to deliver up to 35–40J, which is sufficient to terminate most tachyarrhythmias.

Cardiac resynchronization

LV dyssynchrony exacerbates congestive heart failure (CHF) through inefficient ventricular contraction, ventricular dilatation, increased wall stress, and increased mitral regurgitation. Over the last decade, cardiac resynchronization therapy (CRT) with biventricular pacing has become an important therapeutic means to improve symptoms and survival in appropriately selected patients with CHF.

Lead implantation

To achieve synchronized LV contraction, an RV lead is placed at the apex of the RV against the interventricular septum and a second lead is placed epicardially in a posterolateral position via the coronary sinus, thus leading to simultaneous activation of the LV from two different sites. It may be practically difficult to insert a lateral LV because of difficulties in gaining access to the coronary sinus, but more commonly in finding a suitable lateral branch of the coronary sinus. Therefore, after the coronary sinus is successfully cannulated, a contrast venography is performed to visualize all branching veins that could be targeted for LV lead placement.

Once the lead has been placed, sensing and capture threshold testing is performed. Pacing from the LV lead should be also tested at high output in order to ensure that the phrenic nerve or lateral chest wall are not captured. Pacing from the LV lead should result in a QRS complex with right bundle branch block (RBBB) morphology, whereas pacing both RV and LV leads will likely show a narrow QRS, although this is not an absolute criterion for successful cardiac resynchronization [14].

Pacing modes

For patients in sinus rhythm, biventricular devices are usually programmed to pace in DDD mode with or without rate responsiveness, in order to preserve the beneficial effect of atrial contraction on ventricular filling. However, their hemodynamics of AV sequential pacing may differ from those of patients with spontaneous atrial activity and VDD-like functioning of the device, and the optimal paced AV delay may be much longer than the optimal sensed AV delay. Therefore, the optimal AV delay in a given patient is usually established with the use of several echocardiographic parameters [15–17].

Another important feature of the programmed AV delay is the rate responsiveness. Unlike in traditional dual-chamber pacemaker patients for whom a rate adaptive shortening of the AV delay to mirror the physiological shortening of the PR interval from increased sympathetic tone is of hemodymamic benefit, in CRT patients increased heart rate seems to require a longer AV delay from baseline to maximize cardiac output [18].

Modern CRT devices allow VV programming, with up to 80 ms offset between the LV and RV pacing. The most common programming is simultaneous LV–RV timing (VV interval 0) or a 20-ms LV pre-excitation (given that most patients who undergo CRT implantation have a baseline left bundle branch block [LBBB]). RV pre-excitation should be avoided, due to its association with decreased LV function [19].

For patients in AF, the device is usually programmed in VVIR. In order to maximize the benefit of biventricular pacing, an adequate AVN blockade should be ensured either pharmacologically or non-pharmacologically (AVN ablation).

Indications

The main indication for CRT arose from the CARE-HF study [20], the first large scale randomized study to show significant morbidity and mortality reduction in resynchronized patients with chronic CHF refractory to medical treatment, LV ejection fraction (LVEF) <35%, and LV dyssynchrony. Despite advances in echocardiography, a QRS duration of >120–130 ms is still the most widely used measure of dyssynchrony. The COMPANION (Comparison of Medical therapy, Pacing, and Defibrillation in Heart Failure) trial [21] randomly assigned patients with an LVEF of 35% or less, NYHA class III or IV, and cardiac dyssynchrony (QRS >120 ms) to optimal medical therapy, biventricular pacing alone, or biventricular pacing with a device with ICD capabilities. Patients assigned in either of the CRT arms had improvements in clinical heart failure outcomes, and those assigned to the CRT–ICD arm also had improved overall survival.

Review of key clinical trials

Defibrillators
Worldwide, approximately three million people a year suffer a sudden cardiac arrest with an estimated survival rate of less than 1%. It is estimated that in the US the survival rate for a sudden cardiac arrest is 5% [22]. Although there has been a reduction in total cardiac mortality over the last decade, the number of SCDs still exceeds the total number of deaths from AIDS, breast cancer, lung cancer, and stroke annually.

Secondary prevention of sudden cardiac death
Initial therapies utilizing ICDs were aimed at preventing SCD following the survival of an initial event. Improved technology associated with the implantation of an ICD as well as multiple studies showing dramatic success in preventing SCD led to widespread acceptance of this new therapy. Implantation of ICDs increased from around 10000 per year in 1990 up to 90000 per year in 2000. Studies showing success in secondary prevention of SCDs included: Antiarrhythmic versus Implantable defibrillators (AVID) [23], Cardiac Arrest Study Hamburg (CASH) [24], and Canadian Implantable Defibrillator Study (CIDS) [25] (Table 7.3).

AVID [23] was a large (n = 1016) multicenter trial conducted in the US and Canada comparing ICD versus antiarrhythmic drug (AAD; amiodarone). Patients enrolled into the trial were resuscitated from VT, had sustained VT with syncope or had sustained VT with an LVEF of <40% or symptoms suggesting severe hemodynamic compromise. The trial showed a significant (p < 0.02) relative reduction in all-cause mortality with ICDs after 18 months of follow-up. CIDS [25] and (CASH) [24] also showed a trend towards a lower risk of death with ICD therapy (20%; p = 0.1 and 23%; p = 0.2 relative risk reduction, respectively). Pooled analysis of the three studies demonstrated that mortality is reduced by 27% (p < 0.001) with an ICD compared with amiodarone. Moreover, deaths attributed to an arrhythmia was reduced by 51% (p < 0.001), with no difference between treatment groups in the risk of death from non-arrhythmic causes [26].

Primary prevention of sudden cardiac deaths
With the widespread acceptance of the ICD as a method of treating the survivors of SCD, attention has turned to primary prevention (Table 7.3). The earliest primary prevention trial was the Multicenter Automatic Defibrillator Implantation Trial (MADIT I) [27]. This small trial involved a direct comparison between ICD and best medical management. The patients in this study

Table 7.3 Clinical trials of implantable device therapy.

Study	Inclusion criteria	Number of patients	Study design	Endpoint	Follow-up	Results
ICD therapy in secondary prevention						
AVID [23]	Resuscitated VF, sustained VT and syncope or sustained VT with LVEF ≤0.40%	1016	Multicenter randomized study: ICD vs AAD (amiodarone)	All-cause mortality	18 months	31% relative reduction in primary endpoint with ICD (p < 0.02)
CIDS [25]	Resuscitated VF, sustained VT and syncope, sustained VT with LVEF ≤0.35% or unwitnessed syncope plus inducible VT	659	Multicenter randomized study: ICD vs amiodarone	All-cause mortality	36 months	20% relative reduction in primary endpoint with ICD (p = 0.1)
CASH [24]	Cardiac arrest secondary to VF or VT	228	Multicenter randomized study: ICD vs AAD	All-cause mortality	57 months	23% relative reduction in primary endpoint with ICD (p = 0.2)
ICD therapy for inducible ventricular arrhythmias						
MUSTT [28]	LVEF ≤0.40%, non-recent myocardial infarction (>4 days), spontaneous non-sustained VT, and inducible VT	704	Multicenter randomized study: ICD vs best medical therapy	Cardiac arrest	39 months	28% reduction in sudden cardiac death with ICD (p < 0.001)
MADIT I [27]	LVEF ≤0.35%, non-recent myocardial infarction (>3 weeks) or CABG (>3 months), spontaneous VT, and inducible VT	196	Multicenter randomized trial: ICD vs AAD (amiodarone and class I)	All-cause mortality	27 months	54% risk reduction in primary endpoint with ICD (p = 0.009)

ICD therapy in primary prevention

Trial	Inclusion criteria	n	Study design	Primary endpoint	Follow-up	Results
MADIT II [29]	NYHA class I–III, LVEF ≤0.30%, remote myocardial infarction (>1 month)	1232	Multicenter randomized study: ICD vs best medical therapy	All-cause mortality	20 months	31% relative reduction in primary endpoint with ICD (p = 0.02)
SCD-HeFT [30]	NYHA class II–III, LVEF ≤0.35%, non-recent myocardial infarction or revascularization (>30 days), non-recent heart failure onset (>3 months)	2521	Multicenter randomized study: ICD vs placebo	All-cause mortality	45.5 months	23% relative reduction in primary endpoint with ICD (p < 0.01)

Resynchronization therapy

Trial	Inclusion criteria	n	Study design	Primary endpoint	Follow-up	Results
CARE-HF [20]	NYHA class III–IV, LVEF ≤0.35%, LVEDD 30mm/m (height), QRS >150ms or QRS >120ms and echocardiographic criteria of dyssynchrony; stable optimal medical therapy	813	Multicenter randomized trial: CRT + optimal medical therapy vs optimal medical therapy alone	Composite endpoint of all-cause death and cardiovascular hospitalization	29 months	Primary endpoint reached in 39% of CRT + medical therapy patients vs 55% of medical therapy alone patients; p < 0.001
COMPANION [21]	NYHA class III–IV, LVEF ≤0.35%, non-recent myocardial infarction or cardiac revascularization surgery (>60 days), QRS >120ms, non-recent onset of heart failure (>6 months)	903	Multicenter 1:2:2 randomized trial: optimal medical therapy vs medical therapy + CRT vs medical therapy + CRT + ICD	All-cause death or hospitalization	15 months	20% relative reduction in primary end point (p = 0.01) with CRT + ICD
MADIT-CRT [34]	NYHA class I or II, ischemic or non-ischemic cardiomyopathy, LVEF ≤30%, QRS ≥130ms	1820	Multicenter 3:2 randomized trial: CRT + ICD (1089) vs ICD alone (731)	Death from any cause or a non-fatal heart failure event	28.8 months	34% reduction in primary endpoint with CRT + ICD vs ICD alone (p < 0.001)

AAD, antiarrhythmic drug; CABG, coronary artery bypass graft; CRT, cardiac resynchronization therapy; ICD, implantable cardioverter defibrillator; LVEDD, left ventricular end-diastolic diameter; LVEF, left ventricular fibrillation; VF, ventricular fibrillation;

had coronary artery disease with an LVEF of less than 35% and an abnormal electrophysiological study with inducible, non-suppressible sustained ventricular arrhythmia during programmed ventricular stimulation. This trial was stopped early after it showed a 54% relative reduction in total mortality (p = 0.009) and a 75% reduction in SCD.

In the Multicenter Unsustained Tachycardia Trial (MUSTT) [28], 704 patients with an LVEF of less than or equal to 40% and coronary artery disease were randomized to angiotensin-converting enzyme (ACE) inhibitors and beta-blockers (control group) versus best guided electrophysiological therapy. For most of these patients the best guided therapy was an ICD. This trial also resulted in a statistically significant reduction in SCD of 28% with ICD therapy.

In 2002, the MADIT II trial [29] was published. This study compared ICD versus usual care in patients with severe LV ischemic dysfunction (LVEF of ≤30%), NYHA class I–III, and no other risk stratification criteria. The study enrolled 1232 patients from 71 centers in the US and five centers in Europe, from July 1997 to January 2002. Sixty percent of patients received an ICD. Patients who had experienced a recent MI (<1 month before valuation) or revascularization procedure (≤3 months), as well as patients who had inducible sustained arrhythmia during an invasive electrophysiological study (fulfilling the criteria for MADIT I) were excluded. Patients were followed up for an average of 20 months after which period this trial was stopped when it revealed a 31% relative reduction in total mortality (p < 0.02) associated with ICD therapy. Over the 20 months, 19.8% of patients in the conventional therapy group died compared with 14.2% in the ICD group (5.4% absolute reduction).

The MADIT II researchers noted that the effect of ICD therapy was similar in subgroup analyses stratified by age, gender, ejection fraction, NYHA class, and QRS duration. However, patients with higher QRS values (>120 ms) had a larger absolute and relative risk reduction that trended towards statistical significance. Nevertheless, it has been suggested that the QRS duration should not be used alone, but rather along with other non-invasive risk assessment tools, such T-wave alternance or heart rate, to further stratify patients likely to benefit from an ICD.

In 2004 and early 2005, several trials focused on the primary prevention of SCD in patients with coronary artery disease as well as patients with non-ischemic dilated cardiomyopathy. The Sudden Cardiac Death in Heart Failure (SCD-HeFT) trial [30] enrolled 2521 patients with an LVEF of 35% or less at 148 sites in the US, Canada, and New Zealand from September 1997 until July 2001, and they were followed for a median of 45.5 months. These patients were randomized to best medical therapy (n = 847), amiodarone (n = 845) or ICD (n = 829). A similar proportion of patients with ischemic (52%) and non-ischemic (48%) etiologies of LV dysfunction were enrolled. Twenty-nine percent of patients died in the placebo group, 28% in the amiodarone group, and 22% in the ICD group. As compared with placebo, amiodarone was associated with a similar risk of death, while ICD therapy was associated with a decreased risk of death over a placebo or amiodarone of 23% (p = 0.007) and an absolute decrease in mortality of 7.2% after 5 years in the overall population, indicating that almost 14 patients would need to be treated with an ICD to prevent one death during that time. Results did not vary according to either ischemic or non-ischemic causes of CHF, but they did vary according to the NYHA class: ICD therapy had a significant benefit in patients in NYHA class II but not in those in NYHA class III, whereas amiodarone therapy had no benefit in patients in NYHA class II and decreased survival among patients in NYHA class III, as compared to those who received placebo.

Time-dependent benefit

All of the patients in MADIT I and MADIT II, and almost all of those in MUSTT, were enrolled more than 3 weeks after they had had a MI. The DINAMIT trial [31] specifically addressed the potential benefit of ICD implantation in patients with a reduced LVEF (<35%) in the early period after an MI. Patients were randomly assigned to a study group 6–40 days after an MI, with a mean interval of 18 days between the MI and enrolment. Despite the higher risk of sudden death from cardiac causes in the early period after an MI, there was no reduction in all-cause mortality in the group that received an ICD. These data, along with those derived from MADIT II (no benefit from ICD therapy was evident among patients whose MI occurred <18 months before enrolment) and SCD-HeFT (the survival curves did not diverge until after the first year), suggest that ICD therapy may not be effective early after MI, possibly due to the different mechanisms of death early after MI.

Cardiac resynchronization

When it accompanies heart failure due to systolic dysfunction, QRS delay adds significant morbidity and mortality. Affecting 30–50% of patients with NYHA class III or IV heart failure, QRS duration, especially of LBBB morphology, adversely affects the cardiac function by introducing intraventricular dyssynchrony. Previous studies of cardiac resynchronization therapy devices published between 2001 and 2003 [32,33] showed significant improvements in symptoms, functional status, quality of life, heart failure progression, ventricular function, and morbidity in these patients; subsequent trials (Cardiac Resynchronisation Heart Failure [CARE-HF] and Comparison of Medical therapy, Pacing and Defibrillation in Patients with Chronic Congestive Heart Failure [COMPANION]) demonstrated that CRT not only provides significant symptomatic improvements in these patients but also better prognostic outcomes by reducing total mortality (Table 7.3).

The CARE-HF study [20] enrolled 813 patients with an LVEF of less than or equal to 35%, QRS duration greater than 150 ms or QRS duration greater than 120 ms and echocardiographic criteria of dyssynchrony, NYHA class III or IV, and stable optimal medical therapy. Patients were randomized either to CRT plus optimal medical therapy or to optimal medical therapy alone. Over a mean follow-up of 29 months, CRT resulted in significant reduction in the primary composite endpoint of death or cardiovascular hospitalization. Additionally, reduction in the secondary endpoint of mortality was achieved.

The COMPANION trial [21] included patients with both coronary artery disease and dilated cardiomyopathy with LVEFs equal to or less than 35% and a QRS duration of greater than 120 ms. A total of 1520 patients who had advanced heart failure (NYHA class III or IV) due to ischemic or non-ischemic cardiomyopathies and a QRS interval of at least 120 ms were randomly assigned in a 1:2:2 ratio to receive optimal pharmacological therapy (diuretics, ACE inhibitors, beta-blockers, and spironolactone) alone or in combination with CRT with either a pacemaker or a pacemaker–defibrillator. The primary composite endpoint was the time to death from or hospitalization for any cause. As compared with optimal pharmacological therapy alone, CRT with a pacemaker decreased the risk of the primary endpoint (HR, 0.81; p = 0.014), as did CRT with a pacemaker–defibrillator (HR, 0.80; p = 0.01). The risk of the combined endpoint of death from or hospitalization for heart failure was reduced by 34% in the pacemaker group (p < 0.002) and by 40% in the pacemaker–defibrillator group (p < 0.001 for the comparison with the pharmacological therapy group). A pacemaker reduced the risk of the secondary endpoint of death from any cause by 24% (p = 0.059), and a pacemaker–defibrillator reduced the risk by 36% (p = 0.003). This therapy held true for both dilated cardiomyopathy and coronary artery disease patients.

In light of the SCD-HeFT, COMPANION, and MADIT II data, patients with ischemic or idiopathic dilated cardiomyopathy (diagnosed for at least 9 months) with an LVEF of 35% or less and NYHA class II or III are now indicated for an ICD as a primary prevention strategy for SCD. Class III and IV patients with an LVEF of less than 35% and prolonged QRS duration benefit from CRT–ICD implantation. NYHA class IV patients are now indicated for an ICD if they meet the requirements for CRT.

The Multicenter Automatic Defibrillator Implantation Trial with Cardiac Resynchronization Therapy (MADIT-CRT) [34] was designed to determine whether prophylactic CRT in combination with an ICD would reduce the risk of death or non-fatal heart failure events (whichever occurred first) in patients with ischemic or non-ischemic cardiomyopathy, an LVEF of 30% or less, a QRS duration of 130 ms or more, and NYHA class I or II symptoms, as compared with patients receiving only an ICD. The 1820 enrolled patients were randomly assigned in a 3:2 ratio to receive CRT plus an ICD (1089 patients) or an ICD alone (731 patients). The primary composite endpoint was death from any cause or a non-fatal heart failure event. During an average follow-up of 2.4 years, the primary endpoint occurred in 187 of 1089 patients in the CRT–ICD group (17.2%) and in 185 of 731 patients in the ICD-only group (25.3%) (HR in the CRT–ICD group, 0.66; p = 0.001). The benefit did not differ significantly between those patients with ischemic cardiomyopathy and those with non-ischemic cardiomyopathy. The superiority of CRT was driven by a 41% reduction in the risk of heart failure events, a finding that was evident primarily in a prespecified subgroup of patients with a QRS duration of 150 ms or more. CRT was associated with a significant reduction in LV volumes and improvement in the ejection fraction.

This study provided evidence that preventive CRT–ICD therapy decreases the risk of heart failure events in vulnerable patients with ischemic or non-ischemic heart disease who have minimal heart failure symptoms but a wide QRS complex.

Review of key trials evaluating atrial fibrillation ablation versus medical therapy

AF is the most frequent arrhythmia encountered in clinical practice, affecting 0.4% of the population and associated with increased mortality [35]. Over the last decades, efforts have been made to identify the best treatment strategy that could improve symptoms and mortality in patients with AF. Although rhythm-control and rate-control strategies [36,37] demonstrated similar efficacy in terms of morbidity/mortality, both in patients with normal (Atrial Fibrillation Follow-Up Investigation of Rhythm Management [AFFIRM] study [36]) or impaired LV function (AF-CHF study), 25–35% of patients with AF who are rate-controlled will continue to have activity-limiting symptoms, whereas the use of AADs is hampered by their limited efficacy and potential for toxic effects. Indeed, more than 35% of patients have relapses of AF despite the best AAD regimen and 11–28% of them experience adverse reactions leading to drug discontinuation, as highlighted by the AFFIRM () [36] and Canadian Trial of Atrial Fibrillation (CTAF) [38] results; the overall efficacy of AADs is probably about 39% [36], although the success rate of pharmacological therapy in drug-naïve patients may reach 65% [38]. Moreover, it appears that maintenance of sinus rhythm is associated with a 47% reduction in the risk of death, whereas use of AAD therapy is associated with a 49% increase in mortality [39].

In patients with paroxysmal or short-duration persistent AF who have had limited prior drug exposure, 20–40% of those treated with class I drugs or sotalol and 60–70% of those treated with amiodarone have no recurrence of AF at 1 year [38,40,41]. Interestingly, failure of prior AAD treatment (due to either recurrence or intolerance) has been shown to predict failure of subsequent attempts at pharmacological rhythm control, irrespective of the type of AAD [42]. Circumferential pulmonary vein ablation (CPVA) has emerged as a therapeutic alternative to AADs for maintaining sinus rhythm without exposing patients to the detrimental effects of AADs. Several studies have compared radiofrequency catheter ablation of AF to AADs, some of which are still ongoing (Table 7.4).

The CACAF study (Catheter ablation treatment in patients with drug refractory atrial fibrillation) [43] was a multicenter, prospective, controlled, randomized trial which enrolled 137 patients to investigate the adjunctive role of ablation therapy to AAD therapy in preventing AF relapses in patients with paroxysmal or persistent AF in whom pharmacological treatment had already failed. Overall, one-third of the patients had persistent AF and over 60% had a structural heart disease, although most of them had well-preserved systolic function. Patients were randomized to a single catheter ablation plus AAD

Table 7.4 Clinical trials of radiofrequency ablation versus medical therapy of atrial fibrillation.

Study	Inclusion criteria	Number of patients	Study design	Endpoint	Follow-up	Results (ablation vs AAD)
CACAF [43]	Paroxysmal/persistent AF; at least one AAD failure	137	Multicenter randomized study: ablation +AAD vs AAD alone	AF recurrence	1 year	44.1% vs 91.3% recurrence (p < 0.001)
APAF [44]	Paroxysmal AF; at least one AAD failure	198	Single-center randomized study: ablation vs AAD	AF recurrence	1 year	7% vs 65% recurrence (p < 0.001)
A4 [45]	Paroxysmal AF; at least one AAD failure	112	Randomized multicenter study: ablation vs AAD	AF recurrence	1 year	11% vs 77% recurrence (p < 0.001)
ThermoCool AF [46]	Paroxysmal AF; at least one AAD failure	167	Multicenter, 2:1 randomized trial: ablation vs AAD	Treatment failure (AF recurrence need for repeat ablation, absence of entrance block in the PVs, and/or changes in the drug regimen)	9 months	34% vs 84% recurrence (p < 0.001)
RAAFT (pilot trial) [50]	Paroxysmal AF; drug-naïve patients	70	Randomized trial	AF recurrence	6 months	13% vs 63% recurrence (p < 0.01)

AAD, antiarrhythmic drug; AF, atrial fibrillation; PV, pulmonary vein.

(ablation group; n = 68) or AAD alone (control group; n = 69). After 1 year of follow-up, 91.3% patients in the control group had had at least one AF recurrence, whereas only 44.1% patients (p < 0.001) in ablation group had had a recurrence, thus demonstrating the superiority of the ablative therapy combined with AAD therapy over AAD therapy alone in preventing atrial arrhythmia recurrences. The only identified significant predictor of AF recurrence was the medical therapy (HR for medical therapy/ablation 3.2; 95% CI, 2.0–5.1).

The APAF trial (A randomized trial of circumferential pulmonary vein ablation versus antiarrhythmic drug therapy in paroxysmal atrial fibrillation) [44] was a controlled, randomized, single-center study including 198 patients with paroxysmal AF (mean age, 56 ± 10 years) who had failed at least one AAD designed to compare the relative efficacy of CPVA and AAD in the treatment of patients with paroxysmal AF. Ninety-nine patients were assigned to each group and most of them had a normal underlying heart with preserved LV systolic function. By Kaplan–Meier analysis, 86% of the patients randomized to CPVA needed only a single procedure and were arrhythmia-free at the end of follow-up, as compared to the 22% of patients randomized to AAD (p < 0.001). By monthly rhythm analysis that also took into account the outcome of the second procedure in the ablation group and patients controlled with combined therapy in the AAD group, 93% and 35% of the CPVA and AAD groups, respectively, were free from atrial tachyarrhythmias at 1 year. A second ablation was performed in 9% of patients in the CPVA group for recurrent AF (6%) or atrial tachycardia (3%); 42 patients in the AAD group crossed over to CPVA. Ejection fraction, hypertension, and AF duration independently predicted AF recurrences in the AAD group, with no independent predictors of AF relapses identified in the ablation group.

The A4 study (Atrial fibrillation ablation versus antiarrhythmic drugs) [45] was a randomized multicenter trial comparing ablative therapy versus pharmacological treatment in patients with paroxysmal AF who had failed at least one AAD. The primary endpoint was absence of recurrent AF between months 3 and 12, absence of recurrent AF after up to three ablation procedures, or changes in AADs during the first 3 months. One hundred and twelve patients (16% women; mean age 51.1 ± 11.1 years) were enrolled and randomized to ablation (n = 53) or "new" AAD alone or in combination (n = 59), 24% of whom had background cardiopathy with a mean LVEF of 64.3 ± 9.4%. Crossover between the AAD and ablation groups occurred in 37 (63%) and five patients (9%), respectively. Redo procedures were performed in 23 patients. At the 1-year follow-up, no recurrence of AF was reported in 23% and 89% of the AAD and ablation groups, respectively (p < 0.0001). Symptom score, exercise capacity, and quality of life were significantly improved in the ablation group, probably due to the reduction in AF burden as well as to the discontinuation of AADs. In multivariate analyses, a higher baseline ejection fraction (OR, 1.10; 95% CI, 1.01–1.19; p = 0.02) was the only independent predictor of no AF recurrences after ablation. The baseline LVEF was 56.2 ± 10.4% in the 13 patients who failed catheter ablation compared with $65.3 \pm 10.4\%$ in the 40 patients with a successful outcome ($p = 0.02$).

Results of a prospective, multicenter, randomized (2:1), unblinded, Bayesian-designed study have been recently published [46]. The ThermoCool AF Trial was conducted in 19 centers and enrolled 167 patients who did not respond to at least one AAD and who experienced at least three AF episodes within the 6 months prior to randomization. The clinical profile of these patients was similar to that for patients enrolled in previously outlined studies. The primary endpoint was freedom from protocol-defined treatment failure, which included documented symptomatic paroxysmal AF during the effectiveness evaluation period. Repeated ablation beyond 80 days after the initial ablation, absence of entrance block confirmed in all pulmonary veins at the end of the ablation procedure, or changes in specified drug regimen postblanking (including class I/III drugs, ACE inhibitors, angiotensin II receptor blockers, and AV nodal blockers) were also considered treatment failures, even if they remained free from symptomatic paroxysmal AF. In the AAD group, an adverse event requiring discontinuation of the assigned drug was also considered a treatment failure. At the end of the 9-month effectiveness evaluation period, 66% of patients in the catheter ablation group remained free from protocol-defined treatment failure compared with 16% of patients treated with an AAD. The hazard ratio of catheter ablation to AAD was 0.30 (95% CI, 0.19–0.47; $p < 0.001$). In the AAD group, of the 47 patients who had protocol-defined treatment failures, 36 subsequently underwent catheter ablation. Mean quality of life scores improved significantly in patients treated with catheter ablation compared to an AAD at 3 months and remained so during the course of the study.

Although the results of these studies are encouraging and they all converge towards promising results with radiofrequency catheter ablation of AF with a relatively favorable safety profile, several issues still remain to be answered. First, the results of these trials cannot be extrapolated to patients with significant LV dysfunction, more persistent or permanent forms of AF, and advanced degrees of heart failure, as these categories of patient were generally excluded from these studies. Study patients were relatively young with a lower incidence of cardiovascular comorbidity compared to the general population of patients with AF. Oral *et al.* [47] investigated the benefit of CPVA in addition to amiodarone in a randomized, two-center, controlled study enrolling 146 patients with chronic AF, and demonstrated significantly better outcomes with regard to maintaining sinus rhythm with radiofrequency ablation of AF in addition to amiodarone than with AAD alone after 1-year follow-up. Furthermore, restoration and maintenance of sinus rhythm was associated with a significant increase in LVEF at 12-month follow-up relative to baseline. This finding is consistent with those reported by other studies [48,49], which also showed non-inferior results with regard to maintaining sinus rhythm in patients with AF and impaired LVEF when compared with patients with normal LV systolic function.

Second, different ablation strategies may lead to different outcomes. Although CPVA is the general term used for catheter ablation of AF, different ablation techniques were used in these studies. Wazni *et al.* [50] used electrical isolation of the pulmonary veins (pulmonary vein isolation) as the endpoint of ablation, whereas circumferential anatomical ablation around both ipsilateral veins using 3D mapping was the technique used in other studies [45,44]. The feasibility of circumferential ipsilateral vein ablation using 3D mapping and the double-Lasso technique was previously established [51,52] and the superiority of this strategy compared to individual pulmonary vein isolation subsequently demonstrated [53].

Third, the long-term efficacy of radiofrequency ablation of AF is not currently known. The effectiveness of ablation may decrease with longer follow-up, although short-term efficacy (in most studies the duration of follow-up was 1 year) appears to be reasonably good, even though more than one procedure and adjunctive AAD use are often required. The only longer-term data are from a single-center trial showing good results beyond 2.5 years [54].

Fourth, the role of catheter ablation as first-line therapy for AF remains a matter of debate. The ongoing multicenter, prospective, randomized RAAFT trial (Radiofrequency ablation versus antiarrhythmic drugs as first line treatment of symptomatic atrial fibrillation: A randomised trial) is investigating the feasibility of radiofrequency catheter ablation as first-line therapy for patients with symptomatic AF. The primary endpoint is any recurrence of symptomatic AF or asymptomatic AF lasting longer than 15 s over the 1-year follow-up period. The pilot phase of this trial [50] unraveled some promising prospective data on ablation in drug-naïve patients compared to AAD therapy of AF; it randomized 70 patients, mostly with paroxysmal AF, who had not received AAD therapy prior to ablation (n = 33; mean age, 53 ± 8 years) or AAD (n = 37; mean age, 54 ± 8 years). At the end of the first follow-up year, there was a statistically significant difference in recurrence of symptomatic AF (13% vs 63%; p < 001), and hospital admissions for AF (9% vs 54%; p < 001), favoring radiofrequency ablation. At 6-month follow-up, the improvement in quality of life of patients in the ablation group was significantly better than that noted in the AAD group in five subclasses of the Short-Form 36 health survey.

The main concern in offering a first-line ablation procedure to treat AF is that these procedures are not devoid of potential complications. A recent worldwide survey [55] of more than 8000 AF ablation procedures reported an overall major complication rate of 6%. These complications include femoral pseudoaneurysm, AV fistula, pneumothorax, hemothorax, transient ischemic attack, phrenic nerve paralysis, and cardiac tamponade. The most serious complications resulting in permanent disability were uncommon (death in 0.05% and stroke in 0.28%). Significant pulmonary vein stenosis was reported in 1.3%, but this can be treated with percutaneous interventional procedures. A recently recognized complication of catheter-based AF ablation is left atrial–esophageal fistula, a life-threatening condition. It should also be noted that various ablation techniques have been used over time and the incidence of different complications is likely to decrease with the implementation of more sophisticated techniques and with more experience.

The most recent European Society of Cardiology guidelines for the management of patients with AF [56] recommend second-line catheter ablation in patients with symptomatic paroxysmal/persistent AF who have previously failed a trial of AAD (class IIa indication), whereas ablation as initial treatment may be considered in selected patients with symptomatic paroxysmal AF despite adequate rate control and no significant underlying heart disease (class IIb indication, level of evidence B).

Lastly, there are no long-term follow-up data showing a reduction in the risk of stroke in patients apparently cured of AF with catheter ablation and only few data support a reduction in mortality with AF ablation [54]. Whether long-term maintenance of sinus rhythm post CPVA converts into better survival in this category of patients is yet to be proven.

Some of these unsolved issues will be more definitively addressed in upcoming large-scale clinical trials, such as Catheter Ablation versus Antiarrhythmic Drug Therapy for Atrial Fibrillation (CABANA). The multicenter CABANA trial, with a planned recruitment of 3000 patients in Europe and the US and a primary endpoint of all-cause mortality, is designed to examine specifically the impact of AF ablation on survival. Secondary outcomes will include decrease in the composite endpoint of total mortality, disabling stroke, serious bleeding, and cardiac arrest in patients with untreated or incompletely treated AF warranting therapy, cardiovascular death, freedom from recurrent AF, composite adverse events, cardiovascular hospitalization, arrhythmic death, heart failure death, quality of life, and left atrial size. This trial will include patients with different forms of AF (paroxysmal, persistent, or permanent) either over 65 years old or younger than 65 years with hypertension, low LVEF, prior stroke, or prior transient ischemic attack. Patients will be randomized to catheter ablation or pharmacological therapy (rate or rhythm control) as first-line treatment. All patients will be anticoagulated and crossovers will not be allowed. The planned follow-up is a minimum of 3.5 years. The total trial duration is 6 years. Interestingly, the patient profile is similar to that in the AFFIRM study; although this population represents the majority of patients with AF, data regarding safety and efficacy of the ablative techniques in this category are scarce. As further data from this study become available, we hope to be able to expand the indications for radiofrequency ablation to a broader population in the future.

Conclusion

Over the last decade, treatment strategies for AF have evolved considerably. Pharmacological therapy for rhythm control faces a number of limitations, mainly related to its marginal efficacy and potential for side effects, restricting its utilization. Moreover, several trials directly comparing ablation with pharmacological therapy have demonstrated superiority of ablative therapy with regard to maintaining the sinus rhythm, favoring invasive therapy of AF in patients with persistent or paroxysmal forms. However, there are still questions about the type of population to which these procedures can be offered. Results of several ongoing major trials will hopefully allow us to identify which category of patients with AF may benefit from radiofrequency ablation as first-line therapy, the place for medical treatment, and when a rate-controlling strategy should be considered. The long-term impact of these procedures, particularly on the incidence of stroke and mortality, remains to be proven.

Disclaimer

S.E. is a consultant to Biosense Webster, Siemens, St. Jude Medical, Medtronic, and Stereotaxis.

References

1. Calkins H, Langberg J, Sousa J, et al. Radiofrequency catheter ablation of accessory atrioventricular connections in 250 patients. Abbreviated therapeutic approach to Wolff-Parkinson-White syndrome. *Circulation* 1992;85:1337–1346.
2. Wolf PA, Abbot RD, Kannel WB. Atrial fibrillation as an independent risk factor for stroke: The Framingham Study. *Stroke* 1991;74:236–241.
3. Haïssaguerre M, Jaïs P, Shah DC, et al. Spontaneous initiation of atrial fibrillation by ectopic beats originating in the pulmonary veins. *N Engl J Med* 1998;339:659–666.
4. Guidelines for cardiac pacing and cardiac resynchronisation therapy. *Europace* 2007; 9:959–998.
5. Ernst S, Ouyang F, Linder C, et al. Initial experience with remote catheter ablation using a novel magnetic navigation system: magnetic remote catheter ablation. *Circulation* 2004;109;1472–1475.
6. Calkins H, Yong P, Miller JM, et al. Catheter ablation of accessory pathways, atrioventricular nodal reentrant tachycardia, and the atrioventricular junction: final results of a prospective, multicenter clinical trial. The Atakr Multicenter Investigators Group. *Circulation* 1999;99:262–270.
7. Fuster V, Rydén LE, Cannom DS, et al. ACC/AHA/ESC 2006 Guidelines for the Management of Patients with Atrial Fibrillation: a report of the American College of Cardiology/ American Heart Association Task Force on Practice Guidelines and the European Society of Cardiology Committee for Practice Guidelines (Writing Committee to Revise the 2001 Guidelines for the Management of Patients With Atrial Fibrillation): developed in collaboration with the European Heart Rhythm Association and the Heart Rhythm Society. *Circulation* 2006;114:e257–354.
8. O'Neill MD, Jais P, Hocini M, et al. Catheter ablation for atrial fibrillation. *Circulation* 2007;116:1515–1523.
9. Stabile G, Bertaglia E, Senatore G, et al. Catheter ablation treatment in patients with drug-refractory atrial fibrillation: a prospective, multicentre, randomized, controlled study (Catheter Ablation for the Cure of Atrial Fibrillation Study). *Eur Heart J* 2006; 27:216–221.
10. Cappato R, Calkins H, Chen S-A, et al. Worldwide survey on the methods, efficacy, and safety of catheter ablation for human atrial fibrillation. *Circulation* 2005;111:1100–1105.
11. ACC/AHA/ESC 2006 guidelines for the management of patients with ventricular arrhythmias and the prevention of sudden cardiac death. A report of the American

College of Cardiology / American Heart Association Task Force and the European Society of Cardiology Committee for Practice Guidelines. *Europace* 2006;8:746–837.

12. Horduna I, Khairy P. Discrimination algorithms and arrhythmia detection. In: Al-Ahmad A, Ellenbogen K, Wang P, Natale A. *Pacemakers and Implantable Cardioverter Defibrillators: an Experts Manual*. Cardiotext, 2010.

13. Wathen MS, DeGroot PJ, Sweeney MO, *et al*. Prospective randomized multicenter trial of empirical antitachycardia pacing versus shocks for spontaneous rapid ventricular tachycardia in patients with implantable cardioverter-defibrillators. Pacing Fast Ventricular Tachycardia Reduces Shock Therapies (PainFREE Rx II) trial results. *Circulation* 2004;110:2591–2596.

14. Barold SS, Giudici MC, Herweg B, *et al*. Diagnostic value of 12 lead electrocardiogram during conventional and biventricular pacing for cardiac resynchronisation. *Cardiol Clin* 2006;24:471–490.

15. Ritter P, Daubert C, Mabo P, *et al*. Haemodynamic beneficial benefit of rate-adapted A-V delay in dual chamber pacing. *Eur Heart J* 1989;10:637–646.

16. Lane RE, Chow AWC, Chin D, *et al*. Selection and optimisation of biventricular pacing: the role of echocardiography. *Heart* 2004;90 (Suppl 6):vi10–vi16.

17. Jansen AH, Bracke FA, Van Dantzig JM, *et al*. Correlation of echo-Doppler optimisation of atrioventricular delay in cardiac resynchronisation therapy with invasive hemodynamics in patients with heart failure secondary to ischemic or idiopathic dilated cardiomyopathy. *Am J Cardiol* 2006;97:552–557.

18. Scharf C, Li P, Muntwyler J, *et al*. Rate-dependent AV delay optimisation in cardiac resynchronisation therapy. *Pacing Clin Electrophysiol* 2005;28:279–284.

19. Sogaard P, Ebebald H, Pedersen AK, *et al*. Sequential versus simultaneous biventricular resynchronisation for severe heart failure: evaluation by tissue Doppler imaging. *Circulation* 2002;106:2078–2084.

20. Cleland JG, Daubert JC, Erdmann E, *et al*. Cardiac Resynchronisation Heart Failure (CARE-HF) Study Investigators: the effect of cardiac resynchronisation on morbidity and mortality in heart failure. *N Engl J Med* 2005;352:1539–1549.

21. Salukhe TV, Francis DP, Sutton R. Comparison of medical therapy, pacing and defibrillation in heart failure (COMPANION) trial. *Int J Cardiol* 2003;87:119–120.

22. Zhi-Jie Z, Croft JB, Giles WH, *et al*. Sudden cardiac death in the United States, 1989–1998. *Circulation* 2001;104:2158–2163.

23. The Antiarrhythmics Versus Implantable Defibrillators (AVID) Investigators. A comparison of antiarrhythmic-drug therapy with implantable defibrillators in patients resuscitated from near-fatal ventricular arrhythmias. *N Engl J Med* 1997;337:1576–1584.

24. Kuck KH, Cappato R, Siebels J, Reppel R for the CASH investigators. Randomized comparison of antiarrhythmic drug therapy with implantable defibrillators in patients resuscitated from cardiac arrest. *Circulation* 2000;102:748–754.

25. Connolly SJ, Gent M, Roberts RS, *et al*. Canadian implantable defibrillator study (CIDS): a randomized trial of the implantable cardioverter defibrillator against amiodarone. *Circulation* 2000;101:1297–1302.

26. Connolly SJ, Hallstrom AP, Cappato R, *et al*. Meta-analysis of the implantable cardioverter secondary prevention trials. AVID, CASH and CIDS studies. *Eur Heart J* 2000;21:2071–2078.

27. Moss AJ, Hall WJ, Cannom DS, *et al*. Improved survival with an implanted defibrillator in patients with coronary disease at high risk for ventricular arrhythmia. Multicenter Automatic Defibrillator Implantation Trial Investigators. *N Engl J Med* 1996;335: 1933–1940.

28. Buxton AE, Lee KL, Fisher JD, Josephson ME, Prystowsky EN, Hafley G. A randomized study of the prevention of sudden death in patients with coronary artery disease. Multicenter Unsustained Tachycardia Trial Investigators. *N Engl J Med* 1999;341:1882–1890.
29. Moss AJ, Zareba W, Hall WJ, *et al.* Prophylactic implantation of a defibrillator in patients with myocardial infarction and reduced ejection fraction. *N Engl J Med* 2002;346: 877–883.
30. Bardy GH, Lee KL, Mark DB, *et al.* Amiodarone or an implantable cardioverter-defibrillator for congestive heart failure. *N Engl J Med* 2005:352:225–237.
31. Hohnloser SH, Kuck KH, Dorian P, *et al.* Prophylactic use of an implantable cardioverter–defibrillator after acute myocardial infarction. *N Engl J Med* 2004;351:2481–2488.
32. Higgins SL, Hummel JD, Niazi IK, *et al.* Cardiac resynchronisation therapy for the treatment of heart failure in patients with intraventricular conduction delay and malignant ventricular tachyarrhythmias (CONTAK study). *J Am Coll Cardiol* 2003;42:1454–1459.
33. Abraham WT, Young JB, Leon AR, *et al.*, on behalf of the multicenter InSync ICD II study group (MIRACLE ICD II). Effects of cardiac resynchronization on disease progression in patients with left ventricular systolic dysfunction, an indication for an implantable cardioverter-defibrillator, and mildly symptomatic chronic heart failure. *Circulation* 2004;110:2864–2868.
34. Moss AJ, Hall WJ, Cannom DS, *et al.* for the MADIT-CRT Trial Investigators. Cardiac-Resynchronization Therapy for the Prevention of Heart-Failure Events. *N Engl J Med* 2009;361:1329–1338.
35. Kannel WB, Abbott RD, Savage DD, McNamara PM. Epidemiologic features of chronic atrial fibrillation: the Framingham Study. *N Engl J Med* 1982;306:1018–1022.
36. Wyse DG, Waldo AL, DiMarco JP, *et al.* A comparison of rate control and rhythm control in patients with atrial fibrillation. *N Engl J Med* 2002;347:1825–1833.
37. Roy D, Talajic M, Nattel S, *et al.* Rhythm Control versus Rate Control for Atrial Fibrillation and Heart Failure for the Atrial fibrillation and Congestive Heart Failure Investigators. *N Engl J Med* 2008;358:2667–2677.
38. Roy D, Talajic M, Dorian P, *et al.* Canadian Trial of Atrial Fibrillation Investigators. Amiodarone to prevent recurrence of atrial fibrillation. *N Engl J Med* 2000;342:913–920.
39. Corley SD, Epstein AE, DiMarco JP, *et al.* Relationships between sinus rhythm, treatment, and survival in the Atrial Fibrillation Follow-up Investigation of Rhythm Management (AFFIRM) Study. *Circulation* 2004;109:1509–1513.
40. AFFIRM First Antiarrhythmic Drug Substudy Investigators. Maintenance of sinus rhythm in patients with atrial fibrillation. *J Am Coll Cardiol* 2003;42:20–29.
41. Singh BN, Singh SN, Reda DJ, *et al.* Amiodarone versus Sotalol for atrial fibrillation. *N Engl J Med* 2005;352:1861–1872.
42. Curtis AB, Seals AA, Safford RE, *et al.* Clinical factors associated with abandonment of a rate-control or rhythm-control strategy for the management of atrial fibrillation in the AFFIRM study. *Am Heart J* 2005;149:304–308.
43. Stabile G, Bertaglia E, Senatore G, *et al.* Catheter ablation treatment in patients with drug refractory atrial fibrillation: a prospective, multicentre, randomized, controlled study (Catheter Ablation for the Cure of Atrial Fibrillation study). *Eur Heart J* 2006;27: 216–221.
44. Pappone C, Augello G, Sala S, *et al.* A randomized trial of circumferential pulmonary vein ablation versus antiarrhythmic drug therapy in paroxysmal atrial fibrillation: the APAF Study. *J Am Coll Cardiol* 2006;48:2340–2347.
45. Jais P, Cauchemez B, Macle L, *et al.* Atrial fibrillation ablation versus antiarrhythmic drugs: A multicenter randomized trial. *Circulation* 2008;118:2498–2505.

46. Wilber DJ, Pappone C, Neuzil P, *et al*. Comparison of antiarrhythmic drug therapy and radiofrequency catheter ablation in patients with paroxysmal atrial fibrillation. *JAMA* 2010;303:333–340.

47. Oral H, Pappone C, Chugh A, *et al*. Circumferential pulmonary-vein ablation for chronic atrial fibrillation. *N Engl J Med* 2006;354:934–941.

48. Hsu L-F, Jaïs P, Sanders P, *et al*. Catheter ablation for atrial fibrillation in congestive heart failure. *N Engl J Med* 2004;351:2373–2383.

49. Chen MS, Marrouche NF, Khaykin Y, *et al*. Pulmonary vein isolation for the treatment of atrial fibrillation in patients with impaired systolic function. *J Am Coll Cardiol* 2004;43:1004–1009.

50. Wazni OM, Marrouche NF, Martin DO, *et al*. Radiofrequency ablation vs antiarrhythmic drugs as first-line treatment of symptomatic atrial fibrillation: a randomized trial. *JAMA* 2005;293:2634–2640.

51. Ouyang F, Bänsch D, Ernst S, *et al*. Complete isolation of the left atrium surrounding the pulmonary veins: new insights from the double Lasso technique in paroxysmal atrial fibrillation. *Circulation* 2004;110:2090–2096.

52. Ouyang F, Ernst S, Chun J, *et al*. Electrophysiological findings during ablation of persistent atrial fibrillation with electroanatomical mapping and double Lasso catheter technique. *Circulation* 2005;112:3038–3048.

53. Arentz T, Weber R, Bürkle G, *et al*. Small or Large Isolation Areas Around the Pulmonary Veins for the Treatment of Atrial Fibrillation? Results From a Prospective Randomized Study. *Circulation* 2007;115:3057–3063.

54. Pappone C, Rosanio S, Augello G, *et al*. Mortality, morbidity, and quality of life after circumferential pulmonary vein ablation for atrial fibrillation: outcomes from a controlled nonrandomized long-term study. *J Am Coll Cardiol* 2003;42:185–197.

55. Cappato R, Calkins H, Chen SA, *et al*. Worldwide survey on the methods, efficacy, and safety of catheter ablation for human atrial fibrillation. *Circulation* 2005;111:1100–1105.

56. European Heart Rhythm Association; European Association for Cardio-Thoracic Surgery, Camm AJ, Kirchhof P, Gregory YH, *et al*. Guidelines for the management of atrial fibrillation. The Task Force for the Management of Atrial Fibrillation of the European Society of Cardiology (ESC). *Eur Heart J* 2011;32:1172.

CHAPTER 8

Percutaneous coronary intervention

Dharam J. Kumbhani[1,2] and Deepak L. Bhatt[1-3]
[1]Brigham and Women's Hospital, Boston, MA, USA
[2]Harvard Medical School, Boston, MA, USA
[3]VA Boston Healthcare System, Boston, MA, USA

Introduction

Percutaneous coronary intervention (PCI) broadly refers to percutaneous transluminal coronary angioplasty (PTCA) or balloon angioplasty, usually along with the use of stents or other coronary devices. Historically, the first balloon angioplasty in humans was performed by Dr Andreas Gruentzig in 1977 in Zurich, Switzerland, when he passed a prototype, fixed-wire balloon catheter across a severe lesion in the left anterior descending artery (LAD) [1]. The first randomized trial comparing PTCA with conventional therapy for chronic angina was reported in 1992 [2]. Since then, the field of interventional cardiology has grown in leaps and bounds, and the number of PCI procedures done today for revascularization exceeds the number of coronary artery bypass graft surgeries (CABG) done for the same indication worldwide. Improvements in patient outcomes following PCI are a result not only of significant improvements in the techniques associated with PCI, but also due to improvements and additions to the periprocedural pharmacological armamentarium.

Balloon PTCA

Although once the sole method of coronary intervention, balloon PTCA is seldom employed on its own today. It mechanically expands the coronary lumen by stretching and tearing the atherosclerotic plaque and vessel wall, resulting in a localized dissection of the intima and sometimes the media. The dissection is covered by platelet-rich thrombus and later by new intimal layers. When used alone, abrupt closure rates approximate 5–8%, while 6-month restenosis rates approximate 30–49% [3].

Cardiovascular Clinical Trials: Putting the Evidence into Practice, First Edition.
Edited by Marcus D. Flather, Deepak L. Bhatt, and Tobias Geisler.
© 2013 Blackwell Publishing Ltd. Published 2013 by Blackwell Publishing Ltd.

PTCA versus medical therapy (Table 8.1)

The ACME (Angioplasty Compared to Medicine) trial, the first randomized study comparing PTCA with conventional medical therapy to be published, was reported in 1992. Male patients were enrolled in the study if they had significant stenosis in one major coronary artery, with evidence of exercise-induced myocardial ischemia. They were then randomized to either PTCA or medical therapy, which included nitrates, beta-blockers, and/or calcium channel blockers. The success rate for PTCA was relatively low (78.1% with two emergent CABG surgeries). Patients undergoing PTCA did better with respect to the primary endpoints of this trial: change in exercise duration at 6 months (2.1 ± 3.1 minutes in the PTCA group and 0.5 ± 2.2 minutes in the medical group; $p < 0.0001$) and freedom from angina at 6 months (64% in the PTCA group vs 46% in the medical group; $p < 0.001$). The study was not powered to study mortality or myocardial infarction (MI) rates [2].

In contrast, a subsequent study by the ACME investigators in patients with double-vessel coronary artery disease (CAD) presenting with stable angina, and with evidence of ischemia on nuclear treadmill testing, found no significant difference between PTCA and medical therapy in terms of degree of improvement in exercise duration (1.2 vs 1.3 minutes; $p = 0.89$) or freedom from angina at 6 months (53% vs 36%; $p = 0.09$) [4].

The RITA-2 (Randomized Interventional Treatment of Angina 2) trial included a few patients with left ventricular dysfunction and multivessel disease, with total follow-up of 2.7 years. Angina improved by 16.5% in the PTCA group compared to the medical group at 3 months ($p < 0.001$), which attenuated to 7.6% after 2 years ($p = 0.02$). Similarly, total exercise duration improved initially with PTCA, but this appeared to diminish at late follow-up. Subgroup analyses suggested that the beneficial effects of PTCA on angina and exercise time at 6 months were restricted to patients with class II or worse angina, or baseline exercise time of 9 minutes or less [5].

While these trials studied patients with stable angina predominantly, the TIMI-3B (Thrombolysis in Myocardial Ischemia 3B) and VANQWISH (Veterans Affairs Non–Q-Wave Infarction Strategies In Hospital) trials were landmark studies comparing PTCA with medical therapy in patients presenting with unstable angina. TIMI-3B compared early invasive (coronary angiography within 18–48 hours, with early revascularization with PTCA or CABG) with an early conservative strategy (medical therapy, with angiography performed only for failure of initial therapy) in patients with unstable angina or non–Q-wave MI. No difference was noted between the two strategies for the primary endpoint of the combination of death and non-fatal MI at 6 weeks (2.3% vs 2.0%; $p = 0.74$) or at 1 year (4.1% vs 4.4%; $p = 0.79$) [6,7]. The VANQWISH trial randomized 920 patients presenting with non–Q-wave MI to early invasive versus conservative management. They found that compared with conservative management, the early invasive strategy was associated with a higher incidence of the primary endpoint of death or non-fatal MI (3.3% vs 7.8%; $p = 0.004$) as well as death (1.3% vs 4.5%; $p = 0.007$) at hospital discharge. Similar findings were noted at 1 year for the primary endpoint

Table 8.1 PTCA versus medical therapy trials.

Variable	ACME [2]	ACME [4]	RITA-2 [5]	AVERT [9]	TIMI-3B [6,7]	VANQWISH [8]
Patient population	Stable angina, 1-VD	Stable angina, 2-VD	Stable and unstable angina	Stable angina	Unstable angina	Unstable angina
Years of enrollment	1987–1990	NA	1992–1996	1995–1996	1989–1992	1993–1995
Stents/other	No	No	Yes (4.3%)	Yes (18.7%)	No	Yes (unknown %)
Number of patients (PTCA/medical therapy)	105/107	51/50	504/514	177/164	740/733	462/458
Baseline characteristics						
Median age (years)	63.5	NA	NA	58.5	59.0	61.5
Women (%)	0	NA	18.0	15.8	34.0	2.6
Diabetes mellitus (%)	18.0	NA	9.0	15.8	NA	26.1 (type 1)
3-VD (%)	0	0	7.0	0	NA	44.0
Clinical outcomes (% PTCA group vs % medical therapy group)	6 months	6 months	2.7 years	1.5 years	1 year	1 year
Death	0.9 vs 0	3.9 vs 2.0	2.2 vs 1.4	0.6 vs 0.6†	4.1 vs 4.4	12.6 vs 7.9*
MI	4.8 vs 2.8	3.9 vs 12.0	4.2 vs 1.9	2.8 vs 2.4	8.3 vs 9.3	NA
Revascularization	NA	27.5 vs 18.0	20.2 vs 25.4	17.0 vs 12.2	64.0 vs 58.0*	NA
Repeat PTCA	15.2 vs 9.3	21.6 vs 14.0	12.3 vs 19.6	11.9 vs 11.0	39.0 vs 32.0*	NA
CABG	6.7 vs 0*	5.9 vs 2.0	7.9 vs 5.8	5.1 vs 1.2	30.0 vs 30.0	NA
Freedom from angina	64.0 vs 46.0*	53.0 vs 36.0	NA	54.0 vs 41.0*	71.0 vs 69.0	NA

*p < 0.05.
†Cardiac deaths only.
CABG, coronary artery bypass graft surgery; MI, myocardial infarction; NA, not available; PTCA, percutaneous transluminal coronary angioplasty; VD, vessel disease.

(18.6% vs 24%; p = 0.05), and for death (7.9% vs 12.6%; p = 0.025) [8]. Thus, early data seemed to suggest that in patients with unstable angina or non-Q wave MI, an early conservative strategy was safer and more efficacious than an early invasive one using PTCA. Only a small proportion of these patients received coronary stents.

Current indications for PTCA alone

With the advent of stents, the use of PTCA as a standalone procedure has decreased significantly. There are a few specific situations where PTCA still has great utility:

• Patients presenting with acute coronary syndromes (ACS) found to have multivessel disease suitable for urgent/emergent CABG (e.g., PTCA alone rapidly restores patency to the infarct-related artery yet avoids the need for prolonged antiplatelet therapy, thereby allowing the patient to proceed to surgery without delay).

• Patients found to have significant coronary disease in the preoperative setting (PTCA alone may allow revascularization while avoiding the requirement of prolonged antiplatelet therapy that would delay surgery). However, in most settings, bare metal stenting can provide superior long-term results with only a 4–6-week minimum requirement for antiplatelet therapy.

• Side branch PCI in bifurcation lesions, especially short segments.

• Occasionally, distal disease that is too small to stent is treated with PCTA alone. However, restenosis rates tend to be high.

Bare metal stents

First implemented in the late 1980s for the emergency treatment of coronary dissection after angioplasty, the early era of the intracoronary stent was plagued by high rates of subacute closure (3–5%) despite intensive anticoagulation regimens. Second-generation balloon-expandable stents were introduced towards the late 1990s, with varying amounts of cobalt, chromium, tantalum, or other metals, in addition to stainless steel, along with enhancements in strut design and delivery and deployment systems, among other factors. These soon became the predominant method of PCI, being used in more than 90% of cases. They have proven effective in treating dissections and reducing the incidence of abrupt closure, emergency CABG (<1%), and restenosis, as compared with PTCA. Because these later stents were coated with a pharmacological agent on their abluminal surface (so-called "drug-coated" or "drug-eluting" stents; see below), they are now referred to as "bare metal" stents (BMSs).

Bare metal stents versus PTCA (Table 8.2)

In the BENESTENT (BElgian NEtherlands STENT) trial, 520 patients with stable angina and a single coronary artery lesion (reference vessel diameter ≥3.0 mm) were randomly assigned to either Palmaz–Schatz stent implantation or standard PTCA. The primary clinical endpoint of death, occurrence of a

Table 8.2 Randomized controlled trials of BMS versus PTCA.

Variable	STRESS [12]	BENESTENT [13]	BENESTENT II [14]	REST [15]	SAVED [16]	TOSCA [17]
Lesion type	De novo, native	De novo, native	De novo, native	Restenosis, native	Saphenous vein grafts	Chronic total occlusions
Years of enrollment	1991–1993	1991–1993	1995–1996	1991–1996	1993–1995	1996–1997
Number of patients (PTCA/BMS)	202/205	257/259	410/413	176/178	107/108	208/202
Type of stent	Palmaz–Schatz (stainless steel)	Palmaz–Schatz (stainless steel)	Heparin coated	Palmaz–Schatz (stainless steel)	Palmaz–Schatz (stainless steel)	Heparin coated
Baseline characteristics						
Mean age (years)	60.0	57.5	54.5	59.5	66.0	58.0
Women (%)	22.0	19.0	21.5	19.0	19.5	18.0
Diabetes mellitus (%)	15.5	6.5	12.0	17.5	29.5	16.5
Multivessel disease (%)	34.0	NA	NA	32.5	NA	NA
RVD (mm)	3.01	3.00	2.95	3.03	3.19	3.57
Clinical outcomes (% in PTCA group vs % in BMS group)	8 months	7 months	12 months	6 months	8 months	6 months
Death	1.5 vs 1.5	0.4 vs 0.8	1.2 vs 1.0	1.1 vs 1.1	9.0 vs 7.0	0.5 vs 0.5
MI	6.9 vs 6.3	4.6 vs 3.9	4.6 vs 3.4	1.2 vs 4.5	15.0 vs 11.0	3.8 vs 11.9*
Revascularization	15.4 vs 10.2	NA	NA	NA	26.0 vs 17.0	15.4 vs 8.4*
Repeat PTCA	12.4 vs 11.2	23.3 vs 13.5*	17.8 vs 11.9*	26.6 vs 10.3*	16.0 vs 13.0	14.4 vs 6.9
CABG	8.4 vs 4.9	2.3 vs 3.9	2.2 vs 2.4	0.6 vs 2.2	12.0 vs 7.0	1.4 vs 1.5

*p < 0.05.
BMS, bare metal stent; CABG, coronary artery bypass graft surgery; MI, myocardial infarction; NA, not available; PTCA, percutaneous transluminal coronary angioplasty; RVD, reference vessel diameter.

cerebrovascular accident, MI, need for CABG, or a second percutaneous intervention at 7 months was significantly reduced in the stent arm as compared with the PTCA arm (20% vs 30%; RR, 0.68; 95% CI, 0.50–0.92; p = 0.02). This was predominantly driven by a significant 42% reduction in the need for a second PCI in the stent arm (p = 0.005). Angiographic follow-up demonstrated a higher incidence of restenosis in the PTCA arm (22% vs 32%; p = 0.02). Of note, peripheral vascular complications necessitating surgery, blood transfusion, or both were more frequent after stenting than after PTCA (3.1% vs 13.5%; p < 0.001) [10]. One- (15.2% vs 24.2% 10%; p = 0.01) and 5-year (17.2% vs 27.3%; p = 0.008) follow-up data confirmed a lower rate of repeat revascularization in the stent arm as compared with the PTCA arm [10,11].

In the STRESS (Stent Restenosis Study) trial, 410 patients with stable angina and predominantly single coronary artery lesions (66%) were randomly assigned to either Palmaz–Schatz stent implantation or standard PTCA. At 6 months, the patients with stented lesions had a lower rate of restenosis (31.6% vs 42.1%; p = 0.046) than those treated with PTCA. The incidence of death, MI, CABG, vessel closure, including stent thrombosis, or repeated angioplasty was similar between the two arms (19.5% vs 23.8%; p = 0.16). Revascularization of the original target lesion because of recurrent myocardial ischemia was performed less frequently in the stent group than in the angioplasty group (10.2% vs 15.4%; p = 0.06) [12].

Although BMSs reduce the rate of restenosis and repeat revascularization as compared with PTCA alone, vessel trauma from stent implantation resulted in neointimal hyperplasia, with significant restenosis in 17–30% of patients. This risk is increased in patients with small reference vessel size, smaller post-procedural luminal diameter or high degree of residual stenosis, long lesion length, diabetes, and presence of untreated edge dissection during the procedure.

Drug-eluting stents

Noting the high rate of restenosis with BMSs, and recognizing that this was predominantly due to neointimal hyperplasia and matrix accumulation, a number of systemic antiproliferative approaches were attempted, such as oral rapamycin (sirolimus) [18]. Although a beneficial effect on restenosis was noted, such therapies were limited by their side effect profile. This prompted attempts at local delivery systems for these agents, resulting in the genesis of drug-eluting stent (DESs). DESs thus comprise three principal components: the stent backbone itself, pharmacological agent(s) designed to inhibit neointimal hyperplasia, and a carrier polymer which determines the local kinetics of drug elution. Results of trials of currently available DESs compared with BMSs are briefly discussed below (Figure 8.1 and Tables 8.3 and 8.4).

Sirolimus-eluting stents
Sirolimus is a macrocyclic lactone that blocks smooth muscle proliferation by inhibiting mammalian target of rapamycin (mTOR), and thus acts early in the

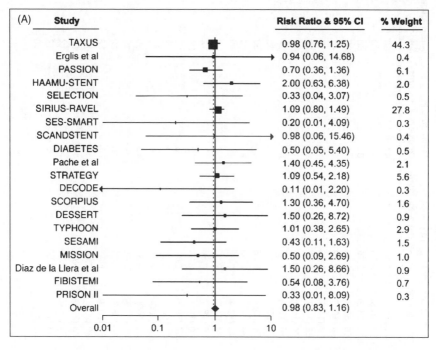

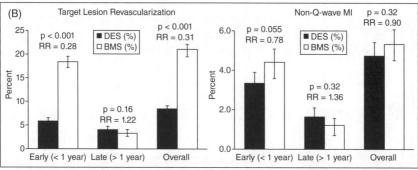

Figure 8.1 (A) Summary plot for all-cause mortality comparing drug-eluting stents (DESs) to bare metal stents (BMSs). (B) Overall risk of target lesion revascularization and non-Q wave myocardial infarction comparing DESs to BMSs. (Reproduced from Roukoz *et al.* [28], with permission.)

cell cycle at G1. This was incorporated into a drug delivery system in which a Bx Velocity stent was coated with a 5-µm thick polymer that was in turn coated with 140 µg of sirolimus/cm^2 (Cypher ®, Cordis, Warren, NJ, USA).

The first trial to report on the use of these stents was the RAVEL (Randomized Study with the Sirolimus-Coated Bx Velocity Balloon-Expandable Stent in the Treatment of Patients with de Novo Native Coronary Artery Lesions) trial. In this trial, 238 patients with a single *de novo* coronary lesion were randomized to either sirolimus-eluting stent (SES) or BMS. The primary

Table 8.3 Baseline characteristics of SES and/or PES versus BMS randomized controlled trials. (Modified from Roukoz et al. [28].)

Trial	DES type	Indication	Number of patients (n)	Mean age (years)	Number of women (%)	Number of diabetics (%)	Mean reference vessel diameter (mm)	Mean duration clopidogrel (months)	Mean follow-up (months)
TAXUS I [29]	PES	Stable	61	65	7 (11.5)	11 (18.0)	2.97	6	60
TAXUS II [30]	PES	Stable	536	60	234 (43.7)	58 (10.8)	2.75	>6	60
TAXUS IV [26]	PES	Stable	1314	62	367 (27.9)	318 (24.2)	2.75	6	60
TAXUS V [31]	PES	Stable	1156	63	353 (30.5)	356 (30.8)	2.69	>6	36
TAXUS VI [32]	PES	Stable	446	63	106 (23.8)	88 (19.7)	2.79	6	48
Erglis et al. [33]	PES	Stable	103	62	17 (16.5)	12 (11.6)	3.26	>6	6
PASSION [34]	PES	STEMI	619	61	149 (24.1)	68 (11.0)	3.17	9	12
HAAMU-STENT [35]	PES	STEMI	164	63	46 (28.0)	24 (14.6)	NA	12	12
SELECTION [36]	PES	STEMI	80	61	14 (17.5)	10 (12.5)	2.86	9	7
SIRIUS [20]	SES	Stable	1058	62	307 (29.0)	275 (26)	2.8	3	60
E-SIRIUS [22]	SES	Stable	352	62	103 (29.3)	81 (23)	2.55	2	60
C-SIRIUS [23]	SES	Stable	100	60	31 (31.0)	24 (24)	2.63	2	60
RAVEL [19]	SES	Stable	238	61	57 (23.9)	45 (18.9)	2.62	2	60
SES-SMART [37]	SES	Stable	257	64	73 (28.4)	64 (24.9)	2.2	>2	8
SCANDSTENT [38]	SES	Stable	322	63	75 (23.3)	58 (18.0)	2.86	12	12
DIABETES [39]	SES	Stable	160	66.5	60 (37.5)	160 (100)	2.34	12	24
Pache et al. [40]	SES	Stable	500	67	109 (21.8)	154 (30.8)	2.7	>6	12
DECODE [41]	SES	Stable	83	61	27 (32.5)	83 (100)	2.51	>3	6
SCORPIUS [42]	SES	Stable	200	66	78 (39.0)	200 (100)	2.6	>6	12
DESSERT [43]	SES	Stable	150	70	67 (44.7)	150 (100)	2.3	>3	36
STRATEGY [44]	SES	STEMI	175	63	47 (26.9)	26 (14.9)	2.66	2–6	12
TYPHOON [45]	SES	STEMI	715	59	157 (22.0)	116 (16.3)	2.81	>6	12
SESAMI [46]	SES	STEMI	320	62	60 (18.7)	66 (20.6)	NA	NA	12
MISSION [47]	SES	STEMI	316	59	38 (12.0)	30 (9.5)	2.84	12	12
Diaz de la Llera et al. [48]	SES	STEMI	120	65	25 (20.8)	33 (27.5)	NA	1–9[†]	12
FIBISTEMI [49]	SES	STEMI	156	58	30 (19.2)	29 (18.6)	2.93	>9	12
PRISON II [50]	SES	Stable	200	59	41 (20.5)	26 (13)	2.56	>6	12
BASKET [51]	Both	Both	826	64	176 (21.3)	153 (19)	NA	6	18
TOTAL			10727						

[†]At least 1 month for BMS and 9 months for SES.

BMS, bare metal stent; CABG, coronary artery bypass grafting; DES, drug-eluting stent; NA, not available; PES, paclitaxel-eluting stent; SES, sirolimus-eluting stent; STEMI, ST elevation.

Table 8.4 Results: overall, early and late outcomes of DES versus BMS meta-analysis. (Modified from Roukoz *et al.* [28].)

	DES (%)	BMS (%)	RR	95% CI	p-value
All-cause mortality					
Early (<1 year)	2.1	2.4	0.91	0.70–1.18	0.47
Late (>1 year)	5.9	5.7	1.03	0.83–1.28	0.79
Overall	5.3	5.5	0.98	0.83–1.16	0.82
Cardiovascular mortality					
Early (<1 year)	1.6	1.7	0.95	0.68–1.31	0.75
Late (>1 year)	2.4	2.1	1.26	0.89–1.77	0.19
Overall	3.1	2.9	1.08	0.86–1.35	0.52
Q-wave MI					
Early (<1 year)	0.8	0.7	1.14	0.60–2.17	0.68
Late (>1 year)	0.8	0.6	1.24	0.64–2.40	0.52
Overall	1.4	1.2	1.23	0.79–1.90	0.36
Non-Q-wave MI					
Early (<1 year)	3.3	4.4	0.78	0.61–1.00	**0.055**
Late (>1 year)	1.6	1.2	1.36	0.74–2.53	0.32
Overall	4.7	5.3	0.90	0.72–1.11	0.32
Target lesion revascularization					
Early (<1 year)	5.8	18.4	0.28	0.21–0.38	**<0.001**
Late (>1 year)	4.0	3.3	1.22	0.92–1.60	0.16
Overall	8.5	21.0	0.31	0.23–0.41	**<0.001**
Stent thrombosis					
Early (< 30 days)	0.8	0.9	0.94	0.61–1.46	0.79
Late (30 days–<1 year)	0.3	0.4	0.92	0.43–1.94	0.82
Very late (>1 year)	0.7	0.1	4.57	1.54–13.57	**0.006**
Overall	1.4	1.3	1.13	0.81–1.58	0.48

BMS, bare metal stent; DES, drug eluting stent; RR, relative risk.

endpoint of late luminal loss (the difference between the minimal luminal diameter immediately after the procedure and the diameter at end of follow-up) at 6 months was significantly lower in the SES arm (–0.01 ± 0.33 mm) than in the BMS arm (0.80 ± 0.53 mm; p < 0.001). This corresponded to a significant difference in the incidence of in-stent restenosis (0% vs 26.6%; p < 0.001). At 1-year follow-up, the incidence of death, MI or revascularization was significantly lower in the SES arm (5.8% vs 28.8%; p < 0.001), driven by a significant reduction in the need for repeat revascularization (0% vs 27%; p < 0.001), with no difference in death or MI [19].

Similar results were noted in the SIRIUS (Sirolimus-coated Bx Velocity Balloon-expandable Stent in the Treatment of Patients with De Novo Coronary Artery Lesions) trial. A total of 1058 patients with a single newly diagnosed target lesion (mean reference vessel diameter, 2.80 mm) in a *de novo* coronary artery were randomized to either SES or BMS. The primary endpoint of target vessel failure (TVF), comprising cardiac death, MI, or repeat target lesion revascularization (TLR), was significantly reduced in the SES arm as compared with the BMS arm (8.6% vs 21.0%; p < 0.001), driven predominantly by a reduction in the need for repeat revascularization (4.1% vs 16.6%; p < 0.001). Commensurate with this, a significant reduction in angiographic restenosis was noted in the SES arm (3.2% vs 35.4%; p < 0.001). The incidence of stent thrombosis was similar (0.4% vs 0.8%) [20]. Five-year results from the SIRIUS trial confirmed the superiority of SES in reducing TVF (22.5% vs 33.5%; p < 0.0001), as compared with BMS, again due to a reduction in the need for TLR (9.4% vs 24.2%; p < 0.0001). Stent thrombosis at 5 years appeared to be similar (3.9% vs 4.2%) [21]. The European (E-SIRIUS) and Canadian (C-SIRIUS) versions of the SIRIUS trial noted similar short-term outcomes [22,23]. A meta-analysis of 14 trials comparing SES to BMS noted a decrease in the need for reintervention with SES, with no difference in death or MI, and a slightly increased risk of late stent thrombosis [24].

Paclitaxel-eluting stents
Paclitaxel inhibits microtubular assembly during cell division, and was studied on both polymeric and non-polymeric platforms. The latter has now fallen out of favor due to a higher rate of restenosis [25]. The Taxus® stent (Boston Scientific, Natick, MA, USA) elutes paclitaxel within 30 days of implantation; however, the majority remains within the polymer and elutes indefinitely.

In the TAXUS-IV (Treatment of *de novo* coronary disease using a single pAclitaXel elUting Stent IV) trial, 1314 patients with a single *de novo* coronary lesion (mean reference vessel diameter, 2.75 mm) were randomized to receive either a paclitaxel-eluting stent (PES) or BMS. The incidence of the primary endpoint of ischemia-driven target vessel revascularization (TVR) at 9 months was significantly lower with PES as compared with BMS (4.7% vs 12.0%; p < 0.001). TLR (3.0% vs 11.3%; p < 0.001) and angiographic restenosis (7.9% vs 26.6%; p < 0.001) were similarly reduced at 9 months, with no difference in death or MI. Stent thrombosis also tended to be similar (0.6% vs 0.8%; p = 0.75) [26]. Similar results for TVR (16.9% vs 27.4%; p < 0.0001) and stent thrombosis (2.2% vs 2.1%; = 0.87) were noted at 5 years [27].

Late stent thrombosis (Table 8.5)
As a result of the above DES trials, the use of DESs skyrocketed, and by 2005, SESs and PESs accounted for 75–85% of all coronary stents placed in the US [52]. Based on these trials, dual antiplatelet therapy (DAT) with aspirin and clopidogrel was recommended for a minimum of 3 months with SES and 6 months with PES [20,26]. Following renewed concerns of late stent thrombosis with DES as compared with BMS, in a meta-analysis, Bavry *et al.* noted that the incidence (per 1000 patients) and risk of a thrombotic event with DESs compared with BMSs for greater than 30 days, greater than 6 months, and greater than 1 year were 5.0 (OR, 1.56; 95% CI, 0.77–3.16; p = 0.22), 4.4 (OR,

Table 8.5 Definitions of stent thrombosis. (Modified from Bavry and Bhatt [56].)

- **Protocol definition:**
  - Acute coronary syndromes (ACS) with angiographic evidence of stent thrombosis
  - Myocardial infarction (MI) within the stented vessel
  - Intervening revascularization procedures censor later stent thromboses

- **Academic Research Consortium definition:**
  - *Definite*: ACS with angiographic or autopsy evidence of stent thrombosis
  - *Probable*: MI within stented vessel
  - *Possible*: unexplained death after 30 days
  - Intervening revascularization procedures do not censor later stent thromboses

3.67, 95% CI, 1.30–10.38; p = 0.014), and 5.0 (OR, 5.02; 95% CI, 1.29–19.52; p = 0.02), respectively, with similar results for SES and PES as compared with BMS. These findings thus demonstrated that DESs were associated with a significantly elevated risk of late and very late stent thrombosis compared with BMSs, with a median thrombosis time that was 11–14 months longer than late BMS thrombosis. The rate of stent thrombosis with DESs also seemed to be constant at about five events per 1000 patients or about 0.5% per year [53]. This and other studies [54,55] prompted the FDA to recommend increasing the minimum duration of DAT with DES to 1 year, in the absence of contraindications [52].

Factors affecting stent thrombosis

Several postulates regarding the pathogenesis of late stent thrombosis have been proposed. Angioscopic and postmortem studies suggest that while DESs effectively reduce in-stent smooth muscle cell hyperplasia, and thereby restenosis, they may also cause slower, less complete arterial healing and endothelial coverage, predisposing to stent thrombosis [57,58]. In addition, delayed endothelialization and healing due to polymer-related hypersensitivity, inflammation, or both, as well as acquired late incomplete stent apposition due to positive vessel remodeling in the stented arterial segment have also been suggested as possible mechanisms [59]. The most common determinant though appears to be premature cessation of dual antiplatelet therapy [60–62]. Other predictors of stent thrombosis include renal failure, bifurcation lesions, diabetes, low ejection fraction, primary stenting for acute MI, total stent length, and "off-label" use of DES [52,60,62,63]. Another entity that has received a lot of attention recently is that of clopidogrel "resistance" or hyporesponsiveness and factors associated with the same [64]. In a genetic analysis of the TRITON-TIMI-38 (Trial to Assess Improvement in Therapeutic Outcomes by Optimizing Platelet Inhibition with Prasugrel - Thrombolysis in Myocardial Infarction-38) Mega *et al.* noted that carriers of a reduced-function cytochrome P-450 (CYP)2C19 allele had significantly lower levels of the active metabolite of clopidogrel, diminished platelet inhibition, and a higher rate of major adverse cardiovascular events, including stent thrombosis, than did non-carriers [65]. However, methods to assess for antiplatelet therapy resistance and genetic analyses to determine CYP2C19 allele status are still considered experimental, and routine testing is not currently recommended.

SES versus PES

A meta-analysis of 16 trials with a total of 8695 patients with CAD who were randomized to receive SES or PES noted that, compared with PES, SES significantly reduced the risk of reintervention (HR, 0.74; 95% CI, 0.63–0.87; $p < 0.001$), and stent thrombosis (HR, 0.66, 95% CI, 0.46–0.94; $p = 0.02$) without significantly impacting on the risk of death (HR, 0.92; 95% CI, 0.74–1.13; $p = 0.43$) or MI (HR, 0.84; 95% CI, 0.69–1.03; $p = 0.10$) (Figure 8.2) [66]. Similar findings have been noted in diabetic patients randomized to SES or PES [67].

Everolimus-eluting stents

Everolimus-eluting stents (EESs) represent the second generation of DESs. Everolimus is a semisynthetic analog of sirolimus (rapamycin), and binds to cytosolic FKBP12 and subsequently to mTOR. The EES is designed such that the drug is released from a thin (7.8-μm), non-adhesive, durable, biocompatible fluoropolymer coated onto a low-profile (0.0032" strut thickness), flexible cobalt–chromium stent (Xience V ®, Abbot Vascular, Santa Clara, CA, USA).

The FUTURE-1 (First Use To Underscore Restenosis Reduction with Everolimus-1) trial was the first trial to compare an EES (stainless steel stent with a bioabsorbable polymer) to BMS in 42 patients with CAD. Major adverse cardiac events (MACE) at 30 days (0%), 6 months (7.7 vs 7.1%; $p > 0.05$), and 12 months (7.7 vs 7.1%; $p > 0.05$) were similar. There was no early or late stent thrombosis in either group. Minimum lumen diameter (MLD) at 6-month angiographic follow-up was larger in the EES group (2.97 mm vs 2.10 mm; $p < 0.0001$), and late loss was smaller (0.11 mm vs 0.85 mm; $p < 0.0001$) [68]. The SPIRIT (Clinical Evaluation of the Xience V Everolimus Eluting Coronary Stent System in the Treatment of Patients With de Novo Native Coronary Artery Lesions) trial randomized 60 patients with significant CAD to either EES (cobalt chromium stent with a durable polymer, Xience V®) or BMS. At 6 months, the incidence of angiographic restenosis was significantly lower in the EES arm (0% vs 25.9%; $p = 0.01$). In-stent late loss was lower as well (0.10 mm vs 0.87 mm; $p < 0.001$). MACE were similar between the two arms [69]. Following promising results from the SPIRIT II trial comparing EES to PES [70], the SPIRIT III trial randomized 1002 patients with CAD to receive EES or PES in a 2:1 ratio. The primary endpoint of angiographic in-segment late loss was significantly lower in the EES arm compared with the PES arm (0.14 mm vs 0.28 mm; p for non-inferiority <0.001; p for superiority = 0.004). EESs were non-inferior to PESs for ischemia-driven TLR at 9 months (7.2% vs 9.0%; p for non-inferiority <0.001; p for superiority = 0.31). MACE at 9 months (4.6% vs 8.1%; $p = 0.03$) and at 1 year (6.0% vs 10.3%; $p = 0.02$) were significantly lower in the EES arm. Rates of death (1.2% vs 1.2%; $p = 1.0$), MI (2.8% vs 4.1%; $p = 0.33$), and stent thrombosis (1.7% vs 1.3%; $p = 0.78$) were similar at 1 year [71]. The reduction in MACE noted with EES was sustained at 2

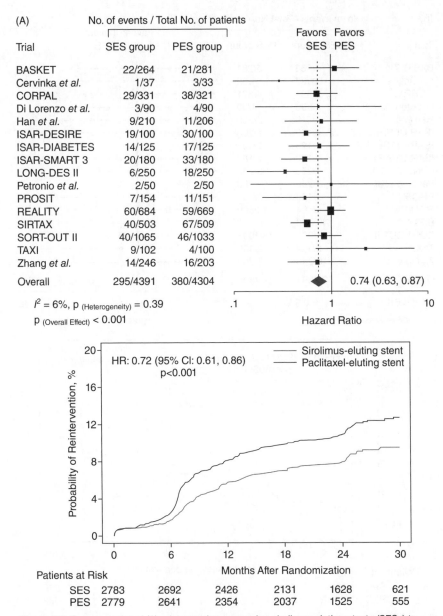

Figure 8.2 Summary plot of (A) reintervention comparing sirolimus-eluting stents (SESs) to paclitaxel-eluting stents (PESs) and (B) stent thrombosis comparing SESs to PESs. (Reproduced from Schomig et al. [66], with permission.)

(B)

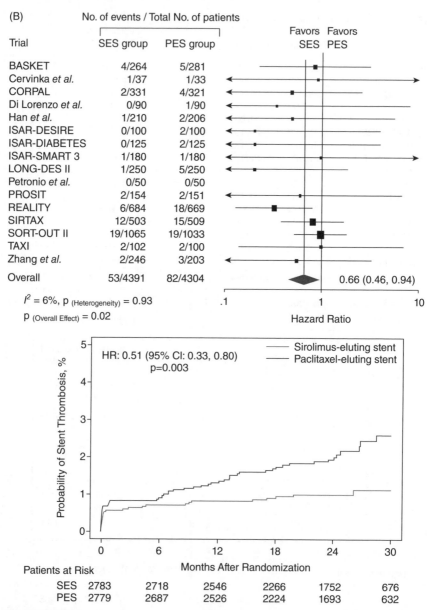

Figure 8.2 (*continued*)

years of follow-up (7.3% vs 12.8%; p = 0.004), with a lower rate of TVF (10.7% vs 15.4%; p = 0.04). Stent thrombosis rates were similar [72]. Since SPIRIT III was primarily powered for non-inferiority, the SPIRIT IV trial was designed to be powered to demonstrate superiority of EES over PES. A total of 3687 patients were randomized to receive EES or PES. The primary endpoint of TVF at 1 year was significantly lower in the EES arm as compared with the

PES arm (4.2% vs 6.8%; p = 0.001). Other endpoints at 1 year such as ischemia-driven TLR (2.5% vs 4.6%; p = 0.001), MI (1.9% vs 3.1%; p = 0.02), and stent thrombosis (0.17% vs 0.85%; p = 0.004) were also lower in the EES arm [73].

Zotarolimus-eluting stents

Zotarolimus is also an analog of sirolimus (rapamycin) (ABT-578), and has been incorporated with a non-erodible polymer, phosphorylcholine, on a thin-strut cobalt–chromium alloy platform (Driver stent) into the Endeavor® stent (Medtronic Inc, Minneapolis, MN, USA). This is also considered to be a second-generation DES.

Following promising results from ENDEAVOR I (The Randomized Comparison of Zotarolimus-Eluting and Paclitaxel-Eluting Stents in Patients with Coronary Artery Disease I) trial, the ENDEAVOR II trial randomized patients with CAD (mean reference vessel diameter [RVD] 2.75 mm) to receive either ZES or BMS. The primary endpoint of TVF at 9 months was significantly lower in the ZES arm as compared with the BMS arm (7.3% vs 15.1%; p = 0.0001). Similarly, in-segment restenosis (13.2% vs 35.0%; p < 0.0001), TLR (4.6% vs 11.8%; p = 0.0001), and MACE (7.3% vs 14.4%; p = 0.0001) at 9 months were lower in the ZES arm [74]. The ENDEAVOR III trial randomized patients with *de novo* CAD to receive ZES or SES in a 3:1 ratio. The primary endpoint of in-segment late loss did not meet the non-inferiority margin of difference of 0.20 mm, with an observed 0.21-mm greater late loss in the Endeavor group (0.34 mm vs 0.13 mm; p = NS for non-inferiority; p < 0.001 for superiority). In-stent restenosis (9.2% vs 2.1%; p = 0.02) was also higher in the ZES arm. At 9 months, TVF was similar between the two arms (12.0% vs 11.5%; p = 1.0) [75]. The SORT OUT III (Efficacy and Safety of Zotarolimus-Eluting and Sirolimus-Eluting Coronary Stents in Routine Clinical Care III) trial randomized all comers with CAD to receive ZES or SES at five high-volume centers in Denmark. At 9 months, patients treated with a ZES were more likely to have met the primary endpoint of cardiovascular death, MI or TLR (6% vs 3%; p = 0.0002). This difference was sustained at 18 months (10% vs 5%; p < 0.0001). There was no difference in the all-cause mortality at 9 months (2% vs 2%), whereas it was higher in the ZES patients at 18 months (4% vs 3%; p = 0.04) [76].

The ENDEAVOR IV trial randomized 1548 patients with single *de novo* coronary lesions to receive ZES or PES. The primary endpoint of TVF at 9 months met the non-inferiority margin of difference, with an event rate of 6.6% in the ZES group and 7.1% in the PES group (p for non-inferiority ≤0.001). In-segment late lumen loss at 8 months was higher in the ZES arm (0.36 mm vs 0.23 mm; p = 0.023), although this did not translate into a higher rate of TLR (4.5% vs 3.2%; = 0.23) or TVR (6.2% vs 6.8%; p = 0.68) at 12 months. MACE rates at 1 year were also similar (6.5% vs 6.7%; p = 0.92). Protocol-defined stent thrombosis at 1 year was numerically higher in the ZES arm (0.8% vs 0.1%; p = 0.12) [77]. At 2 years, rates of MACE (9.8% vs 10.0%; p = 0.93) and TVF (12.4% vs 16.1%; p = 0.052) were still similar, although MI rates were lower with ZES (2% vs 4.1%; p = 0.02). Only one episode of stent thrombosis was noted between years 1 and 2, with cumulative 2-year stent thrombosis rates of 1.9% vs 1.6% (p = 0.84) [78].

EES versus ZES

The Resolute All Comers trial randomized 2292 patients with stable angina or ACS to receive either EES or ZES, with at least one off-label indication for stent placement present in 66% of the patients. ZES was non-inferior to EES for the primary endpoint of TVF (8.2% vs 8.3%; p < 0.001 for non-inferiority). The angiographic endpoint of in-stent percent stenosis was also non-inferior between ZES and EES (21.7% vs 19.8%; p for non-inferiority = 0.04). In-segment late loss tended to be lower with EES (0.15 mm vs 0.06 mm; p = 0.04), although clinical outcomes including clinically indicated TLR (3.9% vs 3.4%; p = 0.5), MACE (8.7% vs 9.7%; p = 0.42), death (1.6% vs 2.8%; p = 0.08), MI (13.5% vs 13.6%; p = 0.95), and stent thrombosis (2.3% vs 1.5%; p = 0.17) were similar between the ZES and EES arms [79].

Biodegradable stents

Biodegradable or bioabsorbable stents represent newer advances in the field of PCI, and are sometimes called third-generation DES. They provide adequate scaffolding for a clinically relevant period, and then disappear. This may avoid some of the disadvantages of permanent metallic stent implantation, such as late stent thrombosis. A number of bioabsorbable polymers are available, and are being tested with different stent delivery platforms. These stents are currently not available in the US.

The LEADERS (Limus Eluted from A Durable versus ERodable Stent coating) trial randomized 1707 patients with stable angina or ACS to a biolimus-eluting stent (from a biodegradable polymer) or SES from a durable polymer. Biolimus is a semi-synthetic analog of sirolimus with enhanced lipophilicity that is coupled to a polylactic acid biodegradable polymer. At 9 months, the primary outcome of death, MI, or urgent revascularization occurred in 9.2% of the biolimus arm versus 10.5% of the sirolimus arm (p for non-inferiority = 0.003; p for superiority = 0.39). Individual components of the composite outcome were similar at 9 months: cardiovascular mortality (1.6% vs 2.5%; p = 0.22), MI (5.7% vs 4.6%; p = 0.30), and urgent TVR (4.4% vs 5.5%; p = 0.29). Cumulative stent thrombosis to 9 months was similar (1.9% vs 2.0%; p = 0.84), as was stent thrombosis from 30 days to 9 months (0.2% vs 0.5%; p = 0.41). In-stent percent diameter stenosis was 20.9% in the biolimus arm versus 23.3% in the sirolimus arm (p for non-inferiority = 0.001; p for superiority = 0.26) [80]. In the ABSORB (Clinical Evaluation of the BVS everolimus eluting stent system) phase II trial, 30 patients with CAD underwent implantation of a bioabsorbable EES system, which is made of a bioabsorbable polylactic acid backbone, and a layer of more rapidly absorbed polylactic acid, that contains and controls the release of the antiproliferative drug, everolimus. One-year MACE rate was 3.3%, with only one MI and no episodes of stent thrombosis. The 6-month late lumen loss was 0.44 mm [81].

Local antiproliferative treatment for in-stent restenosis

Although DESs significantly reduce the incidence of in-stent restenosis as compared with BMSs, the treatment of in-stent restenosis is challenging. The treatment of in-stent restenosis with a DES has also raised concerns about an increased risk of stent thrombosis given the presence of two or more layers of metal in a native coronary artery. Recent trials have sought to study the efficacy of drug-coated angioplasty balloons, primarily paclitaxel-coated balloons, for the treatment of in-stent restenosis. For example, the PACCOCATH ISR (Treatment of In-Stent Restenosis by Paclitaxel-Coated Balloon Catheters) trial studied the safety and efficacy of angioplasty using paclitaxel-coated balloon catheters ($3\,\mu g/mm^2$ of balloon surface area), as compared with angioplasty alone in 52 patients with in-stent restenosis. At 6 months, in-segment late luminal loss was lower in the paclitaxel-coated balloon arm as compared with the uncoated balloon arm ($p = 0.02$). This translated into a significant reduction in the need for TLR at 12 months with the paclitaxel-coated balloon arm as compared with the uncoated balloon arm (0% vs 23%; $p = 0.02$) [82]. These results appeared to be sustained at 2 years of follow-up [83]. The LOCAL TAX (Local intracoronary delivery of paclitaxel after stent implantation for prevention of restenosis in comparison with implantation of a bare metal stent alone or with implantation of a paclitaxel-coated stent) trial compared outcomes in 202 patients with BMS in-stent restenosis, who were randomized to either repeat BMS, DES stenting with a PES, or BMS stenting followed by catheter-based local delivery of fluid paclitaxel. The primary outcome of angiographic in-stent late lumen loss with BMS + local delivery of paclitaxel was significantly lower than with BMS alone ($p = 0.0006$), and non-inferior to PES (p for non-inferiority = 0.023). MACE rates at 6 months were similar between the BMS, BMS + local delivery of paclitaxel, and PES arms (26.8% vs 13.4% vs 13.4%; $p = 0.08$), including the need for TLR (22.1% vs 13.4% vs 11.9%; $p = 0.20$) [84]. Similarly, the PEPCAD II (Paclitaxel-Eluting PTCA Balloon Catheter in Coronary Artery Disease II) trial sought to compare outcomes after PES implantation versus angioplasty using a second-generation paclitaxel-coated balloon in patients with BMS in-stent restenosis. At 6-month follow-up, in-segment late lumen loss was significantly lower in the paclitaxel-coated balloon arm, as compared with the PES arm ($p = 0.03$). This corresponded to a lower rate of binary restenosis in the paclitaxel-coated balloon arm (9% vs 22%; $p = 0.08$) at 6 months. At 12 months, rates of MACE (9% vs 22%; $p = 0.08$) and TLR (6% vs 15%; $p = 0.15$) were similar between the two arms [85].

Directional coronary atherectomy

Directional coronary artherectomy (DCA) involves the utilization of a rotating cup-shaped blade within a windowed cylinder to directionally excise plaque from the vessel wall. It is infrequently employed today, mostly in the setting of in-stent restenosis.

In the CAVEAT I (Coronary Angioplasty vs Excisional Atherectomy trial I) study, 1012 patients with *de novo* lesions in the coronary arteries were randomized to PTCA or PTCA with DCA. Although the acute gain was higher with DCA, the primary endpoint of angiographic restenosis was similar between the DCA and PTCA arms at 6 months (50% vs 57%; p = 0.06), presumably due to a higher late lumen loss with DCA [86]. Similar results were noted in the CCAT (Canadian Coronary Atherectomy CCAT Trial) of 274 patients with proximal lower anterior descending artery (LAD) lesions who were randomized to DCA or PTCA [87]. Given that late lumen loss after DCA is mainly determined by arterial remodeling, the AMIGO (Atherectomy before Multi-link Improves lumen Gain and clinical Outcomes) trial sought to compare outcomes after DCA with stenting versus stenting alone. However, there was no difference in the primary endpoint of angiographic restenosis at 8 months between the two arms (26.7% vs 22.1%; p = 0.24). Similarly, no difference in clinical outcomes was noted between the two arms at 1 year [88]. In a meta-analysis of randomized controlled trials (RCTs) comparing DCA to PTCA or stenting, no difference in 30-day or long-term outcomes was noted (Figure 8.3) [89].

Cutting balloon angioplasty

Cutting balloon angioplasty (CBA) involves the use of a non-compliant balloon with longitudinally mounted microsurgical atherotomes (three or four) to cause scoring of atheromatous plaque, and severing of elastic and fibrotic continuity of the vessel wall, resulting in plaque compression. It is mainly utilized in patients with ostial, non-passable, or bifurcation lesions, which are only mildly calcified. It is also employed in the setting of in-stent restenosis.

Several initial small trials demonstrated a benefit with CBA as compared with PTCA. Ergene *et al.* randomized 71 patients with significant CAD (RVD <3 mm to either CBA or PTCA, and noted a significant reduction in angiographic restenosis with CBA at 6 months, as compared with PTCA (27% vs 47%; p <0.05) [90]. Other single-center studies noted similar positive results [91,92]. On the other hand, the larger, multicenter GRT (Cutting Balloon Global Randomized Trial) of 1238 eligible patients who were randomized to either CBA or PTCA, noted no difference in the primary endpoint of angiographic restenosis at 6 months (31.4% vs 30.4%; p = 0.75). There was a higher rate of coronary perforation with CBA (0.8% vs 0%). Although freedom from TLR was higher in the CBA arm as compared with the PTCA alone arm (88.5% vs 84.6%; p = 0.04), the incidence of MACE at 270 days was higher in the CBA arm (4.7% vs 2.4%; p = 0.03) [93]. Similar results were noted by other randomized trials [94]. The REDUCE III (Restenosis Reduction by Cutting Balloon Evaluation – III) trial randomized 521 patients to either CBA with BMS versus PTCA followed by BMS, and noted lower restenosis rates (11.8% vs 19.6%; p < 0.05) as well as TLR (9.6% vs 15.3%; p < 0.05) with CBA and BMS, as compared with PTCA and BMS, especially in those patients with intravascular ultrasound (IVUS)-guided PCI [95]. In a meta-analysis of RCTs comparing

(A) 30-Day Mortality

Type	Trial	Ablation N	%	PTCA N	%	
CBA	CAPAS	0/114	(0.0)	1/118	(0.8)	
	GRT	4/617	(0.6)	0/621	(0.0)	
	REDUCE 1	0/399	(0.0)	0/403	(0.0)	
	RESCUT	0/214	(0.0)	0/214	(0.0)	
DCA	AMIGO	0/381	(0.0)	0/372	(0.0)	
	BOAT	0/497	(0.0)	2/492	(0.4)	
	CAVEAT-I	0/512	(0.0)	2/500	(0.4)	
	CAVEAT-II	3/149	(2.0)	3/156	(1.9)	
	CCAT	0/138	(0.0)	0/136	(0.0)	
LA	AMRO	0/151	(0.0)	0/157	(0.0)	
	ERBAC ELCA	2/232	(0.9)	2/222	(0.9)	
	LAVA	2/117	(1.7)	0/98	(0.0)	
PTRA	ARTIST	0/152	(0.0)	1/146	(0.7)	*
	COBRA	1/252	(0.4)	4/250	(1.6)	
	DART	1/227	(0.4)	0/219	(0.0)	
	ERBAC PTRA	2/231	(0.9)	2/222	(0.9)	
TOTAL		**15/4383**	**(0.3)**	**15/4104**	**(0.4)**	

(B) 30-Day Major Adverse Cardiac Events

Type	Trial	Ablation N	%	PTCA N	%	
CBA	GRT	23/617	(3.7)	17/621	(2.7)	
	REDUCE 1	1/399	(0.3)	4/403	(1.0)	
	RESCUT	2/214	(0.9)	1/214	(0.5)	
DCA	AMIGO	6/381	(1.6)	4/372	(1.1)	
	BOAT	14/497	(2.8)	16/492	(3.3)	
	CAVEAT-I	57/512	(11.1)	27/500	(5.4)	
	CAVEAT-II	30/149	(20.1)	19/156	(12.2)	
	CCAT	7/138	(5.1)	8/136	(5.9)	
LA	AMRO	9/151	(6.0)	6/157	(3.8)	
	ERBAC ELCA	10/232	(4.3)	6/222	(2.7)	
	LAVA	12/117	(10.3)	4/98	(4.1)	
PTRA	ARTIST	13/152	(8.6)	7/146	(4.8)	*
	COBRA	25/252	(9.9)	19/250	(7.6)	
	DART	12/227	(5.3)	5/219	(2.3)	
	ERBAC PTRA	7/231	(3.0)	6/222	(2.7)	
	SPORT	9/360	(2.5)	5/375	(1.3)	
TOTAL		**237/4629**	**(5.1)**	**148/4361**	**(3.4)**	

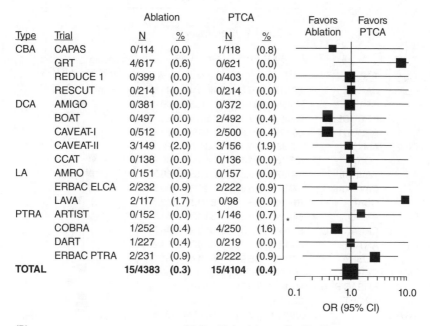

Figure 8.3 (A) 30-day mortality (B) 30-day major adverse cardiac event rates. (C) Angiographic restenosis up to 90–360 days. (D) Cumulative revascularization rates up to 360 days. *The ERBAC control groups are identical. CBA, coronary balloon artherotomy; DCA, directional coronary artherotomy; LA, (eximer or holmium) laser angioplasty; PTRA, percutaneous transluminal rotational atherectomy; PTCA, percutaneous transluminal coronary angioplasty. (Reproduced from Bittl *et al.* [89], with permission.)

(C)

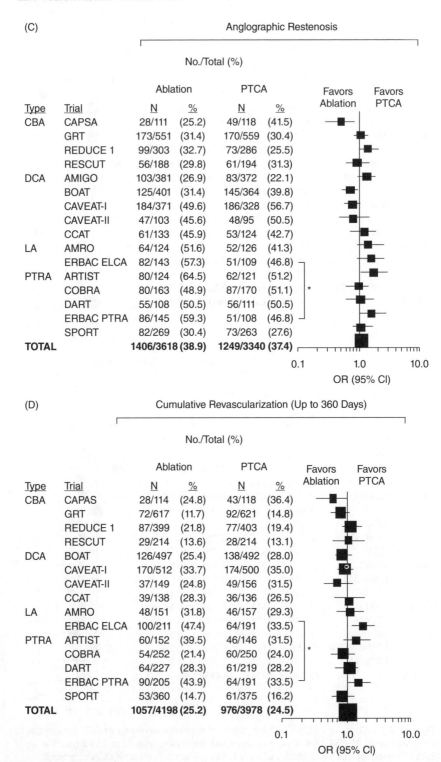

Anglographic Restenosis

No./Total (%)

		Ablation		PTCA		Favors Ablation	Favors PTCA
Type	Trial	N	%	N	%		
CBA	CAPSA	28/111	(25.2)	49/118	(41.5)		
	GRT	173/551	(31.4)	170/559	(30.4)		
	REDUCE 1	99/303	(32.7)	73/286	(25.5)		
	RESCUT	56/188	(29.8)	61/194	(31.3)		
DCA	AMIGO	103/381	(26.9)	83/372	(22.1)		
	BOAT	125/401	(31.4)	145/364	(39.8)		
	CAVEAT-I	184/371	(49.6)	186/328	(56.7)		
	CAVEAT-II	47/103	(45.6)	48/95	(50.5)		
	CCAT	61/133	(45.9)	53/124	(42.7)		
LA	AMRO	64/124	(51.6)	52/126	(41.3)		
	ERBAC ELCA	82/143	(57.3)	51/109	(46.8)		
PTRA	ARTIST	80/124	(64.5)	62/121	(51.2)		
	COBRA	80/163	(48.9)	87/170	(51.1)		
	DART	55/108	(50.5)	56/111	(50.5)		
	ERBAC PTRA	86/145	(59.3)	51/108	(46.8)		
	SPORT	82/269	(30.4)	73/263	(27.6)		
TOTAL		**1406/3618 (38.9)**		**1249/3340 (37.4)**			

0.1   1.0   10.0

OR (95% CI)

(D)

Cumulative Revascularization (Up to 360 Days)

No./Total (%)

		Ablation		PTCA		Favors Ablation	Favors PTCA
Type	Trial	N	%	N	%		
CBA	CAPAS	28/114	(24.8)	43/118	(36.4)		
	GRT	72/617	(11.7)	92/621	(14.8)		
	REDUCE 1	87/399	(21.8)	77/403	(19.4)		
	RESCUT	29/214	(13.6)	28/214	(13.1)		
DCA	BOAT	126/497	(25.4)	138/492	(28.0)		
	CAVEAT-I	170/512	(33.7)	174/500	(35.0)		
	CAVEAT-II	37/149	(24.8)	49/156	(31.5)		
	CCAT	39/138	(28.3)	36/136	(26.5)		
LA	AMRO	48/151	(31.8)	46/157	(29.3)		
	ERBAC ELCA	100/211	(47.4)	64/191	(33.5)		
PTRA	ARTIST	60/152	(39.5)	46/146	(31.5)		
	COBRA	54/252	(21.4)	60/250	(24.0)		
	DART	64/227	(28.3)	61/219	(28.2)		
	ERBAC PTRA	90/205	(43.9)	64/191	(33.5)		
	SPORT	53/360	(14.7)	61/375	(16.2)		
TOTAL		**1057/4198 (25.2)**		**976/3978 (24.5)**			

0.1   1.0   10.0

OR (95% CI)

Figure 8.3 (*continued*)

CBA to PTCA or stenting, no difference in 30-day or long-term outcomes was noted (Figure 8.3) [89].

Rotational atherectomy

This involves the removal or controlled scoring of the obstructing atherosclerotic plaque (rather than its mere displacement), and is usually used for severely calcified lesions, or severe ostial lesions.

The DART (Dilatation vs Ablation Revascularization Trial Targeting Restenosis) trial randomized 446 patients with severe CAD (RVD <3 mm) to either rotational atherectomy (burr-to-artery ratio of 0.70–0.85) followed by no or low-pressure (<1 atm) or high-pressure PTCA. The primary endpoint of TVF at 12 months was similar between the two arms (30.5% vs 31.2%; p = 0.98). Angiographic outcomes such as restenosis and late loss index were also similar [96]. The ARTIST (Angioplasty versus Rotational Atherectomy for Treatment of Diffuse In-stent Restenosis Trial) randomized 298 patients with significant in-stent restenosis (≥70%) to either rotablation followed by low-pressure PTCA (≤6 atm) or PTCA alone. Although short-term outcomes were similar between the two arms, the mean gain in diameter with PTCA was larger than that with rotablation with PTCA (25% vs 17%; p = 0.002), with a resultant lower rate of restenosis of 50% or greater with PTCA alone (51% vs 65%; p = 0.04). Six-month event-free survival was significantly higher in the PTCA alone arm (91.3% vs 79.6%; p = 0.005) [97]. Conversely, the ROSTER (Rotational Atherectomy versus Balloon Angioplasty for Diffuse In-Stent Restenosis) trial in 200 patients with in-stent restenosis who were randomized to rotational atherectomy (burr-to-artery ratio >0.7) followed by low-pressure PTCA (4–6 atm) or high-pressure PTCA (>12 atm) noted a lower incidence of TLR at 12 months with rotational atherectomy and low-pressure PTCA (32% vs 45%; p = 0.04) [98]. In a meta-analysis of RCTs comparing rotational atherectomy to PTCA, the former was associated with a significantly higher rate of 30-day MACE (OR, 1.6; 95% CI, 1.1–2.4), as well as angiographic restenosis (OR, 1.2; 95% CI, 1.0–1.5), as compared with PTCA alone (Figure 8.3) [89].

The STRATUS (Study to Determine Rotablator and Transluminal Angioplasty Strategy) trial compared a strategy of aggressive rotablation (burr-to-artery ratio of 0.7–0.9) followed by no or low-pressure PTCA (<1 atm) or moderate debulking (burr-to-artery ratio <0.7) followed by conventional PTCA. Although clinical success was similar between the two arms, aggressive rotablation was associated with a higher incidence of periprocedural MI (11% vs 7%). At 6 months, the incidence of TLR was similar between the two arms (23.5% vs 21.1%; p = 0.13) [99]. Similar results were noted by the CARAT (Coronary Angioplasty and Rotablator Atherectomy Trial), which compared an aggressive rotablative strategy to a moderate one [100].

Excimer laser angioplasty

Excimer laser angioplasty (ELCA) involves utilizing predominantly the photoacoustic effects of laser energy to cause tissue absorption, and thereby plaque ablation. This technique is currently predominantly used for saphenous vein graft lesions, although it can theoretically be applied in a number of settings.

The LAVA (Laser Angioplasty Versus Angioplasty) trial randomized 208 patients with angina to either ELCA with holmium:YAG or PTCA. ELCA was associated with a higher incidence of procedural complications (18.0% vs 3.1%; p = 0.0004), including major complications such as coronary occlusions, emergency CABG, and sustained ventricular tachycardia/fibrillation. However, 12-month event-free survival was similar between the two arms (64.9% vs 66.5%; p = 0.55) [101]. The AMRO (Amsterdam-Rotterdam) study compared ECLA with an ultraviolet laser followed by PTCA versus PTCA alone in 308 patients with stable angina, and noted no difference in procedural success between the two arms. Late loss tended to be greater with ELCA, with a resultant higher rate of restenosis in the ELCA arm (52% vs 41%; p = 0.13) [102]. The ERBAC (Excimer Laser, Rotational Atherectomy, and Balloon Angioplasty Comparison) trial randomized 685 patients with a complex coronary lesion to ELCA, rotational atherectomy, or PTCA. Patients who underwent rotational atherectomy had a higher rate of procedural success than those who underwent ELCA or PTCA (89% vs 77% vs 80%; p = 0.0019). Six-month TLR was however performed more frequently in the rotational atherectomy and ELCA arms, as compared with PTCA alone (42.4% vs46.0% vs 31.9%; p = 0.01) [103].

Mechanical thrombectomy

Numerous coronary devices have been developed in an attempt to decrease or prevent embolization during PCI. Three main types of devices are available: simple catheter aspiration (such as Export, Pronto, and Diver catheters), mechanical aspiration (such as AngioJet and X-Sizer), and embolic protection devices (EPDs; such as GuardWire and FilterWire). Two potential uses exist in coronary interventions: for primary PCI in patients with ST-elevation MI (STEMI) and for saphenous vein graft (SVG) interventions.

For primary PCI (Table 8.7)

Simple catheter aspiration
Dudek *et al.* randomized 72 patients presenting with STEMI to either PCI with stenting alone or mechanical thrombectomy with the RESCUE system, followed by stent implantation. Although the number of patients with TIMI-3 flow (Table 8.6) and corrected TIMI frame count (cTFC) were similar between the two arms, complete ST-segment resolution was higher in the mechanical thrombectomy arm (68% vs 25%; p = 0.005). Ejection fraction at 3 months was slightly higher in the mechanical thrombectomy arm (60.3% vs 55.3%; p > 0.05) [104]. The multicenter TAPAS (Thrombus Aspiration during Percutaneous Coronary Intervention in Acute Myocardial Infarction Study) trial randomized 1071 patients with STEMI to either routine PCI or thrombus aspiration with an Export catheter followed by PCI. Complete ST-segment resolution

Table 8.6 TIMI grade flow classification.

TIMI 0 flow (no perfusion) refers to the absence of any antegrade flow beyond a coronary occlusion

TIMI 1 flow (penetration without perfusion) is faint antegrade coronary flow beyond the occlusion, with incomplete filling of the distal coronary bed

TIMI 2 flow (partial reperfusion) is delayed or sluggish antegrade flow with complete filling of the distal territory

TIMI 3 flow (complete perfusion) is normal flow which fills the distal coronary bed completely

---

was higher in the thrombus aspiration arm (56.6% vs 44.2%; p < 0.001). Rates of death (2.1% vs 4.0%), MI (0.8% vs 1.9%), and MACE (6.8% vs 9.4%) were similar between the two arms at 30 days. The authors noted that death and MACE at 30 days were both significantly associated with myocardial blush grade and resolution of ST-segment elevation (p < 0.01) [105].

Mechanical aspiration

In the X AMINE ST (X-sizer in AMI for negligible embolization and optimal ST resolution) trial, 201 patients with STEMI presenting within 12 hours after symptom onset were randomized to mechanical thrombectomy with the X-Sizer (ev3, White Bear Lake, MN, USA) device prior to PCI or conventional PCI. The use of the X-Sizer device was associated with a greater magnitude of ST-segment resolution (7.5 vs 4.9 mm; p = 0.03) and a greater reduction in distal embolization (2% vs 10%; p = 0.03). However, the incidence of 6-month major adverse cardiac and cerebrovascular events (MACCE) (13% vs 13%) and death (6% vs 4%) were similar between the two arms [106]. The AIMI (AngioJet Rheolytic Thrombectomy In Patients Undergoing Primary Angioplasty for Acute Myocardial Infarction) trial randomized 480 STEMI patients presenting within 12 hours of symptom onset to rheolytic thrombectomy (RT) using the AngioJet RT catheter (Possis Medical, Inc, now MEDRAD International, Pittsburgh, PA, USA) prior to PCI, or conventional PCI. The primary endpoint of final infarct size (measured by sestamibi imaging after 14–28 days) was higher in the RT arm as compared with the conventional PCI arm (9.8% vs 12.5%; p = 0.03). Final TIMI-3 flow was also lower in the RT arm (91.8% vs 97.0%; p < 0.02), and 30-day MACE rates were higher (6.7% vs 1.7%; p = 0.01), including 30-day mortality (4.6% vs 0.8%; p = 0.02) [107]. The more recent JETSTENT (Comparison of AngioJET Rheolytic Thrombectomy Before Direct Infarct Artery STENTing in Patients with Acute Myocardial Infarction) trial randomized 501 STEMI patients presenting within 12 hours from symptom onset, and who were noted to have thrombus grade 3–5 after angiography and initial wiring, to either mechanical thrombectomy with the AngioJet device, followed by direct stenting, or direct stenting alone. Procedural time was significantly longer in the thrombectomy arm (59.5 minutes vs 46 minutes; p < 0.001). However, the primary endpoint of ST-segment

Table 8.7 Baseline characteristics of randomized controlled trials comparing thrombectomy to PCI alone for primary PCI. (Modified from Bavry et al. [111] by permission of Oxford University Press.)

Study	Year*	Device	Number of patients	Age (years)	Baseline TIMI-0/1 flow (%)	Visible thrombus (%)	Ischemia (hours)§	Follow-up (Months)
Simple catheter aspiration								
VAMPIRE [112]	2008	TVAC	180/175	63/64	75/75	NA	5.4/6.2	8
TAPAS [105]	2007	Export	535/536	63/63	55/60	49 / 44	3.2/3.1	1
DEAR-MI [113]	2006	Pronto	74/74	57/60	81/ 73	NA	3.4/3.3	1
De Luca V[114]	2006	Diver	38/38	67/65	NA	NA	7.2/7.6	6
Kaltoft et al. [115]	2006	Rescue	108/107	65/63	68/69	69/79	4.0/3.5	1
REMEDIA [116]	2005	Diver	50/49	61/60	86/90	58/55†	4.6/5.0§	1
Dudek et al. [104]	2004	Rescue	40/32	NA	NA	NA	4.3/3.9	H
Noel et al. [117]	A	Export	24/26	61/61	NA	NA	4.7/4.7	H
Sardella et al. [118]	A	Diver	28/34	65/65	NA	NA	6.8/6.8	6
NONSTOP [119]	A	Rescue	129/129	64/66	NA	NA	NA	H
Oreglia et al. [120]	A	Pronto	74/74		NA	NA	NA	H
Mechanical aspiration								
AIMI [107]	2006	AngioJet	240/240	60/60	68/63	NA	5.1/5.0	1
X AMINE ST [106]	2005	X-sizer	100/101	61/62	NA	100‡	NA	6
Antoniucci et al. [121]	2004	AngioJet	50/50	63/66	76/80	NA	3.9/4.4	1
Napodano et al. [122]	2003	X-sizer	46/46	61/64	NA	NA	4.0/3.4	1
Beran et al. [123]	2002	X-sizer	30/31	56/54	80/74	NA	4.9/4.7	1
JETSTENT [108]	A	AngioJet	246/240	63/64	84/84	100‡	2.1/2.3	6
Embolic protection								
DEDICATION [110]	2008	FilterWire	312/314	62/63	67/68	68/75	3.9/3.7	1
Tahk et al. [124]	2008	GuardWire	50/46	57/57	67/76	NA	5.7/5.5	6
MICADO [125]	2007	GuardWire	80/74	65/65	78/71	NA	5.2/4.4	6
UpFlow MI [126]	2007	FilterWire	51/49	60/57	78/92	NA	4.5/3.5	1
PREMIAR [127]	2007	SpideRX	70/70	60/60	85/83	90/97	2.5/2.4	6
Ochala et al. [128]	2007	GuardWire	57/63	58/59	84/78	58/71	6.0/6.0	6
ASPARAGUS [129]	2007	Guardwire	173/168	64/65	61/58	NA	NA	6
PROMISE [130]	2005	FilterWire	100/100	63/60	65/57	NA	6.2/7.9	1
EMERALD [109]	2005	GuardWire	252/249	59/60	64/68	72/72	3.9/3.5	6
DIPLOMATE [131]	A	Angioguard	32/28	32/28	70	NA	NA	1
Wang et al. [132]	A	Angioguard	20/20	NA	NA	NA	NA	H
Nanasato et al. [133]	A	GuardWire	34/30	NA	NA	NA	NA	H

*Defined as year of publication.
†Defined as thrombus score of 4.
‡By protocol all study participants were required to have an occluded thrombus containing lesion.
§Defined as onset of ischemic symptoms until percutaneous coronary intervention, except where noted which is onset of symptoms until angiography.
IIDue to the unexpected high rate of mortality in the control arm, mortality was adjudicated at 6 months.
A, abstract; GP, glycoprotein; H, follow-up to hospital discharge, NA, not available; TIMI, thrombolysis in myocardial infarction; TVAC, transvascular aspiration catheter.

resolution of greater than 50% at 30 minutes was significantly better in the thrombectomy arm (85.8% vs 78.8%; p = 0.04). Infarct size was similar between the two arms. The incidence of MACCE at 30 days (3.1% vs 6.9%; p = 0.05) and at 6 months (12.0% vs 20.7%; p = 0.012) was significantly lower in the thrombectomy arm, primarily driven by a reduction in TVR with thrombectomy; rates of death and MI were similar [108].

Embolic protection devices

The EMERALD (Enhanced Myocardial Efficacy and Recovery by Aspiration of Liberated Debris) trial randomized 501 patients with STEMI presenting within 6 hours of symptom onset to either PCI with a balloon occlusion and aspiration distal microcirculatory protection system (GuardWire Plus, Medtronic Corp, Santa Rosa, CA, USA) or angioplasty without distal protection. The primary endpoints of complete ST-segment resolution at 30 minutes (63.3% vs 61.9%; p = 0.78) and left ventricular infarct size, as measured by sestamibi imaging after 5–14 days were similar between the embolic protection device (EPD) and conventional PCI arms (12.0% vs 9.5%; p = 0.15). MACE incidence at 6 months were also similar (10% vs 11%; p = 0.66) [109]. Similarly, the DEDICATION (Drug Elution and Distal protection In ST-elevation Myocardial Infarction) trial randomized 626 STEMI patients presenting within 12 hours of symptom onset to either distal protection with a FilterWire-EZ (Boston Scientific, Natick, MA, USA) or SpiderX protection device (ev3, Minneapolis, MN, USA), followed by PCI or conventional PCI. There was no difference between the EPD and conventional PCI arms in the incidence of the primary endpoint of complete ST-segment resolution (76% vs 72%; p = 0.29). Other parameters such as peak CK-MB (185 vs 184 µg/L; p = 0.99), median left ventricular wall motion index on echocardiography prior to discharge (1.7 vs 1.7; p = 0.35), and MACCE at 1 month after PCI (5.4% vs 3.2%; p = 0.17) were similar between the two arms [110].

A meta-analysis of 6415 patients from 30 studies noted that overall there was no significant improvement in outcomes with the use of mechanical thrombectomy as compared with conventional PCI, including mortality (3.2% vs 3.7%; p = 0.29), MI (1.3% vs 1.9%), and TLR (5.9% vs 6.4%), over a weighted mean duration of follow-up of 5.0 months. Simple catheter aspiration seemed to be associated with a significant reduction in all-cause mortality (2.7% vs 4.4%; p = 0.018), while mechanical thrombectomy devices seemed to be associated with an increase in all-cause mortality (5.3% vs 2.8%; p = 0.05); EPDs seemed to have no significant difference in mortality compared with conventional PCI (3.1% vs 3.4%; p = 0.69) (Figure 8.4) [111].

For SVG interventions

Although mechanical aspiration devices can sometimes be employed for SVG interventions, the vast majority of mechanical thrombectomies during SVG interventions involve the use of EPDs. Three categories of EPDs are employed: distal occlusion devices (e.g., the GuardWire), distal embolic protection filters (e.g., the FilterWire), and proximal occlusion devices (e.g., the Proxis catheter).

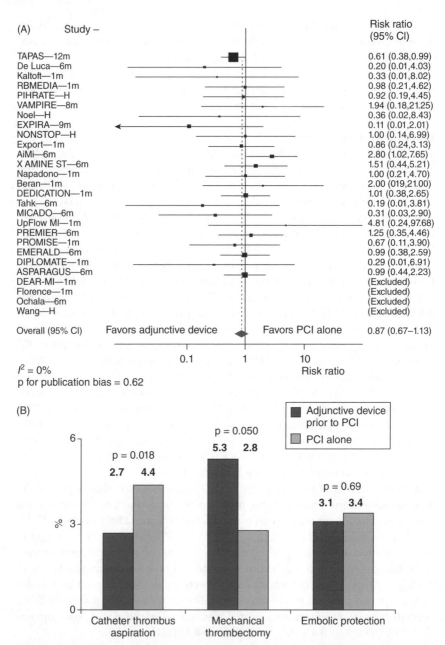

(A)   Study –

	Risk ratio (95% CI)
TAPAS—12m	0.61 (0.38,0.99)
De Luca—6m	0.20 (0.01,4.03)
Kaltoft—1m	0.33 (0.01,8.02)
RBMEDIA—1m	0.98 (0.21,4.62)
PIHRATE—H	0.92 (0.19,4.45)
VAMPIRE—8m	1.94 (0.18,21.25)
Noel—H	0.36 (0.02,8.43)
EXPIRA—9m	0.11 (0.01,2.01)
NONSTOP—H	1.00 (0.14,6.99)
Export—1m	0.86 (0.24,3.13)
AiMi—6m	2.80 (1.02,7.65)
X AMINE ST—6m	1.51 (0.44,5.21)
Napadono—1m	1.00 (0.21,4.70)
Beran—1m	2.00 (019,21.00)
DEDICATION—1m	1.01 (0.38,2.65)
Tahk—6m	0.19 (0.01,3.81)
MICADO—6m	0.31 (0.03,2.90)
UpFlow MI—1m	4.81 (0.24,97.68)
PREMIER—6m	1.25 (0.35,4.46)
PROMISE—1m	0.67 (0.11,3.90)
EMERALD—6m	0.99 (0.38,2.59)
DIPLOMATE—1m	0.29 (0.01,6.91)
ASPARAGUS—6m	0.99 (0.44,2.23)
DEAR-MI—1m	(Excluded)
Florence—1m	(Excluded)
Ochala—6m	(Excluded)
Wang—H	(Excluded)
Overall (95% CI)	0.87 (0.67–1.13)

Favors adjunctive device   Favors PCI alone

0.1   1   10

$I^2 = 0\%$
p for publication bias = 0.62

Risk ratio

(B)

Figure 8.4 (A) Summary plot for mortality comparing percutaneous coronary intervention (PCI) with adjunctive device use versus primary PCI alone. (B) Incidence of mortality with similar type adjunctive thrombectomy devices grouped together (compared with primary PCI alone). (Reproduced from Bavry *et al.* [111] by permission of Oxford University Press.)

The SAFER (Saphenous Vein Graft Angioplasty Free of Emboli Randomized) trial randomized 801 patients with SVG disease to either stent placement over the shaft of the PercuSurge GuardWire device (Medtronic Vascular, Santa Clara, CA, USA) or over a conventional 0.014-inch angioplasty guidewire. The incidence of MACE at 30 days was significantly lower in the EPD arm as compared with the conventional PCI arm (9.6% vs 16.5%; p = 0.004), driven predominantly by a significant reduction in the incidence of periprocedural MI (8.6% vs 14.7%; p = 0.008), and "no reflow" phenomenon (3% vs 9%; p = 0.02) [134]. The FIRE (FilterWire EX Randomized Evaluation) trial randomized 651 patients undergoing SVG interventions to distal protection with the filter-based FilterWire EX (Boston Scientific, Natick, MA, USA) versus the GuardWire balloon occlusion and aspiration system. Device success was similar between the FilterWire EX and GuardWire systems (95.5% vs 97.2%; p = 0.25). FilterWire EX was non-inferior to the GuardWire system for the primary endpoint of 30-day MACE rates (9.9% vs 11.6%; p = 0.0008). Rates of individual outcomes such as death (0.9% vs 0.9%; p = 0.99) and MI (9% vs 10%; p = 0.69) were similar between the two arms [135]. Recently, the Interceptor PLUS Coronary Filter System (Medtronic Vascular, Santa Clara, CA, USA) was shown to be non-inferior to the FilterWire EZ and GuardWire devices in the AMEthyst (Assessment of the Medtronic AVE Interceptor Saphenous Vein Graft Filter System) trial [136].

Special issues

Femoral versus radial access

Femoral access has been the dominant access site for coronary angiography and PCI for the past two decades. However, with increased recognition that bleeding, a common complication of femoral access, is associated with an elevated risk of mortality and morbidity, there has been renewed interest in the role of radial access for diagnostic angiography and PCI to minimize bleeding. A meta-analysis of 23 trials comparing femoral to radial access noted a significant reduction in the incidence of bleeding with radial access (0.05% vs 2.3%; OR, 0.27; 95% CI, 0.16–0.45; p < 0.001), with a trend towards a lower rate of MACE (2.5% vs 3.8%; p = 0.06). Technical difficulties such as inability to cross a lesion with a wire, balloon or stent during PCI were higher with radial access (4.7% vs 3.4%; p = 0.21) [137]. More recently, the landmark RIVAL (RadIal Vs femorAL access for coronary intervention) trial was published, in which 7021 patients with ACS were randomized to either radial or femoral access. The primary outcome of death, MI, stroke, and non-CABG bleeding was similar between radial and femoral access arms (3.7% vs 4.0%; p = 0.5). However, major vascular access site complications (1.4% vs 3.7%; p < 0.0001) and non-CABG major bleeding (1.9% vs 4.5%; p < 0.0001) were significantly lower in the radial access arm. Other outcomes at 30 days were similar. PCI procedure times were similar, but fluoroscopic times were higher. Patient preference for the access site for the next procedure was almost twice as high with radial access. The maximum benefit in this trial was noted in centers with the highest radial access volume [138].

Left main PCI

Although left main (LM) trunk stenosis has long been considered a surgical problem, recent advances in interventional cardiology have prompted renewed interest in the role of unprotected LM PCI as an alternative to CABG. The SYNTAX (Synergy Between Percutaneous Coronary Intervention With TAXUS and Cardiac Surgery) trial attempted to address this issue (see also Chapter 9). In this trial, 1800 patients with three-vessel disease and/or LM disease who were deemed eligible for CABG and PCI were randomized to either DES PCI with a PES or on- or off-pump CABG. The incidence of the primary endpoint of MACCE at 12 months was lower in the CABG arm compared with the PCI arm (12.4% vs 17.8%; p = 0.002), and did not meet the prespecified non-inferiority threshold for PCI. This was driven predominantly by a significant reduction in the incidence of repeat revascularization in the CABG arm compared with PCI (5.9% vs 13.5%; p < 0.001). There was no difference in the incidence of death (3.5% vs 4.4%; p = 0.37) or MI between the two arms (3.3% vs 4.8; p = 0.11). The incidence of cerebrovascular accident was significantly higher in the CABG arm (2.2% vs 0.6%; p = 0.003), whereas the incidence of symptomatic graft occlusion and stent thrombosis was similar between the two arms (3.4% vs 3.3%; p = 0.89) [139]. In subgroup analysis of the LM patients, the overall 12-month MACCE rate was lower with CABG (13.7% vs 15.8%; p = 0.44), although patients with LM only (8.5% vs 7.1%) and LM + one-vessel disease (13.2% vs 7.5%) seemed to do slightly better with PCI. Patients with LM + two-vessel disease (14.4% vs 19.8%), LM + three-vessel disease (15.4% vs 19.3%), or three-vessel disease alone (11.5% vs 19.2%) seemed to do better with CABG than PCI [140]. The ISAR LEFT MAIN (Intra-coronary Stenting and Angiographic Results: Drug-Eluting Stents for Unpro-tected Coronary Left Main Lesions) trial randomized 607 patients with LM disease to either PES or SES, and noted similar rates of MACE (13.6% vs 15.8%; p = 0.44) and stent thrombosis (0.3% vs 0.7%) at 1 year, and similar mortality (10.7% vs 8.7%) and angiographic restenosis (16.0% vs 19.4%) at 2 years [141].

Revascularization of chronic totally occluded lesions

Chronic totally occluded lesions (CTOs) are noted in nearly a third of patients with CAD. The decision to revascularize a CTO revolves around the so-called "open artery" hypothesis. Benefits include improvement of clinical symptoms, normalization of a positive exercise test, reduced left ventricular modeling, lower need for later bypass surgery, and potentially even improved survival. The TOSCA trial randomized 410 patients with non-acute native coronary artery occlusions to either PTCA alone or BMS stenting with a heparin-coated Palmaz–Schatz stent. Although the incidence of MACE at 6 months was similar between the PTCA and BMS arms (23.6% vs 23.3%), there was a significant reduction in the incidence of clinically-driven TVR in the BMS arm at 6 months (15.4% vs 8.4%; p = 0.03). Although lower in the BMS arm as compared with the PTCA arm, restenosis rates were very high overall

(55% vs 70%; p < 0.01) [17]. The PRISON II (Prospective Randomized Trial of Sirolimus-Eluting and Bare Metal Stents in Patients With Chronic Total Occlusions II) trial demonstrated the superiority of SES in reducing in-stent restenosis at 6 months in patients undergoing CTO PCI, as compared with BMS (7% vs 36%; p < 0.001). This translated into a reduction in MACE, primarily due to a reduction in TLR (8% vs 22%; p = 0.009) [50]. Similar results with SES versus BMS were noted in the GISSOC II-GISE (Gruppo Italiano di Studio sullo Stent nelle Occlusioni Coronariche) trial at 8 months angiographically, and at 24 months clinically [142].

Patients in whom an occluded coronary artery is noted post-infarction represent a special subset. In one of the largest studies on this topic, OAT (Occluded Artery Trial) randomized 2166 stable patients with total occlusion of the infarct-related artery 3–28 days after MI, and who met a high-risk criterion (an ejection fraction of <50% or proximal occlusion), to either routine PCI and stenting, or medical management. At 4 years, there was no difference between the PCI and medical management arms in the incidence of the primary endpoint (death, MI or NYHA class IV symptoms) (17.2% vs 15.6%; p = 0.20). No difference was noted in any of the individual endpoints either [143]. Contrary to this, the SWISS II (Swiss Interventional Study on Silent Ischemia Type II) trial randomized 201 patients with a recent MI and evidence of silent ischemia on stress imaging, to either PCI or medical management, and noted a significant reduction in the incidence of MACE with PCI (28.1% vs 63.8%; p < 0.001) over 10.2 years of follow-up. Patients in the PCI arm were more likely than those in the medical management arm to maintain their ejection fraction over the duration of follow-up [144].

Conclusions

PCI has made dramatic advances since its inception. A variety of technologies and techniques have been evaluated through RCTs. Historically, PCI device trials have focused on surrogate endpoints such as late loss, which allows trials to be smaller, but may not provide the most clinically relevant information, especially from the patient's perspective. Additionally, many devices have been approved on the basis of non-randomized studies that demonstrate safety and feasibility, but not efficacy *per se*. Meta-analyses of these trials provide strong evidence for or against the use of specific devices. The infrequency of rare but important events such as stent thrombosis has also been a challenge, but there has been a more recent movement to larger outcome studies that should advance the field, assuming that there will be a funding mechanism for these types of trials.

References

1. Gruntzig A. Transluminal dilatation of coronary-artery stenosis. *Lancet* 1978;1:263.
2. Parisi AF, Folland ED, Hartigan P. A comparison of angioplasty with medical therapy in the treatment of single-vessel coronary artery disease. Veterans Affairs ACME Investigators. *N Engl J Med* 1992;326:10–16.

3. Ellis SG, Cowley MJ, Whitlow PL, *et al.* Prospective case-control comparison of percutaneous transluminal coronary revascularization in patients with multivessel disease treated in 1986–1987 versus 1991: improved in-hospital and 12-month results. Multivessel Angioplasty Prognosis Study (MAPS) Group. *J Am Coll Cardiol* 1995;25: 1137–1142.

4. Folland ED, Hartigan PM, Parisi AF. Percutaneous transluminal coronary angioplasty versus medical therapy for stable angina pectoris: outcomes for patients with double-vessel versus single-vessel coronary artery disease in a Veterans Affairs Cooperative randomized trial. Veterans Affairs ACME InvestigatorS. *J Am Coll Cardiol* 1997;29: 1505–1511.

5. Coronary angioplasty versus medical therapy for angina: the second Randomised Intervention Treatment of Angina (RITA-2) trial. RITA-2 trial participants. *Lancet* 1997;350:461–468.

6. Effects of tissue plasminogen activator and a comparison of early invasive and conservative strategies in unstable angina and non-Q-wave myocardial infarction. Results of the TIMI IIIB Trial. Thrombolysis in Myocardial Ischemia. *Circulation* 1994;89: 1545–2556.

7. Anderson HV, Cannon CP, Stone PH, *et al.* One-year results of the Thrombolysis in Myocardial Infarction (TIMI) IIIB clinical trial. A randomized comparison of tissue-type plasminogen activator versus placebo and early invasive versus early conservative strategies in unstable angina and non-Q wave myocardial infarction. *J Am Coll Cardiol* 1995;26:1643–1650.

8. Boden WE, O'Rourke RA, Crawford MH, *et al.* Outcomes in patients with acute non-Q-wave myocardial infarction randomly assigned to an invasive as compared with a conservative management strategy. Veterans Affairs Non-Q-Wave Infarction Strategies in Hospital (VANQWISH) Trial Investigators. *N Engl J Med* 1998;338:1785–1792.

9. Pitt B, Waters D, Brown WV, *et al.* Aggressive lipid-lowering therapy compared with angioplasty in stable coronary artery disease. Atorvastatin versus Revascularization Treatment Investigators. *N Engl J Med* 1999;341:70–76.

10. Macaya C, Serruys PW, Ruygrok P, *et al.* Continued benefit of coronary stenting versus balloon angioplasty: one-year clinical follow-up of Benestent trial. Benestent Study Group. *J Am Coll Cardiol* 1996;27:255–261.

11. Kiemeneij F, Serruys PW, Macaya C, *et al.* Continued benefit of coronary stenting versus balloon angioplasty: five-year clinical follow-up of Benestent-I trial. *J Am Coll Cardiol* 2001;37:1598–1603.

12. Fischman DL, Leon MB, Baim DS, *et al.* A randomized comparison of coronary-stent placement and balloon angioplasty in the treatment of coronary artery disease. Stent Restenosis Study Investigators. *N Engl J Med* 1994;331:496–501.

13. Serruys PW, de Jaegere P, Kiemeneij F, *et al.* A comparison of balloon-expandable-stent implantation with balloon angioplasty in patients with coronary artery disease. Benestent Study Group. *N Engl J Med* 1994;331:489–495.

14. Serruys PW, van Hout B, Bonnier H, *et al.* Randomised comparison of implantation of heparin-coated stents with balloon angioplasty in selected patients with coronary artery disease (Benestent II). *Lancet* 1998;352:673–681.

15. Erbel R, Haude M, Hopp HW, *et al.* Coronary-artery stenting compared with balloon angioplasty for restenosis after initial balloon angioplasty. Restenosis Stent Study Group. *N Engl J Med* 1998;339:1672–1678.

16. Savage MP, Douglas JS, Jr., Fischman DL, *et al.* Stent placement compared with balloon angioplasty for obstructed coronary bypass grafts. Saphenous Vein De Novo Trial Investigators. *N Engl J Med* 1997;337:740–747.

17. Buller CE, Dzavik V, Carere RG, *et al*. Primary stenting versus balloon angioplasty in occluded coronary arteries: the Total Occlusion Study of Canada (TOSCA). *Circulation* 1999;100:236–242.

18. Rodriguez AE, Granada JF, Rodriguez-Alemparte M, *et al*. Oral rapamycin after coronary bare-metal stent implantation to prevent restenosis: the Prospective, Randomized Oral Rapamycin in Argentina (ORAR II) Study. *J Am Coll Cardiol* 2006;47: 1522–1529.

19. Morice MC, Serruys PW, Sousa JE, *et al*. A randomized comparison of a sirolimus-eluting stent with a standard stent for coronary revascularization. *N Engl J Med* 2002;346:1773–1780.

20. Moses JW, Leon MB, Popma JJ, *et al*. Sirolimus-eluting stents versus standard stents in patients with stenosis in a native coronary artery. *N Engl J Med* 2003;349:1315–1323.

21. Weisz G, Leon MB, Holmes DR Jr, *et al*. Five-year follow-up after sirolimus-eluting stent implantation results of the SIRIUS (Sirolimus-Eluting Stent in De-Novo Native Coronary Lesions) Trial. *J Am Coll Cardiol* 2009;53:1488–1497.

22. Schofer J, Schluter M, Gershlick AH, *et al*. Sirolimus-eluting stents for treatment of patients with long atherosclerotic lesions in small coronary arteries: double-blind, randomised controlled trial (E-SIRIUS). *Lancet* 2003;362:1093–1099.

23. Schampaert E, Cohen EA, Schluter M, *et al*. The Canadian study of the sirolimus-eluting stent in the treatment of patients with long de novo lesions in small native coronary arteries (C-SIRIUS). *J Am Coll Cardiol* 2004;43:1110–1115.

24. Kastrati A, Mehilli J, Pache J, *et al*. Analysis of 14 trials comparing sirolimus-eluting stents with bare-metal stents. *N Engl J Med* 2007;356:1030–1039.

25. Lansky AJ, Costa RA, Mintz GS, *et al*. Non-polymer-based paclitaxel-coated coronary stents for the treatment of patients with de novo coronary lesions: angiographic follow-up of the DELIVER clinical trial. *Circulation* 2004;109:1948–1954.

26. Stone GW, Ellis SG, Cox DA, *et al*. A polymer-based, paclitaxel-eluting stent in patients with coronary artery disease. *N Engl J Med* 2004;350:221–231.

27. Ellis SG, Stone GW, Cox DA, *et al*. Long-term safety and efficacy with paclitaxel-eluting stents: 5-year final results of the TAXUS IV clinical trial (TAXUS IV-SR: Treatment of De Novo Coronary Disease Using a Single Paclitaxel-Eluting Stent). *JACC Cardiovasc Interv* 2009;2:1248–1259.

28. Roukoz H, Bavry AA, Sarkees ML, *et al*. Comprehensive meta-analysis on drug-eluting stents versus bare-metal stents during extended follow-up. *Am J Med* 2009;122: 581e1–10.

29. Grube E, Silber S, Hauptmann KE, *et al*. TAXUS I: six- and twelve-month results from a randomized, double-blind trial on a slow-release paclitaxel-eluting stent for de novo coronary lesions. *Circulation* 2003;107:38–42.

30. Colombo A, Drzewiecki J, Banning A, *et al*. Randomized study to assess the effectiveness of slow- and moderate-release polymer-based paclitaxel-eluting stents for coronary artery lesions. *Circulation* 2003;108:788–794.

31. Stone GW, Ellis SG, Cannon L, *et al*. Comparison of a polymer-based paclitaxel-eluting stent with a bare metal stent in patients with complex coronary artery disease: a randomized controlled trial. *JAMA* 2005;294:1215–1223.

32. Grube E, Dawkins KD, Guagliumi G, *et al*. TAXUS VI 2-year follow-up: randomized comparison of polymer-based paclitaxel-eluting with bare metal stents for treatment of long, complex lesions. *Eur Heart J* 2007;28:2578–2582.

33. Erglis A, Narbute I, Kumsars I, *et al*. A randomized comparison of paclitaxel-eluting stents versus bare-metal stents for treatment of unprotected left main coronary artery stenosis. *J Am Coll Cardiol* 2007;50:491–497.

34. Laarman GJ, Suttorp MJ, Dirksen MT, *et al*. Paclitaxel-eluting versus uncoated stents in primary percutaneous coronary intervention. *N Engl J Med* 2006;355:1105–13.

35. Tierala I SM, Kupari M. The HAAMU-STENT study. Available at: http://www.tctmd.com/Show.aspx?id=56036. Accessed March 26, 2012.

36. Chechi T, Vittori G, Biondi Zoccai GG, *et al*. Single-center randomized evaluation of paclitaxel-eluting versus conventional stent in acute myocardial infarction (SELECTION). *J Interv Cardiol* 2007;20:282–291.

37. Ardissino D, Cavallini C, Bramucci E, *et al*. Sirolimus-eluting vs uncoated stents for prevention of restenosis in small coronary arteries: a randomized trial. *JAMA* 2004;292:2727–34.

38. Kelbaek H, Thuesen L, Helqvist S, *et al*. The Stenting Coronary Arteries in Non-stress/benestent Disease (SCANDSTENT) trial. *J Am Coll Cardiol* 2006;47:449–455.

39. Sabate M, Jimenez-Quevedo P, Angiolillo DJ, *et al*. Randomized comparison of sirolimus-eluting stent versus standard stent for percutaneous coronary revascularization in diabetic patients: the diabetes and sirolimus-eluting stent (DIABETES) trial. *Circulation* 2005;112:2175–2183.

40. Pache J, Dibra A, Mehilli J, Dirschinger J, Schomig A, Kastrati A. Drug-eluting stents compared with thin-strut bare stents for the reduction of restenosis: a prospective, randomized trial. *Eur Heart J* 2005;26:1262–1268.

41. Chan C, Zambahari R, Kaul U, *et al*. A randomized comparison of sirolimus-eluting versus bare metal stents in the treatment of diabetic patients with native coronary artery lesions: the DECODE study. *Catheter Cardiovasc Interv* 2008;72:591–600.

42. Baumgart D, Klauss V, Baer F, *et al*. One-year results of the SCORPIUS study: a German multicenter investigation on the effectiveness of sirolimus-eluting stents in diabetic patients. *J Am Coll Cardiol* 2007;50:1627–1634.

43. Maresta A, Varani E, Balducelli M, *et al*. Comparison of effectiveness and safety of sirolimus-eluting stents versus bare-metal stents in patients with diabetes mellitus (from the Italian Multicenter Randomized DESSERT Study). *Am J Cardiol* 2008;101:1560–1566.

44. Valgimigli M, Percoco G, Malagutti P, *et al*. Tirofiban and sirolimus-eluting stent vs abciximab and bare-metal stent for acute myocardial infarction: a randomized trial. *JAMA* 2005;293:2109–117.

45. Spaulding C, Henry P, Teiger E, *et al*. Sirolimus-eluting versus uncoated stents in acute myocardial infarction. *N Engl J Med* 2006;355:1093–1104.

46. Menichelli M, Parma A, Pucci E, *et al*. Randomized trial of Sirolimus-Eluting Stent Versus Bare-Metal Stent in Acute Myocardial Infarction (SESAMI). *J Am Coll Cardiol* 2007;49:1924–1930.

47. van der Hoeven BL, Liem SS, Jukema JW, *et al*. Sirolimus-eluting stents versus bare-metal stents in patients with ST-segment elevation myocardial infarction: 9-month angiographic and intravascular ultrasound results and 12-month clinical outcome results from the MISSION! Intervention Study. *J Am Coll Cardiol* 2008;51:618–626.

48. Diaz de la Llera LS, Ballesteros S, Nevado J, *et al*. Sirolimus-eluting stents compared with standard stents in the treatment of patients with primary angioplasty. *Am Heart J* 2007;154:164e1–6.

49. Gao H, Yan HB, Zhu XL, *et al*. Firebird sirolimus eluting stent versus bare mental stent in patients with ST-segment elevation myocardial infarction. *Chin Med J (Engl)* 2007;120:863–867.

50. Suttorp MJ, Laarman GJ, Rahel BM, *et al*. Primary Stenting of Totally Occluded Native Coronary Arteries II (PRISON II): a randomized comparison of bare metal stent implantation with sirolimus-eluting stent implantation for the treatment of total coronary occlusions. *Circulation* 2006;114:921–928.

51. Kaiser C, Brunner-La Rocca HP, Buser PT, *et al.* Incremental cost-effectiveness of drug-eluting stents compared with a third-generation bare-metal stent in a real-world setting: randomised Basel Stent Kosten Effektivitats Trial (BASKET). *Lancet* 2005;366: 921–929.

52. Kumbhani DJ, Bavry AA, Bhatt DL. Late stent thrombosis with drug-eluting stents: the price to pay to prevent restenosis? *Indian Heart J* 2007;59:B113–117.

53. Bavry AA, Kumbhani DJ, Helton TJ, Borek PP, Mood GR, Bhatt DL. Late thrombosis of drug-eluting stents: a meta-analysis of randomized clinical trials. *Am J Med* 2006;119: 1056–1061.

54. Stone GW, Moses JW, Ellis SG, *et al.* Safety and efficacy of sirolimus- and paclitaxel-eluting coronary stents. *N Engl J Med* 2007;356:998–1008.

55. Lagerqvist B, James SK, Stenestrand U, Lindback J, Nilsson T, Wallentin L. Long-term outcomes with drug-eluting stents versus bare-metal stents in Sweden. *N Engl J Med* 2007;356:1009–1019.

56. Bavry AA, Bhatt DL. Appropriate use of drug-eluting stents: balancing the reduction in restenosis with the concern of late thrombosis. *Lancet* 2008;371:2134–2143.

57. Kotani J, Awata M, Nanto S, *et al.* Incomplete neointimal coverage of sirolimus-eluting stents: angioscopic findings. *J Am Coll Cardiol* 2006;47:2108–2111.

58. Joner M, Finn AV, Farb A, *et al.* Pathology of drug-eluting stents in humans: delayed healing and late thrombotic risk. *J Am Coll Cardiol* 2006;48:193–202.

59. Kereiakes DJ. Does clopidogrel each day keep stent thrombosis away? *JAMA* 2007;297: 209–211.

60. Iakovou I, Schmidt T, Bonizzoni E, *et al.* Incidence, predictors, and outcome of thrombosis after successful implantation of drug-eluting stents. *JAMA* 2005;293: 2126–2130.

61. Chhatriwalla AK, Bhatt DL. Should dual antiplatelet therapy after drug-eluting stents be continued for more than 1 year?: Dual antiplatelet therapy after drug-eluting stents should be continued for more than one year and preferably indefinitely. *Circ Cardiovasc Interv* 2008;1:217–225.

62. Park DW, Park SW, Park KH, *et al.* Frequency of and risk factors for stent thrombosis after drug-eluting stent implantation during long-term follow-up. *Am J Cardiol* 2006; 98:352–356.

63. Eisenstein EL, Anstrom KJ, Kong DF, *et al.* Clopidogrel use and long-term clinical outcomes after drug-eluting stent implantation. *JAMA* 2007;297:159–168.

64. Michelson AD. Platelet function testing in cardiovascular diseases. *Circulation* 2004; 110:e489–493.

65. Mega JL, Close SL, Wiviott SD, *et al.* Cytochrome p-450 polymorphisms and response to clopidogrel. *N Engl J Med* 2009;360:354–362.

66. Schomig A, Dibra A, Windecker S, *et al.* A meta-analysis of 16 randomized trials of sirolimus-eluting stents versus paclitaxel-eluting stents in patients with coronary artery disease. *J Am Coll Cardiol* 2007;50:1373–1380.

67. Kumbhani DJ, Bavry AA, Kamdar AR, Helton TJ, Bhatt DL. The effect of drug-eluting stents on intermediate angiographic and clinical outcomes in diabetic patients: insights from randomized clinical trials. *Am Heart J* 2008;155:640–647.

68. Grube E, Sonoda S, Ikeno F, *et al.* Six- and twelve-month results from first human experience using everolimus-eluting stents with bioabsorbable polymer. *Circulation* 2004;109:2168–2171.

69. Serruys PW, Ong AT, Piek JJ, *et al.* A randomized comparison of a durable polymer Everolimus-eluting stent with a bare metal coronary stent: The SPIRIT first trial. *EuroIntervention* 2005;1:58–65.

70. Serruys PW, Ruygrok P, Neuzner J, *et al.* A randomised comparison of an everolimus-eluting coronary stent with a paclitaxel-eluting coronary stent:the SPIRIT II trial. *EuroIntervention* 2006;2:286–294.

71. Stone GW, Midei M, Newman W, et al. Comparison of an everolimus-eluting stent and a paclitaxel-eluting stent in patients with coronary artery disease: a randomized trial. *JAMA* 2008;299:1903–1913.

72. Stone GW, Midei M, Newman W, *et al.* Randomized comparison of everolimus-eluting and paclitaxel-eluting stents: two-year clinical follow-up from the Clinical Evaluation of the Xience V Everolimus Eluting Coronary Stent System in the Treatment of Patients with de novo Native Coronary Artery Lesions (SPIRIT) III trial. *Circulation* 2009;119: 680–686.

73. Stone GW, Rizvi A, Newman W, *et al.* Everolimus-eluting versus paclitaxel-eluting stents in coronary artery disease. *N Engl J Med* 2010;362:1663–1674.

74. Fajadet J, Wijns W, Laarman GJ, *et al.* Randomized, double-blind, multicenter study of the Endeavor zotarolimus-eluting phosphorylcholine-encapsulated stent for treatment of native coronary artery lesions: clinical and angiographic results of the ENDEAVOR II trial. *Circulation* 2006;114:798–806.

75. Kandzari DE, Leon MB, Popma JJ, *et al.* Comparison of zotarolimus-eluting and sirolimus-eluting stents in patients with native coronary artery disease: a randomized controlled trial. *J Am Coll Cardiol* 2006;48:2440–2447.

76. Rasmussen K, Maeng M, Kaltoft A, *et al.* Efficacy and safety of zotarolimus-eluting and sirolimus-eluting coronary stents in routine clinical care (SORT OUT III): a randomised controlled superiority trial. *Lancet* 2010;375:1090–1099.

77. Leon MB, Mauri L, Popma JJ, *et al.* A randomized comparison of the ENDEAVOR zotarolimus-eluting stent versus the TAXUS paclitaxel-eluting stent in de novo native coronary lesions 12-month outcomes from the ENDEAVOR IV trial. *J Am Coll Cardiol* 2010;55:543–554.

78. Leon MB, Kandzari DE, Eisenstein EL, *et al.* Late safety, efficacy, and cost-effectiveness of a zotarolimus-eluting stent compared with a paclitaxel-eluting stent in patients with de novo coronary lesions: 2-year follow-up from the ENDEAVOR IV trial (Randomized, Controlled Trial of the Medtronic Endeavor Drug [ABT-578] Eluting Coronary Stent System Versus the Taxus Paclitaxel-Eluting Coronary Stent System in De Novo Native Coronary Artery Lesions). *JACC Cardiovasc Interv* 2009;2: 1208–1218.

79. Serruys PW, Silber S, Garg S, *et al.* Comparison of zotarolimus-eluting and everolimus-eluting coronary stents. *N Engl J Med* 2010;363:136–146.

80. Windecker S, Serruys PW, Wandel S, *et al.* Biolimus-eluting stent with biodegradable polymer versus sirolimus-eluting stent with durable polymer for coronary revascularisation (LEADERS): a randomised non-inferiority trial. *Lancet* 2008;372:1163–1173.

81. Ormiston JA, Serruys PW, Regar E, *et al.* A bioabsorbable everolimus-eluting coronary stent system for patients with single de-novo coronary artery lesions (ABSORB): a prospective open-label trial. *Lancet* 2008;371:899–907.

82. Scheller B, Hehrlein C, Bocksch W, *et al.* Treatment of coronary in-stent restenosis with a paclitaxel-coated balloon catheter. *N Engl J Med* 2006;355:2113–2124.

83. Scheller B, Hehrlein C, Bocksch W, *et al.* Two year follow-up after treatment of coronary in-stent restenosis with a paclitaxel-coated balloon catheter. *Clin Res Cardiol* 2008;97: 773–781.

84. Herdeg C, Gohring-Frischholz K, Haase KK, *et al.* Catheter-based delivery of fluid paclitaxel for prevention of restenosis in native coronary artery lesions after stent implantation. *Circ Cardiovasc Interv* 2009;2:294–301.

85. Unverdorben M, Vallbracht C, Cremers B, *et al.* Paclitaxel-coated balloon catheter versus paclitaxel-coated stent for the treatment of coronary in-stent restenosis. *Circulation* 2009;119:2986–2994.

86. Topol EJ, Leya F, Pinkerton CA, *et al.* A comparison of directional atherectomy with coronary angioplasty in patients with coronary artery disease. The CAVEAT Study Group. *N Engl J Med* 1993;329:221–227.

87. Adelman AG, Cohen EA, Kimball BP, *et al.* A comparison of directional atherectomy with balloon angioplasty for lesions of the left anterior descending coronary artery. *N Engl J Med* 1993;329:228–233.

88. Stankovic G, Colombo A, Bersin R, *et al.* Comparison of directional coronary atherectomy and stenting versus stenting alone for the treatment of de novo and restenotic coronary artery narrowing. *Am J Cardiol* 2004;93:953–958.

89. Bittl JA, Chew DP, Topol EJ, Kong DF, Califf RM. Meta-analysis of randomized trials of percutaneous transluminal coronary angioplasty versus atherectomy, cutting balloon atherotomy, or laser angioplasty. *J Am Coll Cardiol* 2004;43:936–942.

90. Ergene O, Seyithanoglu BY, Tastan A, *et al.* Comparison of Angiographic and Clinical Outcome After Cutting Balloon and Conventional Balloon Angioplasty in Vessels Smaller than 3mm in Diameter: A Randomized Trial. *J Invasive Cardiol* 1998;10:70–75.

91. Molstad P, Myreng Y, Golf S, *et al.* The Barath Cutting Balloon versus conventional angioplasty. A randomized study comparing acute success rate and frequency of late restenosis. *Scand Cardiovasc J* 1998;32:79–85.

92. Izumi M, Tsuchikane E, Funamoto M, *et al.* Final results of the CAPAS trial. *Am Heart J* 2001;142:782–789.

93. Mauri L, Bonan R, Weiner BH, *et al.* Cutting balloon angioplasty for the prevention of restenosis: results of the Cutting Balloon Global Randomized Trial. *Am J Cardiol* 2002;90:1079–1083.

94. Albiero R, Silber S, Di Mario C, *et al.* Cutting balloon versus conventional balloon angioplasty for the treatment of in-stent restenosis: results of the restenosis cutting balloon evaluation trial (RESCUT). *J Am Coll Cardiol* 2004;43:943–949.

95. Ozaki Y, Yamaguchi T, Suzuki T, *et al.* Impact of cutting balloon angioplasty (CBA) prior to bare metal stenting on restenosis. *Circ J* 2007;71:1–8.

96. Mauri L, Reisman M, Buchbinder M, *et al.* Comparison of rotational atherectomy with conventional balloon angioplasty in the prevention of restenosis of small coronary arteries: results of the Dilatation vs Ablation Revascularization Trial Targeting Restenosis (DART). *Am Heart J* 2003;145:847–854.

97. vom Dahl J, Dietz U, Haager PK, *et al.* Rotational atherectomy does not reduce recurrent in-stent restenosis: results of the angioplasty versus rotational atherectomy for treatment of diffuse in-stent restenosis trial (ARTIST). *Circulation* 2002;105:583–588.

98. Sharma SK, Kini A, Mehran R, Lansky A, Kobayashi Y, Marmur JD. Randomized trial of Rotational Atherectomy Versus Balloon Angioplasty for Diffuse In-stent Restenosis (ROSTER). *Am Heart J* 2004;147:16–22.

99. Whitlow PL, Bass TA, Kipperman RM, *et al.* Results of the study to determine rotablator and transluminal angioplasty strategy (STRATAS). *Am J Cardiol* 2001;87:699–705.

100. Safian RD, Feldman T, Muller DW, *et al.* Coronary angioplasty and Rotablator atherectomy trial (CARAT): immediate and late results of a prospective multicenter randomized trial. *Catheter Cardiovasc Interv* 2001;53:213–220.

101. Stone GW, de Marchena E, Dageforde D, *et al.* Prospective, randomized, multicenter comparison of laser-facilitated balloon angioplasty versus stand-alone balloon angioplasty in patients with obstructive coronary artery disease. The Laser Angioplasty Versus Angioplasty (LAVA) Trial Investigators. *J Am Coll Cardiol* 1997;30:1714–1721.

102. Appelman YE, Piek JJ, Strikwerda S, et al. Randomised trial of excimer laser angioplasty versus balloon angioplasty for treatment of obstructive coronary artery disease. *Lancet* 1996;347:79–84.

103. Reifart N, Vandormael M, Krajcar M, et al. Randomized comparison of angioplasty of complex coronary lesions at a single center. Excimer Laser, Rotational Atherectomy, and Balloon Angioplasty Comparison (ERBAC) Study. *Circulation* 1997;96:91–98.

104. Dudek D, Mielecki W, Legutko J, et al. Percutaneous thrombectomy with the RESCUE system in acute myocardial infarction. *Kardiol Pol* 2004;61:523–533.

105. Svilaas T, Vlaar PJ, van der Horst IC, et al. Thrombus aspiration during primary percutaneous coronary intervention. *N Engl J Med* 2008;358:557–567.

106. Lefevre T, Garcia E, Reimers B, et al. X-sizer for thrombectomy in acute myocardial infarction improves ST-segment resolution: results of the X-sizer in AMI for negligible embolization and optimal ST resolution (X AMINE ST) trial. *J Am Coll Cardiol* 2005;46:246–252.

107. Ali A, Cox D, Dib N, et al. Rheolytic thrombectomy with percutaneous coronary intervention for infarct size reduction in acute myocardial infarction: 30-day results from a multicenter randomized study. *J Am Coll Cardiol* 2006;48:244–252.

108. Antoniucci D. *Comparison of AngioJET Rheolytic Thrombectomy Before Direct Infarct Artery STENTing in Patients with Acute Myocardial Infarction: the JETSTENT Trial.* American College of Cardiology. Atlanta, GA, 2010.

109. Stone GW, Webb J, Cox DA, et al. Distal microcirculatory protection during percutaneous coronary intervention in acute ST-segment elevation myocardial infarction: a randomized controlled trial. *JAMA* 2005;293:1063–1072.

110. Kelbaek H, Terkelsen CJ, Helqvist S, et al. Randomized comparison of distal protection versus conventional treatment in primary percutaneous coronary intervention: the drug elution and distal protection in ST-elevation myocardial infarction (DEDICATION) trial. *J Am Coll Cardiol* 2008;51:899–905.

111. Bavry AA, Kumbhani DJ, Bhatt DL. Role of adjunctive thrombectomy and embolic protection devices in acute myocardial infarction: a comprehensive meta-analysis of randomized trials. *Eur Heart J* 2008;29:2989–3001.

112. Ikari Y, Sakurada M, Kozuma K, et al. Upfront thrombus aspiration in primary coronary intervention for patients with ST-segment elevation acute myocardial infarction: report of the VAMPIRE (VAcuuM asPIration thrombus REmoval) trial. *JACC Cardiovasc Interv* 2008;1:424–431.

113. Silva-Orrego P, Colombo P, Bigi R, et al. Thrombus aspiration before primary angioplasty improves myocardial reperfusion in acute myocardial infarction: the DEAR-MI (Dethrombosis to Enhance Acute Reperfusion in Myocardial Infarction) study. *J Am Coll Cardiol* 2006;48:1552–1559.

114. De Luca L, Sardella G, Davidson CJ, et al. Impact of intracoronary aspiration thrombectomy during primary angioplasty on left ventricular remodelling in patients with anterior ST elevation myocardial infarction. *Heart* 2006;92:951–957.

115. Kaltoft A, Bottcher M, Nielsen SS, et al. Routine thrombectomy in percutaneous coronary intervention for acute ST-segment-elevation myocardial infarction: a randomized, controlled trial. *Circulation* 2006;114:40–47.

116. Burzotta F, Trani C, Romagnoli E, et al. Manual thrombus-aspiration improves myocardial reperfusion: the randomized evaluation of the effect of mechanical reduction of distal embolization by thrombus-aspiration in primary and rescue angioplasty (REMEDIA) trial. *J Am Coll Cardiol* 2005;46:371–376.

117. Noel B, Morice MC, Lefevre T, et al. Thromboaspiration in acute ST elevation MI improves myocardial reperfusion. *Circulation* 2005;112 (Suppl II):519.

118. Sardella G, De Luca L, Mancone M, *et al*. Impact of thromboaspiration device during primary angioplasty on left ventricular remodeling in patients with acute anterior myocardial infarction. *Circulation* 2005;112 (Suppl II):519.

119. Kunii H, Kijima M, Araki T, *et al*. Lack of benefit of intracoronary thrombus aspiration before coronary stenting in patients with acute myocardial infarction: a multicenter randomized trial. *J Am Coll Cardiol* 2004;43 (Suppl A):245A.

120. Oreglia JA, Silva-Orrego P, Colombo A, *et al*. Impact of thrombus aspiration in acute myocardial infarction on procedural aspects of primary percutaneous intervention. *Am J Cardiol* 2006;98(Suppl 1):25M.

121. Antoniucci D, Valenti R, Migliorini A, *et al*. Comparison of rheolytic thrombectomy before direct infarct artery stenting versus direct stenting alone in patients undergoing percutaneous coronary intervention for acute myocardial infarction. *Am J Cardiol* 2004; 93:1033–1035.

122. Napodano M, Pasquetto G, Sacca S, *et al*. Intracoronary thrombectomy improves myocardial reperfusion in patients undergoing direct angioplasty for acute myocardial infarction. *J Am Coll Cardiol* 2003;42:1395–1402.

123. Beran G, Lang I, Schreiber W, *et al*. Intracoronary thrombectomy with the X-sizer catheter system improves epicardial flow and accelerates ST-segment resolution in patients with acute coronary syndrome: a prospective, randomized, controlled study. *Circulation* 2002;105:2355–2360.

124. Tahk SJ, Choi BJ, Choi SY, *et al*. Distal protection device protects microvascular integrity during primary percutaneous intervention in acute myocardial infarction: a prospective, randomized, multicenter trial. *Int J Cardiol* 2008;123:162–168.

125. Matsuo A, Inoue N, Suzuki K, *et al*. Limitations of using a GuardWire temporary occlusion and aspiration system in patients with acute myocardial infarction: multicenter investigation of coronary artery protection with a distal occlusion device in acute myocardial infarction (MICADO). *J Invasive Cardiol* 2007;19:132–138.

126. Guetta V, Mosseri M, Shechter M, *et al*. Safety and efficacy of the FilterWire EZ in acute ST-segment elevation myocardial infarction. *Am J Cardiol* 2007;99:911–915.

127. Cura FA, Escudero AG, Berrocal D, *et al*. Protection of Distal Embolization in High-Risk Patients with Acute ST-Segment Elevation Myocardial Infarction (PREMIAR). *Am J Cardiol* 2007;99:357–363.

128. Ochala A, Smolka G, Wojakowski W, Gabrylewicz B, Garbocz P, Tendera M. Prospective randomised study to evaluate effectiveness of distal embolic protection compared to abciximab administration in reduction of microembolic complications of primary coronary angioplasty. *Kardiol Pol* 2007;65:672–680; discussion 681–683.

129. Muramatsu T, Kozuma K, Tsukahara R, *et al*. Comparison of myocardial perfusion by distal protection before and after primary stenting for acute myocardial infarction: angiographic and clinical results of a randomized controlled trial. *Catheter Cardiovasc Interv* 2007;70:677–682.

130. Gick M, Jander N, Bestehorn HP, *et al*. Randomized evaluation of the effects of filter-based distal protection on myocardial perfusion and infarct size after primary percutaneous catheter intervention in myocardial infarction with and without ST-segment elevation. *Circulation* 2005;112:1462–1469.

131. Lefevre T, Guyon P, Reimers B, Fauvel JM, Pansieri M, Dewez MP. Distal protection in acute myocardial infarction: final results of the randomized DIPLOMATE study. *Eur Heart J* 2004;25 (Suppl):420.

132. Wang L, Nguyen T, Yang X, Yang C. Distal protection with Angioguard during PCI for acute myocardial infarction. *Am J Cardiol* 2003;92 (Suppl 6A):38L.

133. Nanasato M, Hirayama H, Muramatsu T, *et al.* Impact of angioplasty with distal protection device on myocardial reperfusion. *J Am Coll Cardiol* 2004;43 (Suppl 1):246A.

134. Baim DS, Wahr D, George B, *et al.* Randomized trial of a distal embolic protection device during percutaneous intervention of saphenous vein aorto-coronary bypass grafts. *Circulation* 2002;105:1285–1290.

135. Stone GW, Rogers C, Hermiller J, *et al.* Randomized comparison of distal protection with a filter-based catheter and a balloon occlusion and aspiration system during percutaneous intervention of diseased saphenous vein aorto-coronary bypass grafts. *Circulation* 2003;108:548–553.

136. Kereiakes DJ, Turco MA, Breall J, *et al.* A novel filter-based distal embolic protection device for percutaneous intervention of saphenous vein graft lesions: results of the AMEthyst randomized controlled trial. *JACC Cardiovasc Interv* 2008;1:248–257.

137. Jolly SS, Amlani S, Hamon M, Yusuf S, Mehta SR. Radial versus femoral access for coronary angiography or intervention and the impact on major bleeding and ischemic events: a systematic review and meta-analysis of randomized trials. *Am Heart J* 2009; 157:132–140.

138. Jolly SS, Yusuf S, Cairns J, *et al.* Radial versus femoral access for coronary angiography and intervention in patients with acute coronary syndromes (RIVAL): a randomised, parallel group, multicentre trial. *Lancet* 2011;377:1409–1420.

139. Serruys PW, Morice MC, Kappetein AP, *et al.* Percutaneous coronary intervention versus coronary-artery bypass grafting for severe coronary artery disease. *N Engl J Med* 2009;360:961–972.

140. Morice MC, Serruys PW, Kappetein AP, *et al.* Outcomes in patients with de novo left main disease treated with either percutaneous coronary intervention using paclitaxel-eluting stents or coronary artery bypass graft treatment in the Synergy Between Percutaneous Coronary Intervention with TAXUS and Cardiac Surgery (SYNTAX) trial. *Circulation* 2010;121:2645–2653.

141. Mehilli J, Kastrati A, Byrne RA, *et al.* Paclitaxel- versus sirolimus-eluting stents for unprotected left main coronary artery disease. *J Am Coll Cardiol* 2009;53:1760–1768.

142. Rubartelli P, Petronio AS, Guiducci V, *et al.* Comparison of sirolimus-eluting and bare metal stent for treatment of patients with total coronary occlusions: results of the GISSOC II-GISE multicentre randomized trial. *Eur Heart J* 2010;31:2014–2020.

143. Hochman JS, Lamas GA, Buller CE, *et al.* Coronary intervention for persistent occlusion after myocardial infarction. *N Engl J Med* 2006;355:2395–2407.

144. Erne P, Schoenenberger AW, Burckhardt D, *et al.* Effects of percutaneous coronary interventions in silent ischemia after myocardial infarction: the SWISSI II randomized controlled trial. *JAMA* 2007;297:1985–1991.

CHAPTER 9

Randomized controlled trials in cardiac surgery: is there any alternative?

Thanos Athanasiou,[1] Amir Sepehripour,[2] and John Pepper[3]
[1]Hammersmith Hospital, London, UK
[2]Imperial College, London, UK
[3]Royal Brompton Hospital, London, UK

Controversies and uncertainties in cardiac surgery

Optimal judgment in cardiac surgery depends upon the successful integration of evidence, careful inference based on our biological understanding of the disease, and our experience taking into account patient preference and the capability of the surgeon. The balanced application of evidence is considered the central point of practicing evidence-based clinical practice (EBCP), and involves integration of clinical expertise and judgment, patient and societal values, and the best available evidence. Unfortunately, systematic reviews of randomized controlled trials (RCTs) are rarely available to guide the practice of cardiac surgery and, if available, mainly address pharmacological interventions. In the absence of systematic reviews, individual high-quality RCTs or well-designed observational studies with sufficiently large and consistent sizes of effect are the next best choices to inform clinical decision-making. The large randomized trial is one of our most reliable sources of evidence for assessment of intervention effects. Disagreements often occur between meta-analyses and large trials, and between large trials on the same topic. Discordance rates seem to depend on whether primary or secondary outcomes are assessed. *The most common scenario in cardiac surgery decision-making is that there are no large trials but several small trials with low statistical power.*

In a leading article in the cardiac surgery literature, Dr Blackstone pointed out the following: "often, a cursory glance at patient characteristics in each group reveals important differences that lead medical and statistical reviewers and readers alike to scoff, they're comparing 'apples and oranges'" [1]. This very important point causes cardiovascular physicians to be skeptical that the difference in outcome attributed to a difference in treatment (or patient condition) may not be a real one. It is important to keep in mind that randomized trials go against one of the fundamental things that surgeons do

Cardiovascular Clinical Trials: Putting the Evidence into Practice, First Edition.
Edited by Marcus D. Flather, Deepak L. Bhatt, and Tobias Geisler.

in their practice: select an appropriate operation for the appropriate patient. *We call this "indication" not "bias." RCTs seek to erase selection "bias."*

Need for a hierarchical system to stratify the evidence

EBCP has been defined as the "conscientious, explicit, and judicious use of current best evidence in making decisions about the care of individual patients." Basic components of EBCP include the awareness of the need for evidence, the formulation of a focused and answerable question to address a clinical problem, the search for and critical appraisal of appropriate studies in the literature, and the judicious application of the best available evidence to the individual patient [2]. Another important principle of EBCP is the integration of individual patient values and circumstances with the evidence. The evidence cycle is subsequently completed by a critical reflection of one's own decision-making process. Advocates of "evidence-based medicine" classify studies according to "grades of evidence" on the basis of the research design, using internal validity (i.e., the correctness of the results) as the criterion for hierarchical rankings. The highest grade is reserved for research involving "at least one properly randomized controlled trial" and the lowest grade is applied to descriptive studies (e.g., case series) and expert opinion; observational studies, both cohort studies and case–control studies, fall at intermediate levels. Although the quality of studies is sometimes evaluated within each grade, each category is considered methodologically superior to those below it. This hierarchical approach to study design has been promoted widely in individual reports, meta-analyses, consensus statements, and educational materials for clinicians. When comparison is made in the context of a properly designed, appropriate, ethical, feasible, well-analyzed, generalizable randomized trial, most cardiac surgeons would accept a cause-and-effect linkage between treatment and difference in outcome. In contrast, when the comparison is based on studies of clinical experience, cause-and-effect attribution is considered "speculative" at best.

What are the most common difficulties encountered in performing RCTs in cardiac surgery?

Potential difficulties associated with the application of RCTs to cardiac surgical problems include the difficulty in successfully blinding patients, investigators, and assessors; the variability of surgical techniques and operator skills; and the "learning curve," which influences the efficacy of many interventions under study [3,4].

Randomization and blinding

Two criteria are given particular weight in the critical appraisal process of RCTs: randomization protocol and blinding [5–7]. Random assignment is a cornerstone of clinical trial design. Baseline characteristics that could confound an observed outcome are distributed equally, except for chance variation, among randomized groups. Notably, randomization intends to create groups of equal prognosis by providing similar distributions not only for known variables, but also for unknown prognostic variables. For instance, assuming that randomization was done properly and provides no opportunity for unintentional or intentional tampering.

The second hallmark of an RCT is blinding. Studies have shown that non-randomized trials and RCTs that do not incorporate blinding are more likely to show advantages of a new intervention over the standard treatment. Blinding safeguards a trial against bias, defined as the systematic deviation of the study results away from "truth in the universe," by guarding against placebo effects, co-interventions, and biased outcome assessment. Blinding applies not only to the study subject and the investigator, but also to multiple levels of study personnel (i.e., the surgeon, nurse, study coordinator) and outcome assessors (i.e., cardiologist, radiologist, pathologist, etc.). Furthermore, blinding can be achieved at levels other than participants and assessors, such as treatment providers, analysts, and reporters. Blinding of study personnel is usually feasible in studies of pharmaceutical interventions but may be less feasible in trials of surgical procedures and interventions. Blinding of outcome assessors is nearly always possible and particularly important when the outcome assessment of a study involves some degree of subjectivity. Blinding of outcome assessors is less important if the outcome can be assessed in a fairly objective and reproducible manner (e.g., time to death from all causes). Terms such as double- or triple-blind are poorly defined and should be avoided.

Methodological issues

Aside from randomization and blinding there are several methodological issues that affect study validity, such as completeness of follow-up or the adequacy of the statistical analysis. Pre-study sample size calculations based on a clearly defined outcome are considered essential for both scientific and ethical reasons. Studies with small sample sizes are often inadequately powered to detect small but clinically significant differences between interventions and are therefore not a valid justification to establish the usefulness of new treatments.

"Intention-to-treat" analyses are usually favored over "per-protocol" analyses as they avoid bias associated with non-random loss of participants. Intention-to-treat analyses include all patients, whereas per-protocol analyses exclude data from patients with protocol deviations. Therefore, intention-to-treat analyses must deal with missing data. Suggested strategies include carrying forward the last observed response or calculating the most likely outcome based on the outcome of other patients. Per-protocol analyses exclude patients with missing data from the analyses. If patients with missing data are mainly outliers, per-protocol analyses may increase homogeneity and precision. On the other hand, if losses to follow-up are related to prognostic factors, adverse events, or lack of treatment response, per-protocol analyses may overestimate the intervention effects. *In general, the intention-to-treat analysis is the most reliable type for analyzing data from randomized trials* [8]. However, discrepancies between intention-to-treat and per-protocol analyses as part of sensitivity analysis may provide important additional information, and using both analytical strategies may be considered.

Recruitment process

Another difficulty with RCTs in cardiac surgery is recruitment. The process of recruiting patients into any clinical study is fundamentally critical for the implementation, execution, and completion of any project. Simply put, if the study does not have the required number of patients, then no adequate conclusions regarding outcomes and results can be attained. The completion of such a critical process for a RCT costs more and consumes more time than any other aspect of the project.

The successful recruitment of subjects within a surgical trial involves adequate planning, effective teamwork, and a multimodal approach in selection. Specifically trained recruiters should be equipped with a broad knowledge base and skills with which to effectively inform and select patients. Subjects can be recruited from a large source of patient groups within a variety of healthcare systems, but recruitment should be targeted to the specific research area of the trial.

The role of recruitment is a fundamental necessity to the ultimate completion of a trial, and if successful can greatly strengthen the quality of the data eventually assessed. Surgeons have been criticized for a lack of adequate scientific assessment of new and old techniques and technology. In response, it has been argued that the problems of surgery in general lie not with the quality of clinical research but with doctor–patient communication, which significantly affects the recruitment process, and that more science and more clinical trials cannot heal the deep rifts in communication between surgeons and their patients.

Even when there is indecision among competent experts faced with competing therapies (equipoise), there may be specific methodological and feasibility problems in cardiac surgery that make randomization difficult. There seem to be important differences in compliance with randomized allocation of treatment, irrespective of patient preferences, when comparing drugs with cardiac surgery interventions. The most poorly understood variable is patient preference. Whether a patient elects to enter a clinical trial may reflect a principled view of trials themselves, but may also result from differences in the "magnitude" of competing therapies. Also, surgeons, when asked to choose from competing therapies as expert "surrogates" for their patients, show a low and variable acceptance of trials and their preferences for therapies depend on their specialty training and geographical differences (rural vs. urban) in their practices. Another major barrier may be that surgeons perceive randomization of therapies as creating uncertainty, both for themselves and their patients.

Funding

It is well recognized that funding of RCTs is problematic in cardiac surgery. Few surgeons appear to obtain funding for trials, although how many apply for funding is unknown. This may reflect a lack of interest in cardiac surgical trials among potential funders (industry, community organizations, and government bodies); training on the part of surgeons; or a controlling body like the US Food and Drug Administration (FDA). Good trial design and quality assurance (internal validity) are clearly major issues in surgical RCTs, and it is possible that the qualitative weaknesses of surgical RCTs (which may have a lower standard of research protocol) influence funding allocations from major grant bodies. However, many surgeons feel that the lack of funding for surgical RCTs is because physicians and laboratory researchers are overrepresented on granting bodies selection committees.

Need for a variety of endpoints and patient-reported based outcomes

The design of the study will also vary according to the type of endpoint being used in the study (i.e., what is actually being measured). The most valuable endpoints may be "hard" clinical events, such as death, stroke, or myocardial infarction. The results from studies that use these types of endpoints can be applied directly and with confidence to clinical practice. Other studies may measure clinical findings such as ejection fraction (EF) or patency of coronary grafts. Trials that use such surrogate endpoints can be much smaller than those that require clinical endpoints, and they often require a shorter time to complete. If a trial has shown, for example, a comparable degree of graft patency between two surgical techniques (a surrogate endpoint), one would hope that mortality (a clinical endpoint) would also be comparable. This, unfortunately, is not always true, which highlights the importance of the trials that use clinical endpoints. *However, smaller studies that establish mechanisms and efficacy are the necessary building blocks for larger trials with clinical endpoints, and well-designed registries have generated much useful data; all should therefore be considered valuable to the potential investigator.*

Not all trials measure purely clinical endpoints; many include an economic component that measures such factors as length of hospital stay, overall cost of treatment, quality of life, patient satisfaction or other patient-reported based outcomes (PROMS), including quality-adjusted life years (QALY). Because the economic and social circumstances of real-world medical care often introduce factors not evident in a controlled trial setting, these types of analyses frequently provide a valuable look not just at which therapy is superior in the clinical setting, but which therapy would be superior as medicine is actually practiced.

It has become increasingly common for clinical trials in cardiovascular medicine to use composite primary endpoints that often have varying clinical importance [9,10]. Time-to-event analyses, in which mortality is but one of several outcomes, are particularly problematic as the impact of death is clearly not equivalent to other non-fatal outcomes such as readmission to hospital. Another concern is that indiscriminately combining mortality with other outcomes in survival analyses may lead to biases related to "competing risk." Specifically, patients dying early in a clinical trial are unable to experience future non-fatal outcomes. To overcome these concerns, a different approach can be used that relies on a composite outcome, namely "days lost due to death or hospitalization," over the follow-up period. By developing this composite outcome, investigators have avoided directly equating readmission to hospital with death as in a traditional event-free survival analysis, while at the same time allowing for patients to have repeated readmission to hospital.

Another argument is that because of recent advances in cardiovascular medicine and lower short-term mortality rates, it has become necessary for many clinical trials to incorporate composite endpoints into their protocols as a primary outcome in order to demonstrate biological efficacy and statistical significance. Of course, we wonder whether additional methodologies such as "weighting" individual components of a composite endpoint—days dead are counted more heavily than days hospitalized, for example—may further improve these approaches. Perhaps at a minimum, separate reporting of individual components of a composite primary endpoint should become routine and even integrated into the CONSORT (Consolidated Standards of Reporting Trials) guidelines.

Need to improve reporting of RCTs in cardiac surgery

"Surgical research or comic opera?" queried a Lancet editorial in 1996, stimulating a heated debate and serving to highlight the lack of RCTs in surgery and the limitations and difficulties of conducting them. Reports of RCTs should ideally convey relevant information to enable the reader to make an informed judgment concerning the validity of the trial and the effectiveness of the treatment. Furthermore, assessing the validity of the primary studies has been defined as one of the most important steps of the peer-review process.

The need to improve the quality of reporting of RCTs has been highlighted in several specialties across healthcare [11,12]. It was shown that the quality of reporting of general surgical RCTs leaves considerable room for improvement. The quality of reporting in surgical journals is clearly inferior to the quality of reporting of surgical trials in medical journals as assessed by allocation concealment, Jadad score, and modified CONSORT score. Although the reporting of RCTs can give some clues on the quality of the methodology, poor reporting does not necessarily mean that the trials were poorly designed and executed. Well-conducted trials may be reported badly, and studies with poor methodologies can be reported in such a way as to hide important deficiencies.

The significant article by Tiruvoipati et al. [13] demonstrated substantive deficiencies in the reporting of randomized trials in the cardiac surgical literature. Among other things, the authors of that report indicate that lack of awareness of the CONSORT guidelines contributes to the deficiencies they observed (>60% of the authors who reported their studies in the principal cardiothoracic journals were not aware of them).

We cannot know for sure whether the problems in the cardiac surgical literature are worse than in other contexts, but we consider they are because of the infrequent application of rigorous experimental design methods for clinical questions in surgery. The two elements that could potentially improve the reporting of RCTs in cardiothoracic surgery may be awareness of the CONSORT statement among authors and, more importantly, endorsement of the CONSORT statement by the cardiothoracic surgical journals. The CONSORT statement tends to be published in general medical journals but not the specialist surgical journals.

It is therefore important that RCTs are reported in a high quality manner so the readers have a clear view on why the study was conducted, how it was conducted, and how it was analyzed. This would be helpful not only in the immediate appraisal of trials, but also in the long term, when performing further analyses such as in systematic reviews and meta-analyses. *A uniform reporting format about the design and methodology of a trial is vital, so that results of subsequent trials can be compared with those of previously published reports or so that trial results can be appropriately compared in a meta-analysis.* If this is not done, there is a real risk that trial results will not be compared in a valid manner and, as a consequence, that a potentially effective therapy in surgical patients might be either discarded (because of false-negative results) or applied improperly (because of false-positive results). Towards this registries of RCT trials play an important role.

A palliative treatment for the problem: the need for progress in statistical methodology of non-randomized designs

There is evidence that observational studies can be designed with rigorous methods that mimic those of clinical trials, and that well-designed observational studies do not consistently overestimate the effectiveness of therapeutic agents. Comparison of randomized and observational studies shows that treatment effects may differ according to research design, but that "one method does not give a consistently greater effect than the other." The treatment effects are most similar when the exclusion criteria are similar and when the prognostic factors were accounted for in observational studies [14].

A specific method used to strengthen observational studies (the "restricted cohort" design) adapts principles of the design of RCTs to the design of an observational study as follows: it identifies a "zero time" for determining a patient's eligibility and base-line features; uses inclusion and exclusion criteria similar to those of clinical trials; adjusts for differences in baseline susceptibility to the outcome; and uses statistical methods (e.g., intention-to-treat analysis) similar to those of RCTs.

Data in the literature of other scientific disciplines support our contention that research design should not be considered a rigid hierarchy.

One possible explanation for the finding that observational studies may be less prone to heterogeneity in results than RCTs is that each observational study is more likely to include a broad representation of the population at risk. In addition, there is less opportunity for differences in the management of subjects among observational studies. For example, although there is general agreement that physicians do not use therapeutic agents in a uniform way, an observational study would usually include patients with coexisting illnesses and a wide spectrum of disease severity, and treatment would be tailored to the individual patient. In contrast, each RCT may have a distinct group of patients as a result of specific inclusion and exclusion criteria regarding coexisting illnesses and severity of disease, and the experimental protocol for therapy may not be representative of clinical practice.

In the past, several statistical techniques were used to increase the credibility of non-randomized study designs, including:

- Matching
- Multivariate logistic regression analysis and adjustment
- Use of multilevel and hierarchical modeling
- Use of Bayesian methods and statistical simulation techniques
- Use of balancing scores.

Matching

Matching is a method used to ensure that two study groups are similar with regards to "nuisance" factors that might distort or confound a relationship that is being studied. Matching can be implemented using two main approaches:

- Pair (individual) matching, and
- Frequency matching.

Frequency matching can be implemented in various ways, including category matching, caliper matching, stratified random sampling, or a variant of pair matching.

Matching is most commonly used in case–control studies, although it can be used in cohort studies. Theoretical analysis has shown that matching in cohort studies completely controls for any potential confounding by the matching factors without requiring any special statistical methods, and is associated with loss of statistical power. On the other hand, in case–control studies matching does not completely control for confounding, thus requiring the use of statistical methods such as the Mantel Hanzel approach, standardization, or logistic regression. There can be substantial loss of power if a case–control study matches on a factor that is not actually a confounder. It is obvious that with matching, selection factor effects (called bias), which case matching are intended to reduce, may increase bias if unmatched cases are simply eliminated.

Multivariable logistic regression analysis and adjustment

For more than three decades, multivariable risk factor analysis has been the main statistical technique for identifying and quantifying treatment outcome differences adjusted for patient characteristics. *These differences are treated as associations with outcomes, not causes.* There is no guarantee that risk factor analysis is an effective strategy for discovery of a cause-and-effect mechanism [15,16].

Multivariable logistic regression appears to be very suitable for epidemiological research, especially for dichotomous outcomes such as mortality, as disease occurrence has multiple risk factors which can be mutually correlated. Therefore, to determine the independent effect of a risk factor on a disease, the confounding effects attributed to other factors must be held constant. For two or three confounding factors it is possible to statistically adjust for them by performing the analysis on a stratified sample, but with more confounders multiple logistic regression is the most efficient technique of achieving adjustment for them. The mathematical model known as a multiple logistic regression assumes that the dependent variable (the outcome of interest, such as death in this case) is linearly and additively related to the independent variables (patient risk factors) on the logistic scale. Logistic transformation has the ability to transform an S-shaped relationship between two variables into a linear one. This S-shaped pattern is prevalent in real clinical practice, in which there is a large number of cases with risk close to zero at a variable low exposure to a risk factor. Similarly at the other extreme of the spectrum, there is a significant number of cases with increasingly higher exposure to a risk factor, but not much change in their risk of death. The technique is useful primarily because it produces a direct estimate of the odds ratio of any risk factor, which reflects the dose–response relationship between these and the outcome. However, if this actual relationship is non-linear, then an adequate fit can usually be achieved by adding polynomial and product interaction terms to the model, although the meaning of the odds ratios in such an interaction model would be severely circumscribed. An essential step in risk stratification modeling is to evaluate whether there is evidence of an interaction between the variables used in a model. This interaction would imply that the effect of one of the variables is not constant over levels of the other. An important drawback of logistic regression is that it can increase bias due to misclassification and measurement errors in confounding variables and differences between conditional and unconditional odds ratio estimates of treatment effects.

Use of multilevel and hierarchical modeling

Shahian *et al.* [17] have suggested the use of hierarchical models in cardiac surgery risk modeling. Statistical models, such as hierarchical models, have been developed for data that are clustered in nature. Patients within a cardiac center are likely to be more similar than patients across centers, due to similarity in treatments and perhaps socioeconomic characteristics, and may be considered as clustered within a center. Incorrect statistical inferences may be obtained if clustering is ignored in the analysis. These models are appropriate when data from a large number of centers are used for model development and not necessary when a model is developed using data from a single center. They may provide imprecise estimates when the data are from a small number of centers. Although some have used data from a large number of centers for model development, they have not taken into account the clustering aspect.

If interaction terms are considered for inclusion in a risk model, they should be chosen on the basis of clinical plausibility as well as statistical significance. The size of the developmental data would need to be increased to accommodate these terms and interpretations made cautiously.

Conventional single-level models assume that all patients are randomly drawn from the same population. When a sample comprises statistically independent patients, then logistic regression of the patients' variables can be used for "predicting" a binary outcome. However, when the patients have a degree of autocorrelation among them, i.e., patients are clustered within groups, the assumption of statistical independence may not hold. Multilevel or "hierarchical" models are specifically used in observations that may have a clustered structure.

In a well-known study of primary school children carried out in the 1970s, it was claimed that children exposed to a particular style of teaching benefited more than those who were not. The analysis was done using single-level logistic regression techniques which used the individual children as the units of analysis, ignoring their "clustering" within classes (sharing the same teachers). However, it was subsequently demonstrated that when the analysis accounted properly for the clustering into a higher level of grouping (into classes), there were no significant differences between the children. Children within any one cluster (class) tended to have a similar performance because they were taught by the same teachers. Consequently, the "information" provided by children from the same class should be "weighted" less than would have been the case if the same number of students had been taught separately by different teachers. That is, the basic unit for comparison should have been the classes instead of the students. By increasing the number of students (Level 1 units) analyzed per class, one would achieve a more precise estimate of the measure of the teachers' effectiveness (the Level 1 measure). Increasing the number of classes (Level 2 units) to be compared, with the same or an even smaller number of students per class, one would improve the precision of the teachers' comparisons (the Level 2 measure). A multilevel analysis provides more "conservative" standard errors, confidence intervals, and significance tests than a traditional single-level analysis, which is obtained simply by ignoring the presence of clustering. In addition, it enables the researcher to explore the extent to which differences in the students' performance (the Level 1 measure or outcome) between schools are accounted for by factors such as organizational practice (Level 2 covariates). Finally, the methodology would allow the relative ranking of individual schools, using the performances of their students after adjusting for both Level 1 and Level 2 covariates.

The above example for data analysis with hierarchical structure is very common in cardiac surgery if we think that patients with different risk profiles undergo an operation by surgeons with different surgical experience and skills in different institutions and different regions, and our aim is to identify the reasons for variations in outcome.

Use of Bayesian methods and statistical simulation techniques

Bayesian methods can be considered as an alternative to the classical approach to statistical analysis. Such methods have being used in an increasing frequency due to the increased feasibility of their implementation, made possible by recent advances in computation and software technology. An important difference between the two approaches is that Bayesian methodology allows the incorporation into the analysis of information external to the study being analyzed. Such information is specified in a prior distribution and is combined with the study data, in the form of the likelihood, to produce a posterior distribution on which inferences are based. In several studies the incorporation of prior information is not of primary interest, and all prior distributions placed on model parameters are intended to be "vague"; however, sensitivity analysis can be used to check the stability of the results to different prior distributions. The computation of the posterior distributions for parameters in a Bayesian model are often complex, requiring the evaluation of numerous high-dimensional integrals that have no closed form solution.

Within the broad range of Monte Carlo simulation methods (MCMC), one method, Gibbs sampling, has been increasingly used in applied Bayesian analyses. The appeal of Gibbs sampling is that it can be used to estimate posterior distributions by drawing sample values randomly from the full conditional distributions of each parameter conditional on all others and the data. The samples will converge to the marginal distribution. A final word of warning regarding use of MCMC methods is in order: Although they offer great flexibility, issues such as convergence of the simulations need to be established before they are used for estimation and inference; otherwise, biased estimates will be produced.

Bayesian statistics have now permeated all the major areas of medical statistics, including clinical trials, epidemiology, meta-analyses and evidence synthesis, performance comparison, spatial modeling, case–control studies and measurement error longitudinal modeling, survival modeling, and decision-making in respect of new technologies.

Use of balancing scores

Balancing scores are a class of multivariable statistical methods that identify patients with similar chances of receiving one or the other treatment, permitting non-randomized comparisons of treatment outcomes. The developers of balancing score methods claim that the difference in outcome between patients who have a similar balancing score, but receive different treatments, provides an unbiased estimate of the effect attributable to the comparison variable of interest.

In 1983, Rosenbaum and Rubin introduced propensity score analysis (PS) as an alternative tool to control for confounding [18–22]. The PS is the probability of a patient receiving treatment, or more generally any exposure of interest, conditional on the patient's observed pretreatment covariates. PS analysis is a two-step approach in which a model is first built to predict the exposure (treatment model), and second, a model incorporating the information on PS is constructed to evaluate the exposure–outcome association (outcome model). To estimate the PS, usually a logistic regression model is fitted that predicts the exposure and may include a large number of measured pretreatment covariates. From this model, the summary of each study subject's pretreatment covariates yields the expected probability of receiving the treatment or exposure of interest for that individual. This expected probability is the patient's PS. In theory, it is expected that with increasing sample size the pretreatment covariates are balanced between study subjects from the two exposure groups who have nearly identical PS.

The three most common techniques that use the propensity score are *matching, stratification, and regression adjustment*. Each of these techniques is a way to make an adjustment for covariates before calculation of the treatment effect (matching and stratification) or during calculation of treatment effect (stratification and regression adjustment). With all three techniques, the propensity score is calculated in the same way, but once estimated it is applied differently. Propensity scores are useful for these techniques because by definition the propensity score is the conditional probability of treatment given the observed covariates; thus, subjects in treatment and control groups with equal (or nearly equal) propensity scores will tend to have the same (or nearly the same) distributions on their background covariates. Exact adjustments made with the propensity score will, on average, remove all the bias in the background covariates. Therefore, bias-removing adjustments can be made with the propensity scores rather than all the background covariates individually.

Despite the broad utility of propensity score methods, when addressing causal questions from non-randomized studies, it is important to keep in mind that even propensity score methods *can only adjust for observed confounding covariates and not for unobserved ones*. This is always a limitation of non-randomized studies compared with randomized studies, where the randomization tends to balance the distribution of all covariates, observed and unobserved.

In observational studies, confidence in causal conclusions must be built by seeing how consistent the obtained answers are with other evidence (such as results from related experiments) and how sensitive the conclusions are to reasonable deviations from assumptions. Such sensitivity analyses suppose that a relevant but unobserved covariate has been left out of the propensity score model. By explicating how this hypothetical unmeasured covariate is related to treatment assignment and outcome, we can obtain an estimate of the treatment effect that adjusts for it as well as for measured covariates, and investigate how answers might change if such a covariate was available for adjustment. Of course, medical knowledge is needed when assessing whether the proposed relations involving the hypothetical unmeasured covariate are realistic or extreme.

Another limitation of propensity score methods is that they work better in larger samples for the following reason. The distributional balance of observed covariates created by sub-classifying on the propensity score is an expected balance, just as the balance of all covariates in a randomized experiment is an expected balance. In a small randomized experiment, random imbalances of some covariates can be substantial despite randomization; analogously, in a small observational study, substantial imbalances of some covariates may be unavoidable despite sub-classification using a sensibly estimated propensity score. The larger the study, the more minor are such imbalances.

A final possible limitation of propensity score methods is that a covariate related to treatment assignment but not to outcome is handled the same as a covariate with the same relation to treatment assignment but strongly related to outcome. This feature can be a limitation of propensity scores because inclusion of irrelevant covariates reduces the efficiency of the control on the relevant covariates. However, recent work suggests that, at least in modest or large studies, the biasing effects of leaving out even a weakly predictive covariate dominate the efficiency gains from not using such a covariate. Thus, in practice, this limitation may not be substantial if investigators use some judgment.

Recent clinical trials in cardiac surgery: where are we?

There is an ever growing wealth of new technology in cardiac surgery providing enhanced techniques for the surgical treatment of cardiovascular disease. These novel and unfamiliar techniques will require time and experience to become established methods in cardiac surgery, and this highlights the need for surgical trials analyzing the success and potential pitfalls of such techniques. There is subsequently a need for critical appraisal of these trials, dissecting the methods used, the true nature and the potential reliability of the findings, and finally the implications that these findings could have on future practice. Here we focus on several recent trials that have the potential to be hugely influential on the future of cardiac surgery.

The STICH trial

The STICH (Surgical Treatment for Ischaemic Heart Failure) trial was an international multicenter, non-blinded, randomized trial involving 127 clinical sites in 26 countries [23], sponsored by the National Heart, Lung, and Blood Institute (NHLBI) of the National Institutes of Health (NIH). The trial was conducted to investigate the efficacy of medical versus surgical therapy and whether surgical ventricular reconstruction (SVR) plus coronary artery bypass grafting (CABG) would decrease the rate of death or hospitalization for cardiac causes, compared with CABG alone for patients with ischemic cardiomyopathy. There was one medical arm and two surgical arms: CABG and CABG + SVR. Two primary hypotheses were considered: (1) the revascularization hypothesis stated that CABG combined with intensive medical therapy improves long-term survival compared to medical therapy alone; and (2) the reconstruction hypothesis stated that SVR of left ventricular (LV) shape and size combined with CABG improves survival free of subsequent hospitalization for cardiac cause in comparison to CABG alone [24].

Coronary artery disease (CAD) is the predominant cause of heart failure, which has become a major public health problem in the western world, attributed partly to an aging population and more effective treatment of acute myocardial infarction (MI) [25]. After MI the ventricle undergoes a pathological and physiological adaptation process known as ventricular remodeling. In its advanced stages this process can leave the ventricle enlarged and spherical, and consequently with diminished function in both the areas of the infarction and in viable distant areas of myocardium. The enlarged ventricle suffers mechanically, namely as a result of mitral regurgitation due to leaflet restriction [26,27], as well as electrically due to post-infarction differential timing of left and right ventricular contraction [28]. The end result of this ventricular remodeling is ischemic cardiomyopathy, which is the leading cause of heart failure in the western world [29].

Surgical ventricular reconstruction or restoration (SVR) is the term used for a group of surgical procedures designed to counter the effects of this ventricular remodeling. These techniques were originally used to repair ventricular aneurysms [30–32] and were referred to as the Dor procedure as first described by Dor and colleagues to improve geometric reconstruction as compared with standard linear repair in left ventricular aneurysm surgery [33] (Figure 9.1). The aims of these techniques are to "reduce the size and sphericity of the left ventricle by excluding akinetic and dyskinetic areas, in conjunction with complete revascularization and repair of any valvular defects. The goal is to revascularize ischemic myocardium; reduce end-diastolic pressure; reduce ventricular dysynchrony; improve ventricular function, including that of viable but poorly functioning remote areas; and have a positive impact on measurable parameters of heart failure and survival" [28].

Eligibility for enrolment was on the basis of patients having CAD amenable to CABG, symptomatic heart failure defined as NYHA class II–IV (within 3 months of entry), LVEF of 35% or less defined by cardiac magnetic resonance (CMR) or gated single photon emission computed tomography (SPECT), and older than 18 years of age and competent to give informed consent. Exclusion criteria included clearly defined primary valvular heart disease indicating the need for valve repair or replacement, patients with concurrent cardiogenic shock or requiring inotropic or intra-aortic balloon support, planned percutaneous coronary intervention (PCI), acute MI within 30 days, more than one prior cardiac operation, non-cardiac illness with life expectancy of less than 3 years, and non-cardiac illness imposing substantial operative mortality [34]. Patients with 50% or greater stenosis of the left main coronary artery or suffering from angina of Canadian Cardiovascular Society (CCS) class III or IV whilst on medical therapy were deemed ineligible for medical therapy alone. All patients had assessment of LV function and wall motion by cardiac imaging and those found to have dominant anterior akinesia or dyskinesia of the left ventricle were considered amenable for SVR.

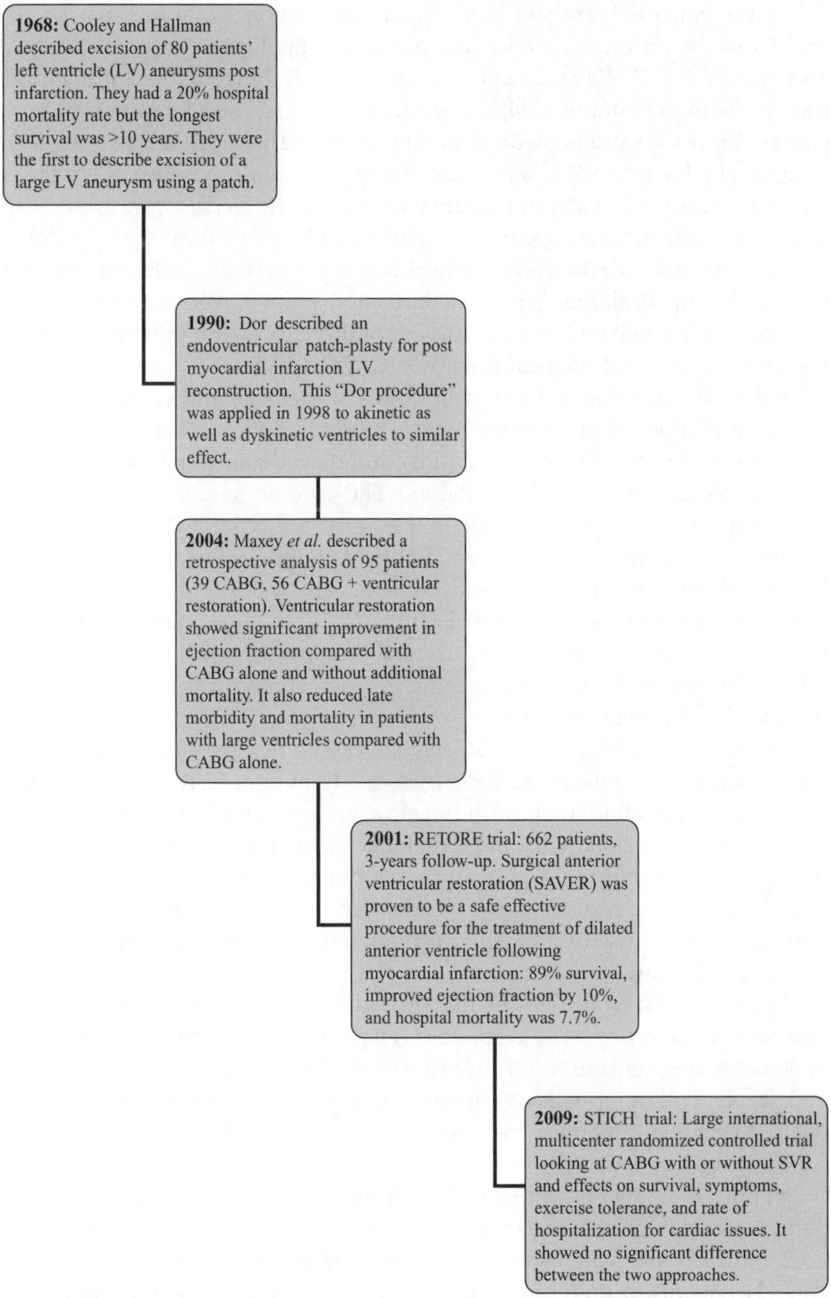

1968: Cooley and Hallman described excision of 80 patients' left ventricle (LV) aneurysms post infarction. They had a 20% hospital mortality rate but the longest survival was >10 years. They were the first to describe excision of a large LV aneurysm using a patch.

1990: Dor described an endoventricular patch-plasty for post myocardial infarction LV reconstruction. This "Dor procedure" was applied in 1998 to akinetic as well as dyskinetic ventricles to similar effect.

2004: Maxey *et al.* described a retrospective analysis of 95 patients (39 CABG, 56 CABG + ventricular restoration). Ventricular restoration showed significant improvement in ejection fraction compared with CABG alone and without additional mortality. It also reduced late morbidity and mortality in patients with large ventricles compared with CABG alone.

2001: RETORE trial: 662 patients, 3-years follow-up. Surgical anterior ventricular restoration (SAVER) was proven to be a safe effective procedure for the treatment of dilated anterior ventricle following myocardial infarction: 89% survival, improved ejection fraction by 10%, and hospital mortality was 7.7%.

2009: STICH trial: Large international, multicenter randomized controlled trial looking at CABG with or without SVR and effects on survival, symptoms, exercise tolerance, and rate of hospitalization for cardiac issues. It showed no significant difference between the two approaches.

Figure 9.1 Timeline of milestones in SVR trials.

Eligible patients were stratified for randomization in three strata (A, B, and C) based on protocol criteria regarding eligibility for medical therapy and for SVR [34]. Patients not eligible for SVR but eligible for medical therapy with or without CABG were randomly assigned within stratum A comprising of the subsets: medical therapy alone and medical therapy + CABG. Patients eligible for SVR and medical therapy due to the absence of left main coronary artery stenosis and angina CCS class III or IV were randomly assigned within stratum B, comprising of the subsets: medical therapy alone, medical therapy + CABG, and medical therapy + CABG + SVR. Patients not eligible for medical therapy alone but eligible for CABG and SVR were randomly assigned within stratum C, comprising of the subsets: medical therapy + CABG and medical therapy + CABG + SVR.

Medical therapy was led by cardiologists at each site and entailed the use of ACE inhibitors, angiotensin-receptors blockers, beta-blockers, aldosterone antagonists, antiplatelet agents, statins, diuretics, digitalis, pacemakers, and implantable cardioverter–defibrillators. The cardiac surgeons at each site were required to meet prespecified performance criteria. For CABG this required providing data on at least 25 patients with LVEF of 40% or less who had undergone the operation, with a death rate of 5% or less. For SVR the requirement was evidence of a consistent postoperative decrease in LV volume in five consecutive patients who survived the operation [23]. During CABG, arterial bypass grafting of the left anterior descending coronary artery was required in all patients with the use of additional arterial conduits and venous grafts for revascularization of all major vessels. Regurgitant mitral valves were repaired or replaced at the surgeons' discretion. SVR was performed after revascularization, with cardioplegic arrest or on the beating heart to aid identification of the akinetic and dyskinetic areas, with an anterior left ventriculotomy centered in the zone of asynergy and a suture placed to encircle the scar and bring healthy viable portions of the ventricular walls together, with the possible use of a patch to optimize the chamber size on closure of the ventriculotomy.

The primary outcome was the time to death from any cause or hospitalization for cardiac causes. The secondary outcomes were death from any cause at 30 days, hospitalization for any cause and for cardiovascular causes, MI, and stroke. Follow-up was at 4-month intervals after randomization during the first year and 6-monthly thereafter with a median follow-up of 48 months for all surviving patients.

Overall 2136 patients were enrolled in the STICH trial with 1000 of these patients enrolled in the Hypothesis 2 component at 96 clinical sites between 2002 and 2006; 499 patients were randomly assigned to undergo CABG alone and 501 patients to undergo CABG + SVR. There were no significant differences between the baseline demographic or clinical characteristics.

The primary outcome occurred in 59% of patients undergoing CABG and 58% of patients undergoing CABG + SVR, with fatal events of any cause occurring in 28% of patients in each group. Hospitalization for cardiac causes occurred in 42% of the CABG group and 41% of the CABG + SVR group.

There were no significant differences in the secondary outcomes between the two groups.

The STICH trial concluded that the addition of SVR resulted in a significantly greater reduction in LV volume in comparison to what was achieved with revascularization alone; however, this did not correlate with a tangible improvement in patient symptomatology. The two study groups had similar symptomatic improvement after surgery and there were no significant differences between the two groups in terms of the primary outcomes of death, hospitalization for cardiac causes or any other clinical outcome. Two possible reasons for the negative outcomes were offered by the investigators. One was that selection bias incurred by the experienced surgeons' opinions of whether patients required or would have benefited from SVR may have influenced their decision to enroll these patients in the trial. The second reason was the idea that a reduction of LV volume may have led to a reduction in diastolic distensibility and hence end-diastolic volume, hence impeding the enhanced filling response of the ventricle to the demand for increased cardiac output.

The one limitation that the STICH investigators placed upon their trial was its non-blinded nature. They speculated that the decision to hospitalize a patient during follow-up may have been influenced by the physicians' knowledge of the procedure performed, and they sought to alleviate this problem by seeking complete follow-up and using non-subjective trial endpoints.

The outcomes of the STICH trial were greeted with mixed opinions and overriding skepticism [28]. One area of criticism was the failure to uphold the rigid entry criteria into the trial. The original grant funded by the NIH required that "all patients be evaluated for appropriateness of surgical ventricular reconstruction indicated by evidence of absent viability in the anterior ventricle by nuclear scan determination, an end-systolic volume index of >60 mL/m² and akinesis of >30% of the anterior LV wall" [34]. However, the trial does not make any mention of viability testing.

Another area of criticism was the lack of a specific requirement for the trial centers to demonstrate a multidisciplinary heart failure team or to have any experience in heart failure surgery. The surgeons were required to have an operative mortality of less than 5% in 25 patients who had undergone CABG with an EF of less than 40% and to provide evidence of a consistent postoperative decrease in LV volume in five consecutive patients who survived SVR. There was no scrutiny of surgical results throughout the trial to determine if the operations were being performed successfully.

There are several different surgical techniques to achieve the same morphological results with SVR. The Surgical Therapy Committee of the trial did not request a specific surgical technique, but rather defined an "acceptable STICH procedure," and it was later stated that, "the two criteria used by the Surgical Therapy Committee to define the acceptable range of specific operative maneuvers essential to be considered an acceptable technical SVR operation for the STICH trial will be any ventricular reconstruction method that consistently results in (1) a low operative mortality and (2) an average EF increase of 10% and average LVESVI [left ventricular end systolic volume index] decrease of 30% as assessed on the 4-month postoperative CMR [cardiovascular magnetic resonance] measurement" [34]. The trial reports an average ESVI reduction of 19% and an ESVI of 67 mL/m², which is far below what was originally deemed an acceptable SVR procedure and furthermore far below the standard in the published literature [23,35–44].

There were other areas of concern regarding the trial. There was an expansion to 127 sites from the original intended 50 sites, with assessment of 10 cases per site, presumably to overcome poor enrolment [45]. Taking the 501 patients who were randomly assigned to undergo CABG + SVR under Hypothesis 2, only an average of four procedures were done per site, which is a very limited number for a technically challenging surgical procedure. Of the cohort of patients studied for SVR, fewer than 50% were NYHA class III or IV. This represents a disproportionately healthy group of patients for such a study. The need for a follow-up period longer than 3 years has also been emphasized and it has been suggested that perhaps 10-year data would be more representative [46].

Surgery versus stent trials

Since the advent of PCI in 1977, the question of whether with the aid of medical treatment of risk factors it could potentially replace CABG, which since its inception in 1968 has been the definitive treatment for CAD, has been heatedly debated. With this question came arguably some of the most closely followed and influential cardiac surgical trials of recent decades comparing PCI and stenting versus CABG for patients with CAD (Tables 9.1 and 9.2).

The SYNTAX trial

The SYNTAX (Synergy between PCI with TAXUS and Cardiac Surgery) trial was a large internationally coordinated cardiac surgical trial designed to assess the optimal revascularization strategy in patients with previously untreated three-vessel or left main CAD, and was perhaps the most significant of the PCI + stent versus CABG trials [65]. It was a prospective RCT conducted over 85 sites in 17 countries in Europe and the US. There was an "all-comers" design with consecutive enrolment of all eligible patients with previously untreated three-vessel or left main CAD. Inclusion criteria included *de novo* and previously untreated lesions of 50% or greater stenosis, stable/unstable angina or atypical chest pain, and positive evidence of MI if asymptomatic. Exclusion criteria included previous PCI or CABG, acute MI, or the need for concomitant cardiac surgery [66]. Patients who were deemed eligible for either therapy and in whom it was determined by the local cardiac surgeon and interventional cardiologist that equivalent anatomical revascularization could be achieved with either treatment were randomized to undergo either CABG or PCI with TAXUS Express paclitaxel-eluting stents. Simultaneously, patients in whom it was felt that only one of these treatments was suitable were entered into a parallel nested registry: the PCI registry for CABG-ineligible patients and the CABG registry for PCI-ineligible patients. Preoperative cardiac investigations were reviewed by an independent core

Table 9.1 Early trials of PCI versus CABG (prior to the use of stents).

Trial	Date	Extent of CAD	Type of trial	Number of patients	Follow-up period (years)	Conclusion
Emory Angioplasty versus Surgery trial (EAST) [47]	1994	Two- or three-vessel disease	Single center randomized trial	392 CABG 194 PCI 198	8	No significant difference in survival between the two approaches
Bypass Angioplasty Revascularization Investigation (BARI) [48,49]	2002 then 2007	Two- or three-vessel disease	Large multicenter RCT	1829 CABG 94 PCI 915	10	No significant difference in non-diabetic. CABG; significantly better survival in diabetic patients
French Monocentric Study [50]	1997	Two- or three-vessel disease	Prospective single-center trial	152 CABG 76 PCI 76	5	PCI effective alternative to CABG but more likely to require further interventions to achieve similar clinical outcomes
Coronary Artery versus Bypass Revascularization Investigation (CABRI) [51]	1999	Two- or three-vessel disease	Multicenter international RCT	1054 CABG 543 PCI 541	1	CABG fewer deaths, revascularization and medication requirements in patients at 1 year compared to PCI
German Angioplasty Bypass Surgery Investigation [52]	1994	Two- or three-vessel disease	Multicenter RCT	Total 8981 only 359 randomized CABG 117 PCI 182	13	No significant difference in survival and symptomatic efficacy
Randomized Intervention Treatment of Angina (RITA-I) [53]	1998	Single or multivessel disease	Multicenter RCT	1011 CABG 511 PCI 500	6.5 mean	No significant difference in death or MI but CABG favored

CABG, coronary artery bypass graft; CAD, coronary artery disease; MI, myocardial infarction; PCI, percutaneous coronary intervention; RCT, randomized controlled trial.

Table 9.2 Trials of PCI vs. CABG following the introduction of stents.

Trial	Stent type	Trial type	Number of patients	Follow-up	Outcome
Arterial Revascularization Therapies Study (ARTS) [54]	BMS	RCT	1205 CABG 605 PCI 600	5 years	No difference between stenting and surgery for multivessel disease Similar incidence of stroke and MI Higher revascularization rate in PCI group
Stent or Surgery (SoS) [55]	BMS	RCT	998 CABG 500 PCI 488	6 years	Lower survival rate in PCI group compare to CABG group
Coronary Angioplasty with Stenting versus Coronary Bypass Surgery (ERACI II) [56]	BMS	RCT	450 CABG 225 PCI 225	5 years	At 5 years no survival benefits for either revascularization procedure but fewer repeat revascularization in 10 patients in the initial period in CABG group and fewer major adverse conditions
Medicine Angioplasty or Surgery Study (MASS II) [57]	BMS	RCT	611 CABG 203 PCI 205 Medical treatment 203	5 years	All three treatments yield compatible relatively low rates of death but significantly less MI, mortality, repeat revascularization with CABG
Chieffo et al. [58]	DES	Non-randomized single center	249 CABG 142 PCI 107	1 year	No significant difference in major adverse events

Study	Stent	Design	Numbers	Duration	Findings
Angina with Extremely Serious Operative Mortality/ Evaluation (AWESOME) Morrison et al. [59]	± BMS	RCT	2431 454 patients in RCT (142 had prior CABG)	36 months for survival rates	PCI comparable to CABG in these patients with medically refractory myocardial ischemia and high risk of adverse outcomes with CABG
Malenka et al. [60]	± BMS	Retrospective study using registries	14 493 CABG 10 198 PCI 4295	3.61 years mean	Adjusted survival for two-vessel disease was comparable but for three-vessel disease, CABG better than PCI
Brener et al. [61]	± BMS	Non- randomized single center	6033 PCI 872 CABG 5161	5 years	Mortality lower with CABG than PCI
Hannan et al. [62]	± BMS	Retrospective analysis using registries	N59 314 CABG 37 212 PCI 22 102	706 days CABG 585 days PCI (mean)	Higher survival rates and lower revascularization rates in those who underwent CABG
Bair et al. (2007) [63]	DES/BMS	Single-center experience	6369 CABG 4581 PCI 1788	7 years average	CABG less death and major adverse events than PCI and stenting
Hannan et al. (2008) [64]	DES	Multicenter retrospective trial	17 400 DES 9963 CABG 7437	1 year	CABG associated with lower 1-month death rate/MI and revascularization

BMS, bare metal stent; drug-eluting stent; CABG, coronary artery bypass graft; CAD, coronary artery disease; MI, myocardial infarction; PCI, percutaneous coronary intervention; RCT, randomized controlled trial.

laboratory blinded to the treatment assignments, and were used to generate a SYNTAX score according to a predefined algorithm [67] designed to predict outcomes related to anatomical characteristics and to a lesser extent the functional risk of occlusion for any segment of the coronary artery bed in patients undergoing PCI.

The primary endpoint was a composite of major adverse cardiac and cerebrovascular events (MACCE; i.e., death from any cause, stroke, MI, or repeated revascularization) throughout the 12-month period after randomization. In total 4337 patients with previously untreated three-vessel or left main CAD were screened between 2005 and 2007, of which 1800 were randomly assigned to undergo CABG (897 patients) or PCI with drug-eluting stents (903 patients). In the remaining group of 1275 patients only one suitable treatment was deemed possible and 1077 were enrolled to undergo CABG and 198 PCI.

A total of 38.8% of patients in the CABG group and 39.5% of patients in the PCI group had left main CAD. Over 20% of patients in both groups were considered to be at high surgical risk on the basis of a euroSCORE [68] value of 6 or more (24.9% in the CABG group and 24.7% in the PCI group).

There were no significant differences between the preprocedural rates of MACCE between the two groups, as was the case with the preprocedural rates of the individual components of the primary outcome, stroke and MI. At 12 months the rates of MACCE were significantly higher in the PCI group than the CABG group (17.8% vs. 12.4%), contributed to by an increased rate of repeat revascularization in the PCI group (13.5% vs. 5.9%). Conversely the rate of stroke was significantly elevated with the CABG group (2.2% vs. 0.6%).

With regards to the SYNTAX score, it was found that PCI patients with higher scores had a particularly high rate of major adverse events and it was therefore concluded that the percutaneous approach should be avoided in these patients.

This trial ultimately concluded that CABG, as compared with PCI, is associated with a lower rate of MACCE at 1 year among patients with three-vessel or left main CAD, and should therefore remain the standard of care for such patients.

Several limitations were placed on the trial by the SYNTAX investigators. First, they speculated that the 12-month follow-up period may not have been sufficiently long to reflect the true long-terms effects of CABG as compared with PCI with drug-eluting stents; however, they emphasized that their results were similar to those of a meta-analysis of trials comparing CABG and PCI, albeit using bare metal stents with longer follow-up periods [69]. Another limitation was the use of different medication between the two groups, reflecting variations in the standard of care. A third limitation was the self-withdrawal of patients after randomization, which was higher for the CABG group than the PCI group. Finally, the investigators eluded to the fact that their definition of MI was based on a surgical definition (the finding of a new Q-wave on electrocardiography in association with a value for the creatine kinase MB fraction that was five times the upper limit of the normal range), and consequently less severe cases of MI may have been overlooked.

The SYNTAX trial was generally well received by peer review. One very significant comment regarding the validity of the results of the trial was made at a perspective roundtable published in the *New England Journal of Medicine* [70]: there were no differences between the two groups in terms of the endpoints of death, MI and stroke at 1 year and the ultimate findings of the trial were really driven by an increased need for revascularization in the PCI group. It was debated whether the softer endpoint of revascularization should have been considered as a secondary outcome with the hard endpoints of death, MI and stroke remaining as the primary outcomes, and impact this may have had in the interpretation of the results.

Transcatheter versus surgical aortic valve replacement

Over the last few years the development of transcatheter aortic valve replacement (TAVR) has enabled patients previously considered too high risk to undergo aortic valve implantation, whilst avoiding sternotomy, cardioplegic arrest, and cardiopulmonary bypass [71]. The concept of TAVR was first established by Anderson *et al.* [72] in 1992 where stented porcine bioprosthetic aortic valves were successfully implanted in the ascending aorta or aortic root of seven pigs. The first successful TAVR in humans was reported by Cribier *et al.* [73] in 2002 using the percutaneous heart valve (Percutaneous Valve Technologies, Fort Lee, NJ, USA) and implanting the stented bovine bioprosthetic valve using the antegrade trans-septal approach in a patient with severe aortic stenosis and cardiogenic shock. The same group later reported successful TAVR in five of six patients who had been denied open heart surgery [74].

Given that TAVR is a relatively new procedure and that it is applicable to a significantly higher risk subgroup of patients, there have been very few trials comparing it with surgical aortic valve replacement (SAVR). Those that have however, have acknowledged the difficulty in designing such a study and the limiting confounding factors.

One such study by Piazza *et al.* compared 30-day mortality and patient characteristics between TAVR and SAVR. Whilst it called for a randomized control trial to begin, it itself was not one and took the format of a two-center prospective cohort study which was neither randomized nor blinded, limiting to some extent, as we have mentioned, the value of the results. A further weakness was in the discrepancy between the two groups with, out of a total of 1122 patients included in the study, just 114 undergoing TAVR and 1008 SAVR. To optimize analysis of the results, odds ratios were adjusted and attempts made to limit confounding given that the TAVR group had much higher EuroSCOREs, more comorbidities, and the patients were generally older. However, in the end the authors felt unable to draw a firm conclusion, stating that "both measured and unmeasured confounding factors limit the conclusions that can be drawn from observational comparisons. TAVR could be associated with ether substantial benefits or harms. Randomized comparisons of TAVR versus SAVR are warranted" [75].

Another interesting study looked specifically at acute kidney injury (AKI) following TAVR versus SAVR. Again a non-randomized, single-center prospective trial included 119 patients undergoing TAVR and 104 SAVR, all of whom had chronic kidney disease pre-procedure [76]. Inevitably those selected to undergo TAVR were older with more comorbidities, as well as higher baseline estimated glomerular filtration rate (eGFR) and creatinine levels. Results however showed that TAVR patients in this trial had less post-operative acute kidney injury compared to those who had SAVR (9.2% vs 25.9%), with a significant reduction in the need for hemodialysis. It was concluded that the amount of contrast media used in TAVR was not associated with AKI and that the well-known deleterious effects of cardiopulmonary bypass were likely to cause much more significant injury. The study again acknowledged that since it was a *post-hoc* non-prespecified analysis, they could not rule out the possibility of other confounding variables, calling again for more definitive evidence in the form of randomized trials to determine whether TAVR should be favored in this particular subset of patients.

A recent publication by Guarracino *et al.* compared the effects on left ventricular diastole and neuroendocrine response (B naturetic peptide [BNP] production) from TAVR versus SAVR [71]. A prospective single-center trial again, yet in this study the two groups were matched in terms of numbers (30 patients each); however, those undergoing TAVR had a much lower Euro-SCORE as expected. Patients were additionally matched for age, sex, body surface area, chronic renal failure, diabetes, blood pressure, aortic valve area and mitral flow propagation velocity, mitral annulus early diastolic velocity, and preoperative BNP measurement. Results showed that BNP increased postoperatively in 100% of SAVR patients but only in 20% of TAVR patients. TAVR patient also showed an acute improvement in left diastolic function, whereas this worsened in SAVR patients. Conversely however, of the four in-hospital deaths during the study, three were from the TAVR group and only one from the SAVR group. This study concluded therefore that TAVR is likely to play an increasingly important role in treating high-risk patients considered too unwell for surgical AVR.

Vassilades *et al.* also described the importance and need for RCTs with regards to TAVR procedures and specified a number of ways in which these should ideally be carried out [77]. They dictated that each study should include a cardiac surgeon, an interventionalist, a non-interventional clinical investigator charged with monitoring patient welfare, and an echocardiographer. They advocated careful and proper patient selection to ensure patient safety and objectivity, and the setting to be restricted to a small number of high volume centers with experienced practitioners where at least 100–150 surgical valve operations are performed per year, with the surgeon doing 40–50 and the interventionalist doing at least 100 procedures per year. Suggested endpoints included: death, stroke, MI, para-prosthetic leak, device migration, symptom status, angiographic gradient, and rehospitalization. We agree that this would form a solid basis for a trial with perhaps a few additions such as patient-related factors, quality of life, and patient satisfaction to take a more holistic approach.

The Cribier group performed compassionate-use implantation of the Cribier–Edwards stented valve under the I-REVIVE (Initial Registry of Endovascular Implantation of Valves in Europe) trial, which was later continued as the RECAST (Registry of Endovascular Critical Aortic Stenosis Treatment) trial. Implantation was attempted using the trans-septal technique in 26 and using the retrograde approach in seven of the 36 patients selected. Implantation was not attempted in three patients due to sudden cardiac death, death during balloon valvuloplasty, or inappropriate native valve size. Successful implantation was demonstrated in 82% of patients, with greater success using the antegrade approach (85% vs 57%). Aortic valve area increased to $1.7\,cm^2$ and mean transvalvular gradient was decreased to $10\,mmHg$, with resultant improvements in LVEF and NYHA class. There were six deaths (23%) at 30-day follow-up.

The REVIVAL-II (Transcatheter Endovascular Implantation of Valves II) and REVIVE-II (Registry of Endovascular Implantation of Valves in Europe II) trials were multicenter registries set up in the US, Europe, and Canada to recruit patients to evaluate the feasibility of implantation of the Cribier–Edwards valve. In the US registry, 161 patients undergoing transfemoral implantation experienced a device success rate of 88% and 30-day survival of 89%. The Canadian experience included a total of 168 patients for transfemoral TAVR and demonstrated procedural success in 90.5%, with 30-day stroke and mortality rates of 3.0% and 9.5%, respectively. Permanent pacemaker implantation was necessary in 3.6% and 13% of patients suffered a major access site complication.

The PARTNER EU (Placement of Aortic Transcatheter Valve) registry began as a feasibility trial and continued as a post-marketing evaluation of transfemoral and transapical TAVR using the Edwards SAPIEN valve [78]. In the transfemoral group, valve implantation was successful in 91% of 61 patients, with sustained improvements in LVEF and NYHA functional class at 6-month follow-up. In this period survival was 90% and three patients suffered strokes.

The SOURCE (A European Registry of Transcatheter Aortic Valve Implantation Using the Edwards SAPIEN Valve) registry was a postmarketing evaluation of the SAPIEN valve with 463 patients in the transfemoral arm and an overall logistic EuroSCORE of 26%. Appropriate device placement was achieved in 92.4% of cases with a 30-day mortality of 6.3% and stroke rate of 2.4% [79]. Interestingly, the investigators found that the vascular access complications which were a significant source of mortality in the early transfemoral TAVR studies were no longer a significant predictor of death.

On the whole, like in other areas of cardiac surgery but particularly perhaps in the field of TAVR versus SAVR, systematic reviews of RCTs, and the trials themselves are not yet available to guide practice. In their absence, as we described earlier, well-designed observational studies of sufficiently large and consistent sizes have become the next best course of action to enable evidence-based decision-making (Table 9.3). Through the integration of evidence gained from such studies with individual patient values and local circumstances,

Table 9.3 Summary of clinical outcome data with transcatheter aortic valve replacement from studies of different valve types. (Reproduced from Patel JH et al [80], with permission.)

Valve	Study/(year)	Number of patients	Approach	Procedural success rate (%)	30-day outcome	Clinical improvement
Cribier-Edwards	Webb et al. (2006)	18	Retrograde	77	11% mortality rate	
	Webb et al. (2007)	50	Retrograde	86	12% mortality rate	Significant NYHA class improvement at 30 days maintained through 1 year
	Leichtstein et al. (2006)	7	Transapical	100	14% mortality rate	NYHA class well maintained at 6-month follow-up
CoreValve (first-generation)	Grube et al. (2006)	25	Retrograde	88	32% MACE rate	NYHA class improved by 1 to 2 grades in all patients
CoreValve (second- and third-generation)	Grube et al. (2007)	86	Retrograde	88	12% mortality rate	NYHA class improvement from 2.85 + 0.73 before and 1.85 + 0.60 after procedure (p < 0.001)
	Presentation at EuroPCR 2008 by M Buchbinder	536	Retrograde	97	8% mortality rate	Percent of patients categorized in NYHA class III–IV improved from 86% to 8% at 30 days
SAPIEN valve	PARTNER Trial (unpublished) Pasupati et al. (2007)	100	Retrograde and Transapical	First 25 patients: 76 Following 75 patients: 96	15% mortality rate	NYHA class decreased from a mean of >3 to ~1.5 at 12 months in the 31 patients with 1-year follow-up
	Svensson et al. (2008)	40	Transapical	90	17.5% mortality rate	NYHA class improved from 3.33 to 2.25 (p < 0.0001) at 30-day follow-up
	Walther et al. (2008)	59	Transapical	90	13.6% mortality rate	

NYHA, New York Heart Association; PARTNER, Placement of Aortic Transcatheter Valve; PCR, Paris Course on Revascularisation; TAVR, transcetheter aortic valve replacement.

robust evidence-based clinical practice can drive forward this relatively new development in cardiac surgery safely and effectively.

Conclusions

Whether the lack of good surgical RCTs is because surgeons lack the necessary training, expertise, and desire to perform RCTs, inadequate funding from granting agencies, or methodological problems is not entirely clear. If problems preclude an RCT to answer a significant proportion of clinical treatment effectiveness questions, then alternative research designs, such as prospective matched-pair trials, may need to be better developed and used. If RCTs can be performed, other strategies to increase the number and quality of RCTs need to be adopted, including continuing education of surgeons in clinical research methods, compulsory evaluation of new techniques and technology by governing bodies, and more funding for clinical research.

References

1. Blackstone EH. Comparing apples and oranges. *J Thorac Cardiovasc Surg* 2002;123:8–15.
2. Scales CD Jr, Preminger GM, Keitz SA, Dahm P. Evidence based clinical practice: a primer for urologists. *J Urol* 2007;178:775–782.
3. Loop FD. A surgeon's view of randomized prospective studies. *J Thorac Cardiovasc Surg* 1979;78:161–165.
4. Cook A, Ramsay CR, Fayers P, *et al.* Statistical evaluation of learning curve effects in surgical trials. *Clin Trials* 2004;1:421–427.
5. Schulz KF, Grimes DA. Blinding in randomised trials: hiding who got what. *Lancet* 2002;359:696–700.
6. Schulz KF, Grimes DA. Generation of allocation sequences in randomised trials: chance, not choice. *Lancet* 2002;359:515–519.
7. Kunz R, Vist G, Oxman AD. Randomisation to protect against selection bias in healthcare trials. *Cochrane Database Syst Rev* 2007:18.
8. Lachin JM. Statistical considerations in the intent-to-treat principle. *Control Clin Trials* 2000;21:167–189.
9. Freemantle N, Calvert M, Wood J, Eastaugh J, Griffin C. Composite outcomes in randomized trials greater precision but with greater uncertainty? *JAMA* 2003;289: 2554–2559.
10. Lauer MS, Topol EJ. Clinical trials—multiple treatments, multiple end points, and multiple lessons. *JAMA* 2003;289:2575–2577.
11. Moher D, Schulz KF, Altman DG. The CONSORT statement revised recommendations for improving the quality of reports of parallel-group randomised trials. *Lancet* 2001;357: 1191–1194.
12. Huwiler-Muntener K, Juni P, Junker C, Egger M, Quality of reporting of randomized trials as a measure of methodologic quality. *JAMA* 2002;287:2801–2804.
13. Tiruvoipati R, Balasubramanian SP, Atturu G, Peek GJ, Elbourne D. Improving the quality of reporting randomized controlled trials in cardiothoracic surgery: the way forward. *J Thorac Cardiovasc Surg* 2006;132:233–240.
14. Schlesselman JJ. *Case-Control Studies*. Oxford University Press, New York, 1982.
15. Hosmer DW, Lemeshow S. Polytomous logistic regression. In: *Applied Logistic Regression*. John Wiley, New York, 1989.

16. Little RJ, Rubin DB, Causal effects in clinical and epidemiological studies via potential outcomes: concepts and analytic approaches. *Ann Rev Public Health* 2000;21:121–145.

17. Shahian DM, Normand S, Torchiana DF *et al.* Cardiac surgery report cards: comprehensive review and statistical critique. *Ann Thorac Surg* 2001;72:2155–2168.

18. Rosenbaum PR, Rubin DB, The central role of the propensity score in observational studies for causal effects. *Biometrika* 1983;70:41–55.

19. Cologne JB, Shibata Y, Optimal case-control matching in practice. *Epidemiology* 1995;6: 271–275.

20. Rubin DB. Bias reduction using Mahalanobis metric matching. *Biometrics* 1980;36: 393–398.

21. Rosenbaum PR. Optimal matching for observational studies. *J Am Stat Assoc* 1989;84: 1024–1032.

22. D'Agostino RB Jr. Propensity score methods for bias reduction in the comparison of a treatment to a non-randomized control group. *Stat Med* 1998;17: 2265–2281.

23. Jones RH, Velazquez EJ, Michler RE, *et al.*; STICH Hypothesis 2 Investigators. Coronary bypass surgery with or without surgical ventricular reconstruction. *N Engl J Med* 2009; 360:1705–1717.

24. Menicanti L, Di Donato M. Surgical left ventricle reconstruction, pathophysiologic insights, results and expectation from the STICH trial. *Eur J Cardiothorac Surg* 2004; 26:42–47.

25. Califf RM, Adams KF, McKenna WJ, *et al.* A randomized controlled trial of epoprostenol therapy for severe congestive heart failure: the Flolan International Randomized Survival Trial (FIRST). *Am Heart J* 1997;134:44–54.

26. Gaudron P, Eilles C, Kugler I, *et al.* Progressive left ventricular dysfunction and remodeling after myocardial infarction: potential mechanisms and early predictors. *Circulation* 1993;87:755–763.

27. Di Donato M, Sabatier M, Toso A, *et al.* Regional myocardial performance of non-ischemic zones remote from anterior wall left ventricular aneurysm. *Eur Heart J* 1995; 16:1285–1292.

28. Conte J. An indictment of the STICH trial: "True, true, and unrelated". *J Heart Lung Transplant* 2010;29:491–496.

29. Gheorghiade M, Bonow RO. Chronic heart failure in the United States: a manifestation of coronary artery disease. *Circulation* 1998;97:282–289.

30. Cooley DA, Collins HA, Hall GA, *et al.* Ventricular aneurysm after myocardial infarction: surgical excision with use of temporary cardiopulmonary bypass. *JAMA* 1958;167:557.

31. Jatene AD. Left ventricular aneurysmectomy: resection or reconstruction? *J Thorac Cardiovasc Surg* 1985;89:321–331.

32. Fontan F. Transplantation of knowledge. *J Thorac Cardiovasc Surg* 1990;99:387–395.

33. Dor V, Kreitmann P, Jourdan J. Interest of "physiological" closure of left ventricle after resection and endocardiectomy for aneurysm or akinetic zone comparison with classical technique about a series of 209 left ventricular resections [abstract]. *J Cardiovascular Surg* 1985;26:73.

34. http://clinicaltrials.gov/archive/NCT00023595/2005_06_23

35. Di Donato M, Castelvecchio S, Kukulski T, *et al.* Surgical ventricular restoration: left ventricular shape influence on cardiac function, clinical status, and survival. *Ann Thorac Surg* 2009;87:455–461.

36. Suma H, Tanabe H, Uejima T, *et al.* Surgical ventricular restoration combined with mitral valve procedure for endstage ischemic cardiomyopathy. *Eur J Cardiothorac Surg* 2009;36: 280–284.

37. Dor V, Civaia F, Alexandrescu C, *et al*. The post-myocardial infarction scarred ventricle and congestive heart failure: the preeminence of magnetic resonance imaging for preoperative, intraoperative, and postoperative assessment. *J Thorac Cardiovasc Surg* 2008; 136:1405–1412.

38. O'Neill JO, Starling RC, McCarthy PM, *et al*. The impact of left ventricular reconstruction on survival in patients with ischemic cardiomyopathy. *Eur J Cardiothorac Surg* 2006; 30:753–759.

39. Adams JD, Fedoruk LM, Tache-Leon CA, *et al*. Does preoperative ejection fraction predict operative mortality with left ventricular restoration? *Ann Thorac Surg* 2006; 82:1715–1719.

40. Schreuder JJ, Castiglioni A, Maisano F, *et al*. Acute decrease of left ventricular mechanical dyssynchrony and improvement of contractile state and energy efficiency after left ventricular restoration. *J Thorac Cardiovasc Surg* 2005;129:138–145.

41. Tulner SA, Steendijk P, Klautz RJ, *et al*. Surgical ventricular restoration in patients with ischemic dilated cardiomyopathy: evaluation of systolic and diastolic ventricular function, wall stress, dyssynchrony, and mechanical efficiency by pressure–volume loops. *J Thorac Cardiovasc Surg* 2006;132:610–620.

42. Yamaguchi A, Adachi H, Kawahito K, *et al*. Left ventricular reconstruction benefits patients with dilated ischemic cardiomyopathy. *Ann Thorac Surg* 2005;79:456–461.

43. Mickleborough LL, Merchant N, Ivanov J, *et al*. Left ventricular reconstruction: early and late results. *J Thorac Cardiovasc Surg* 2004;128:27–37.

44. Athanasuleas CL, Buckberg GD, Stanley AH, *et al*. RESTORE group surgical ventricular restoration in the treatment of congestive heart failure due to post-infarction ventricular dilation. *J Am Coll Cardiol* 2004;44:1439–1442.

45. Doenst T, Velazquez EJ, Beyersdorf F, *et al.*; STICH investigators. To STICH or not to STICH: we know the answer, but do we understand the question? *J Thorac Cardiovasc Surg* 2005;129:246–249.

46. Buckberg GD. Questions and answers about the STICH trial: a different perspective. *J Thorac Cardiovasc Surg* 2005;130:245–249.

47. King SB 3rd, Lembo NJ, Weintraub WS, *et al*. A randomized trial comparing coronary angioplasty with coronary bypass surgery. Emory Angioplasty versus Surgery Trial (EAST). *N Engl J Med* 1994;331:1044–1050.

48. The BARI Investigators. Comparison of coronary bypass surgery with angioplasty in patients with multivessel disease. *N Engl J Med* 1996;335:217–225.

49. The BARI Investigators. The final 10 year follow up results from the BARI randomized trial. *J Am Coll Cardiol* 2007;49:1600–1606.

50. Carrié D, Elbaz M, Puel J, *et al*. Five-year outcome after coronary angioplasty versus bypass surgery in multivessel coronary artery disease: results from the French Monocentric Study. *Circulation* 1997;96 (9 Suppl):II-1–6.

51. Währborg P. Quality of life after coronary angioplasty or bypass surgery. 1-year follow-up in the Coronary Angioplasty versus Bypass Revascularization investigation (CABRI) trial. *Eur Heart J* 1999;20:653–658.

52. Hamm CW, Reimers J, Ischinger T, Rupprecht HJ, Berger J, Bleifeld W. A randomized study of coronary angioplasty compared with bypass surgery in patients with symptomatic multivessel coronary disease. German Angioplasty Bypass Surgery Investigation (GABI). *N Engl J Med* 1994;331:1037–1043.

53. Henderson RA, Pocock SJ, Sharp SJ, *et al*. Long-term results of RITA-1 trial: clinical and cost comparisons of coronary angioplasty and coronary-artery bypass grafting. Randomised Intervention Treatment of Angina. *Lancet* 1998;352:1419–1425.

54. Serruys PW, Ong AT, van Herwerden LA, *et al.* Five year outcome after the coronary stenting versus bypass surgery for treatment of multivessel disease: the final analysis of the Arterial Revascularization Therapies Study (ARTS) randomized trial. *J Am Coll Cardiol* 2005;46:575–581.

55. Booth J, Clayton T, Pepper J, *et al.*; SoS Investigators Randomized Controlled trial of coronary artery bypass surgery versus percutaneous coronary intervention in patients with multivessel coronary artery disease: six year follow up from the Stent or Surgery Trial (SoS). *Circulation* 2008;118:381–388.

56. Rodriguez AE, Baldi J, Fernandez Pereira C, *et al.*; ERACI Investigators. Five Year Follow up of the Argentine randomized trial of coronary angioplasty with stenting versus coronary artery bypass surgery in patients with multiple vessel disease (ERACI II). *J Am Coll Cardiol* 2005;4:582–588.

57. Hueb W, Lopes NH, Gersh BJ, *et al.* Five year follow up of the Medicine Angiolpasty or Surgery Study (MASS II): a randomized controlled clinical trial of 3 therapeutic strategies for multivessel coronary artery disease. *Circulation* 2007;115:1082–1089.

58. Chieffo A, Morici N, Maisano F, *et al.* Percutaneous treatment with drug-eluting stent implantation versus bypass surgery for unprotected left main stenosis: a single-center experience. *Circulation* 2006;113:2542–2547.

59. Morrison DA, Sethi G, Sacks J, *et al.* Percutaneous coronary intervention versus repeat bypass surgery for patients with medically refractory myocardial ischemia: AWESOME randomized trial and registry experience with post-CABG patients. Investigators of the Department of Veterans Affairs Cooperative Study #385, Angina With Extremely Serious Operative Mortality Evaluation. *J Am Coll Cardiol* 2002;40:1951–1954.

60. Malenka DJ, Leavitt BJ, Hearne MJ, *et al.* Comparing long-term survival of patients with multivessel coronary disease after CABG or PCI: analysis of BARI-like patients in northern New England. Northern New England Cardiovascular Disease Study Group. *Circulation* 2005;112 (9 Suppl):I371–376.

61. Brener SJ, Lytle BW, Casserly IP, Schneider P, Topol EJ, Lauer MS. Propensity analysis of long term survival after surgical or percutaneous revascularization inpatients with multivessel coronary artery disease and high risk features. *Circulation* 2004;109: e9043–9044.

62. Hannan EL, Racz, MJ, Walford G, *et al.* Long term outcomes of coronary –artery bypass grafting versus stent implantation. *N Engl J Med* 2005;235:2174–2183.

63. Bair, T, Muhlestein JB, May HT, *et al.* Surgical revascularization is associated with improved long term outcomes compared with percutaneous stenting in most subgroups of patients with multivessel coronary artery disease: results from the Intermountain Heart Registry. *Circulation* 2007;116:1126–1123.

64. Hannan EL, Wu C, Walford G, *et al.* Drug eluting stents vs. coronary-artery bypass grafting in multivessel coronary disease. *N Engl J Med* 2008;358:331–341.

65. Serruys PW, Morice M-C, Kappetein AP, *et al.*; for the SYNTAX Investigators. Percutaneous Coronary Intervention versus Coronary-Artery Bypass Grafting for Severe Coronary Artery Disease. *N Engl J Med* 2009;360:961–972.

66. Supplement to: Serruys PW, Morice M-C, Kappetein AP, *et al.* Percutaneous coronary intervention versus coronary-artery bypass grafting for severe coronary artery disease. *N Engl J Med* 2009;360:961–972.

67. Sianos G, Morel MA, Kappetein AP, *et al.* The SYNTAX score: an angiographic tool grading the complexity of coronary artery disease. *EuroIntervention* 2005;1:219–227.

68. Parsonnet V, Dean D, Bernstein AD. A method of uniform stratification of risk for evaluating the results of surgery in acquired adult heart disease. *Circulation* 1989;79:I–3. Erratum. *Circulation* 1990;82:1078.

69. Bravata DM, Gienger AL, McDonald KM, *et al*. Systematic review: the comparative effectiveness of percutaneous coronary interventions and coronary artery bypass graft surgery. *Ann Intern Med* 2007;147:703–716.

70. Perspective Roundtable: CABG vs. Stenting: Clinical Implications of the SYNTAX Trial. *N Engl J Med* 2009;390:961–972.

71. Guarracino F, Talini E, Landoni G, Petronio S, Giannini C, Di Bello V. Effect of aortic valve surgery on left ventricular diastole assessed by echocardiography and neuroendocrine response: percutaneous versus surgical approach. *J Cardiothorac Vasc Anesth* 2010;24:25–29.

72. Andersen HR, Knudsen LL, Hasenkam JM. Transluminal implantation of artificial heart valves. Description of a new expandable aortic valve and initial results with implantation by catheter technique in closed chest pigs. *Eur Heart J* 1992;13:704–708.

73. Cribier A, Eltchaninoff H, Bash A, *et al*. Percutaneous transcatheter implantation of an aortic valve prosthesis for calcific aortic stenosis: first human case description. *Circulation* 2002;106:3006–3008.

74. Cribier A, Eltchaninoff H, Tron C, *et al*. Early experience with percutaneous transcatheter implantation of heart valve prosthesis for the treatment of end-stage inoperable patients with calcific aortic stenosis. *J Am Coll Cardiol* 2004;43:698–703.

75. Piazza N, van Gameren M, Jüni P, *et al*. A comparison of patient characteristics and 30-day mortality outcomes after transcatheter aortic valve implantation and surgical aortic valve replacement for the treatment of aortic stenosis: a two-centre study. *EuroIntervention* 2009;5:580–588.

76. Bagur R, Webb JG, Nietlispach F, *et al*. Acute kidney injury following transcatheter aortic valve implantation: predictive factors, prognostic value, and comparison with surgical aortic valve replacement. *Eur Heart J* 2010;31:865–874.

77. Vassiliades TA Jr, Block PC, Cohn LH, *et al*. The clinical development of percutaneous heart valve technology: a position statement of the Society of Thoracic Surgeons (STS), the American Association for Thoracic Surgery (AATS), and the Society for Cardiovascular Angiography and Interventions (SCAI) Endorsed by the American College of Cardiology Foundation (ACCF) and the American Heart Association (AHA). Society of Thoracic Surgeons; American Association for Thoracic Surgery; Society for Cardiovascular Angiography and Interventions; American College of Cardiology Foundation; American Heart Association. *J Am Coll Cardiol* 2005;45:1554–1560.

78. theheart.org: Low 30-day and six-month mortality for transfemoral valve implantation in PARTNERS EU and SOURCE. Available at http://www.theheart.org/article/910857.do. Accessed November 2, 2009.

79. Tuzcu EM, Kapadia SR, Schoenhagen P. Multimodality quantitative imaging of aortic root for transcatheter aortic valve implantation: more complex than it appears. *J Am Coll Cardiol* 2010;55:195–197.

80. Patel JH, Mathew ST, Hennebry TA. Transcatheter valve replacement: A potential option for the nonsurgical patient. *Clin Cardiol* 2009;32:296–301.

CHAPTER 10

Adult congenital heart disease

Cary Ward, J. Kevin Harrison, and Thomas M. Bashore
Duke University Medical Center, Durham, NC, USA

Introduction

Since the advent of congenital heart surgery in 1944 with the first Blalock–Taussig shunt, the survival of children with congenital heart disease (CHD) has steadily increased. Many factors have contributed to the improved outcomes among this patient population, including earlier diagnosis with echocardiography, advances in surgical technique, and the increasing success of percutaneous interventions. The result of this increased survival, however, is that we now have a growing population of *adults* with CHD. A population study by Marelli *et al.* documents that since 1985, there have been more adults than children with CHD [1]. In fact, the prevalence of severe CHD (defined as lesions most likely to be associated with cyanosis) increased in adults by 85% from 1985 to 2000, while it only increased in children by 22% [1].

While this burgeoning population is a testament to the success of pediatric cardiologists and surgeons, the medical issues and problems that arise as they enter adulthood are not well studied, and data as to the optimal care of these patients are lacking when compared to the vast database that exists for adult-onset heart disease. In addition, adult cardiologists specially trained in this population are based predominately at academic centers and may not be easily accessible to some patients. To address these issues, American College of Cardiology (ACC)/American Heart Association (AHA) guidelines for the management of adults with CHD have been published [2]. Remarkably none of the specific recommendations in this document is supported by Level A evidence (i.e., data derived from multiple randomized controlled trials [RCTs] or meta-analyses) and only rarely was there Level B evidence (i.e., data derived from a single randomized trial or from non-randomized studies). In this chapter, we will review the literature for the care of this patient population and focus on the congenital lesions that have been the best studied. However, the reader should be aware that there are many clinical situations for which very little data are available.

Cardiovascular Clinical Trials: Putting the Evidence into Practice, First Edition.
Edited by Marcus D. Flather, Deepak L. Bhatt, and Tobias Geisler.
© 2013 Blackwell Publishing Ltd. Published 2013 by Blackwell Publishing Ltd.

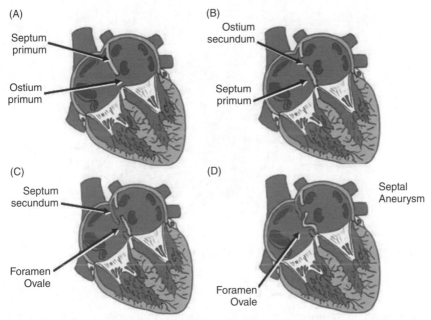

(A)

Septum primum

Ostium primum

(B)

Ostium secundum

Septum primum

(C)

Septum secundum

Foramen Ovale

(D)

Septal Aneurysm

Foramen Ovale

Figure 10.1 Formation of the atrial septum. (A) Formation of the septum primum. The ostium primum precedes the septal wall formation. (B) Occurrence of the ostium secundum defect within the septum primum. (C) Formation of the septum secundum covering the septum primum and ostium secundum. An oval defect within the septum secundum is called the foramen ovale. (D) A patent foramen ovale with redundant atrial septal tissue (septal aneurysm).

Atrial septal defects

Anatomy
Atrial septal defects (ASDs) may occur when there is incomplete formation of one or both of the atrial septal tissue planes during fetal cardiac development, leaving a true opening between the two atrial chambers and allowing persistent shunting of blood. The formation of the atrial septum is schematically shown in Figure 10.1. The initial septation occurs as a result of the septum primum extending inferiorly between the left and right atria. This septum primum is preceded by the ostium primum (Figure 10.1A). In the normal situation, the ostium primum closes and a new fenestration or fenestrations appear in the septum primum. This hole constitutes the ostium secundum (Figure 10.1B). Then, a second septum (septum secundum) migrates inferiorly to cover the right side of the septum primum. Within the septum secundum a large oval hole forms (fossa ovalis) toward its distal end (Figure 10.1C). The two septae normally fuse after birth with the increase in left atrial pressure pushing the septum primum toward the septum secundum. If the ostium secundum is covered, but there remains a path through the fossa ovalis, a patent foramen ovale is defined. If either septum is redundant and floppy, then a septal aneurysm is said to be present (Figure 10.1D). Most often

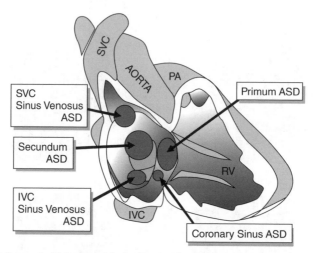

Figure 10.2 Types of atrial septal defects. See text for details.

the redundant septum is the septum primum, but either or both may be affected.

There are five anatomically distinct types of ASDs (Figure 10.2), the most common being the secundum ASD. A secundum ASD is a defect located in the area of the ostium secundum within the septum primum. It occurs when the hole is not completely covered by the septum secundum. Multiple fenestrations in the septum primum may also occur and result in shunting. A sinus venosus defect is located at the junction of either the superior vena cava (SVC) or inferior vena cava (IVC) and the right atrium. The IVC sinus venosus defect is extremely rare. The sinus venosus defect related to the SVC is, in reality, a defect in the posterior floor of the SVC. This anatomy commits the right upper pulmonary vein, which travels posterior to the SVC, into the defect and forms an extracardiac (anomalous vein) plus an interatrial communication between the right atrium and left atrium.

The most inferiorly located true ASD is the primum ASD. This can exist alone, or in conjunction with a membranous ventricular septal defect (VSD) as part of an atrioventricular canal defect and is commonly associated with trisomy 21 (Down syndrome). An atrioventricular canal defect may present with only a primum ASD, only a VSD or both defects. When both defects are present, the atrioventricular valves may straddle the common opening between the atria and ventricles. A primum ASD is frequently associated with abnormalities of the atrioventricular valves, most commonly a cleft in the anterior leaflet of the mitral valve. This can result in mitral valve regurgitation. The tricuspid valve may also be affected.

Finally, the least common type of ASD is not actually a defect in the atrial septum but rather a defect in the roof of the coronary sinus and left atrium—the so-called coronary sinus ASD. Physiologically this allows left atrial blood to enter the "unroofed" coronary sinus and exit through the normal coronary sinus ostium into the right atrium [3].

Clinical implications

Although ASDs always result in some bidirectional shunting, the major direction of the shunt flow is governed by the differential compliance characteristics of the right and left sides of the heart. The right atrial wall is thinner and the chamber has less stiffness and greater compliance than the left atrium. This results in a lower pressure at any particular volume, when compared with the left atrium, and the predominant direction of the interatrial shunt is left to right. Although this left-to-right shunting leads to progressive right atrial and ventricular enlargement, the volume load on the right heart is well tolerated for decades in most patients. Over time, however, the right atrium may become hypertrophied and less compliant, and this results in a reduction in the left-to-right shunting through the same size defect. Eventually, the compliance of the right atrium may worsen to become less than that of the left atrium, and there is even a reversal of the majority of the shunt flow. Cyanosis then occurs. Pulmonary vascular resistance typically remains normal or mildly elevated and there is usually only a modest increase in right ventricular and pulmonary arterial systolic pressure related to high pulmonary blood flow. Pulmonary hypertension eventually develops in only about 15% of patients and is progressive over time.

In 1970, Campbell followed 100 patients with unrepaired ASDs and found all but three of 52 patients did well in the first two decades of life and remained asymptomatic. By his calculations the mortality rates during the first and second decades of life were 0.7% and 0.6% per year, respectively [4]. However, once patients entered the third decade of life complications began to appear, including congestive heart failure, atrial fibrillation, and cyanosis from shunt reversal. During the fourth decade the mortality rate increases to 6.3% per year and continues to increase with each decade that the ASD is left unrepaired [4]. These data have suggested that early repair of this defect should always be considered.

Treatment

Until recently, the repair of ASDs required open heart surgery and usually cardiopulmonary bypass, both of which carry additional risk in adult patients who may have more comorbidities than pediatric patients. In order to investigate if there was a mortality benefit to offset this increased risk, Konstantinides et al. evaluated 179 patients with isolated ASDs, all of whom were over the age of 40 years [5]. Eighty-four of these patients underwent surgical repair, while 95 were treated medically based on the decision of their cardiologists and cardiac surgeons (medical therapy consisted of digitalis, diuretics, and nitrates). Although all types of ASDs were included, 91% were secundum defects. Both groups were followed for an average of 9 years. At baseline, the two groups were very similar with regards to NYHA class, mean pulmonary artery pressure, and incidence of atrial fibrillation. The medically treated group was slightly older in age: 55% were over 55 years compared to 31% in the surgical arm, and had slightly higher pulmonary vascular resistance (141 vs. 113 dyn-sec-cm⁵). However, the patients in the surgical arm had significantly higher shunt ratios with a mean Qp:Qs of 2.9 versus 2.3 in the medical arm [5]. The results of this study demonstrated a strikingly lower mortality rate in the surgical arm with the relative risk of death being 0.31 for patients who underwent surgical closure. The rate of survival was 95% at 10 years for the surgical arm, but only 84% at 10 years for the medical arm [5]. The deaths in the medical arm were predominately secondary to congestive heart failure (21 of 23 patients). There were no perioperative deaths. In addition, there was a significant improvement in the functional capacity of patients who underwent repair, with 32% of patients improving with respect to NYHA class. In the medical arm, 34% experienced worsening symptoms and a decline in their functional class [5].

In 2001, Attie *et al.* randomized 473 patients older than 40 years with isolated ASDs to medical or surgical therapy on a 1:1 basis. Patients with a pulmonary systolic pressure of over 70 mmHg or a shunt ratio of less than 1.5:1 were excluded [6]. Patients were followed for a mean of 7.1 years. The primary endpoint was a composite of cardiovascular events, including cardiac-related death, heart failure, progression of pulmonary hypertension, ventricular arrhythmias or systemic or pulmonary embolism. In contrast to the study by Konstantinides *et al.*, there was no significant difference in the mortality rate between the surgical and medical arms (5.8% vs. 4.3%). However, the primary endpoint was significantly different with 20.7% experiencing a cardiac event in the medical arm and only 11.1% in the surgical arm. When evaluating the study population as a whole, risk factors for the primary endpoint were older age at diagnosis, higher mean pulmonary pressure, and medical treatment [6]. Taken together, these data clearly suggest that ASDs in adult patients associated with a significant shunt ratio can be safely repaired surgically and that repair is beneficial. Current practice guidelines recommend that any ASD associated with right atrial or ventricular enlargement be closed, regardless of whether the patient is symptomatic. This concept is particularly germane to adult patients in that, as described above, the direction of the left-to-right shunt may decline over time as the right heart becomes less compliant. A shunt that began as a 3:1 left-to-right shunt in childhood may present as only a 1.5:1 left-to-right shunt as an older adult. Because one cannot simply use the shunt ratio to decide the significance of the shunt in the adult situation, any patient in whom the right heart is enlarged should be assumed to have a "significant" shunt.

Pulmonary hypertension occurs in only about 15% of patients with a defect proximal to the tricuspid valve (ASD or anomalous pulmonary veins). Normal pulmonary vascular resistance (PVR) is about one-tenth to one-fifteenth that of systemic vascular resistance (SVR). In the high-volume state of a left-to-right shunt, the PVR is usually normal or even low. If the measured PVR is more than two-thirds the SVR, then closing the defect may actually be harmful, since right ventricular function may be quite compromised and the associate right-to-left shunt in this situation may be helping decompress the right heart. In patients with right-to-left shunt and an increase in PVR, temporary occlusion of the defect with a balloon catheter can be performed to transiently test whether acute right ventricular failure would occur with permanent closure.

Device closure

Surgical closure of ASDs has been successfully accomplished over the last half century. Current techniques have evolved to offer patients surgical correction via smaller incisions, such as a right thoracotomy or partial lower sternotomy. The closure of the primum ASD, the sinus venosus ASD, and the coronary sinus ASD requires surgical intervention. However, many patients with a secundum ASD can now be safely and effectively corrected via a percutaneous approach using devices specifically designed to close these ASDs. The first attempt at percutaneous ASD closure was reported over 30 years ago [7]. Over the subsequent decades, multiple device designs and deployment strategies were developed and examined [8–11]. In 2001, the first FDA approval of an ASD device occurred for the Amplatzer ASO device and multiple studies since have proven this device to be safe and effective. Du *et al.* followed 596 patients with secundum ASDs—442 underwent device closure and 154 surgical repair. Although most of the patients enrolled were children (mean age 9.8 years in the device arm and 4.1 years in the surgical arm), the age range included patients as old as 82 years [12]. The device arm achieved a successful closure rate of 97.6% immediately after the procedure and 98.5% at 12 months' follow-up. The surgical arm achieved a 100% closure rate at both time points. However, the surgical arm had more complications with 5.4% of patients experiencing a major complication, including pericardial tamponade (1.9%), pulmonary edema (0.6%), repeat surgery (1.3%), and wound complications (1.3%). Major complications in the device arm occurred at a rate of 1.6% and included arrhythmias and device embolization in two patients, which required surgery [12]. A similar trial done a few years later in Italy evaluated 1268 secundum ASD patients (751 with device closure and 533 with surgical repair) [13]. Again, the complication rate was higher in the surgical group (16% vs 3.6% in the device arm). In addition, the duration of hospital stay was shorter in the device arm [13]. Taken together, these studies indicate that device closure is at least equivalent to surgery in the rate of successful closure and is associated with fewer major complications and shorter hospital stays.

Khan *et al.* recently demonstrated the benefits of device closure in an older population in a prospective study of patients aged 40 years or older with secundum ASDs between 18 and 24 mm in diameter [14]. All patients received the Amplatzer ASO device and there were no procedure-related complications. Patients were evaluated at 6 weeks and 1 year post device implantation by echocardiography, 6-minute walk test, and quality-of-life surveys. As expected, right ventricular diastolic dimensions decreased by an average of 10 mm; interestingly, most of this decrease occurred between the 6-week and 1-year time points. This is in contrast to a younger ASD population in which the majority of right ventricular remodeling occurred in the first few weeks after ASD closure. In addition, these patients experienced an improvement in their 6-minute walk test (average 94 meters), as well as a significant improvement in their quality-of-life scores [14]. Therefore, in adult patients with appropriate anatomy, device closure is now preferred because of its excellent risk–benefit ratio.

Patent foramen ovale

Embryology

During fetal development, oxygenated blood from the maternal circulation is delivered to the fetus via the umbilical vessels. The umbilical arteries connect to the distal aorta, while the umbilical vein joins the IVC. As in the adult, the IVC delivers blood to the right atrium; however, due to the high fetal pulmonary resistance *in utero*, only a small portion of the blood from the right atrium travels through the pulmonary circulation. Two-thirds of the oxygenated fetal blood enters the right ventricle, then the pulmonary artery, and travels out of the patent ductus arteriosus (PDA) to the aorta. One-third of the oxygenated right atrium blood crosses the patent foramen ovale (PFO). After birth, the pulmonary resistance decreases as the baby begins to breathe on his/her own and the left atrium fills with oxygenated blood from the lungs. Left atrial pressure quickly exceeds right atrial pressure. This pressure differential prevents right-to-left shunting through the foramen ovale, and eventually the foramen is sealed shut. However, in a small number of adults, the septum secundum never completely bonds to the septum primum and a potential path from the right atrium to the left atrium occurs through the PFO. A PFO is thought to exist in anywhere from 10% to 25% of the adult population. The degree of right-to-left shunt in these patients is determined by the pressure differential in the atria, the characteristics of the tissues that make up the atrial septum (whether a floppy or redundant atrial septum is present, i.e., a septal aneurysm), and sometimes position or activity. It is assumed that when there is an atrial septal aneurysm, the flopping of the aneurysmal tissue periodically opens the PFO pathway and increases the chances of right-to-left shunting.

Clinical implications

Paradoxical embolus and stroke

As a source of right-to-left shunting, a PFO provides a possible route for paradoxical embolus and has therefore been implicated as an etiology for cryptogenic stroke. Studies have attempted to define the role of PFO in cerebrovascular disease by evaluating the risk of recurrent stroke in patients with a PFO. From 1996 to 2000, Mas *et al.* followed 581 patients younger than 55 years of age who had suffered a cryptogenic stroke. All patients were treated with aspirin and all underwent transesophageal echocardiograms; 48% were found to have a PFO. At a follow-up of 3 years, the rate of recurrent stroke was 2.3% in patients with a PFO and 4.3% in patients without a PFO. However, in patients with a PFO and an atrial septal aneurysm (ASA), defined as movement of the atrial septum more than 10 mm in either direction, the rate of recurrent stroke was slightly higher at 6.3%. When the authors examined the combined endpoint of recurrent stroke and transient ischemic attack (TIA), the group with PFO and ASA stood out further with a recurrence rate of 10.3%, compared with a rate of 5.2% in the group with no evidence of a PFO and 5.6% in the group with a PFO alone. Although these data demonstrate no increased risk in patients with a PFO alone, they are suggestive of an increased risk in patients with a PFO and ASA [15].

This study was followed by the PICCS (PFO in Cryptogenic Stroke Study), a substudy of the WARRS (Warfarin-Aspirin Recurrent Stroke Study), which was designed to investigate the appropriate treatment of patients with recurrent ischemic stroke. In the substudy, 601 of these patients underwent transesophageal echocardiography (TEE). Of the 250 patients who had a history of cryptogenic stroke, 39% were found to have a PFO. Only 30% of the group with stroke from other causes was found to have a PFO. When the rate of recurrent cerebrovascular accident (CVA) in those with a history of cryptogenic stroke was examined, there was a slight increase in the rate of recurrent stroke for those with a PFO (14.5%) and for a PFO and ASA (15.9%) versus those without a PFO (12.7%). Again, these data are suggestive of a role for PFO in cryptogenic stroke [16]. PFO has also been implicated as a possible source of arterial emboli to the gut or lower extremities, although these cases are much less common.

Hypoxemia

In addition to providing a possible mechanism for clot to reach the left heart, a PFO also provides a route for deoxygenated blood from the venous side to reach the systemic circulation. This is especially true in situations in which the pressures in the right atrium exceed those in the left atrium. For example, a patient with idiopathic pulmonary hypertension may have secondary poor right ventricular and right atrial compliance, leading to an elevation in right atrial pressure. If a PFO is present, a right-to-left shunt may occur and worsen the hypoxemia. In addition, this right-to-left shunting may be positional in some patients: when they stand up they stretch their atrial septum and pull the tissue planes of the PFO apart, leading to an increase in the amount of right-to-left shunt and a decrease in their oxygen level. This positional nature of the right-to-left shunt via a PFO is one etiology of the platypnea–orthodeoxia syndrome, and may be secondary to a dilated aortic root or other distortions in atrial anatomy that occur as people age [17]. Diagnostic measures include an echocardiogram during the injection of agitated saline to create microbubbles that can be shown to cross the interatrial septum. At times in patients with orthodeoxia these microbubbles cross more readily when injected from the femoral vein rather than the arm (due to the baffling effect of the Eustachian valve in the right atrium).

Special case of migraine headaches

The possible association between PFO and migraine headache was first noted by Lamy *et al.* during a prospective study of 581 patients with cryptogenic stroke: migraines were almost twice as common in patients with a PFO (27%) than in those with normal atrial septal anatomy (14%) [18]. This curious association was even stronger in patients with a PFO and ASA [19]. The mechanism by which a PFO might lead to migraines is not clear, but proposed mechanisms include vasoactive substances that are not cleared when blood bypasses the lungs, microscopic paradoxical emboli causing brain ischemia, and vasoconstriction or endothelial dysfunction in the cerebral vasculature caused by intermittent right-to-left shunting via a PFO. Anzola *et al.* quantified right-to-left shunting by transcranial Doppler and found that larger shunts were present in patients with migraine and stroke than in patients with migraine alone or stroke alone [19], suggesting that there may be a common mechanism for both migraine and stroke in patients with a PFO. In a recent meta-analysis, some support can be gathered for PFO closure in migraine patients [20], but other work including a recent case–control study has suggested no relationship between migraines and a PFO [21]. The only randomized controlled trial to investigate the role of PFO in migraine examined 432 patients who were randomized to closure versus a sham procedure group. There was a reduction in the frequency of migraines in the closure group, but no significant difference in the primary endpoint of complete migraine cessation [22]. Thus, a review by Tepper *et al.* [23] concluded that "Patent foramen ovale appears to be associated with migraine with aura, probably through cardiac shunting. PFOs may also be comorbid with cryptogenic strokes. Although multiple open-label, retrospective, and case-controlled studies have noted sometimes dramatic reductions in migraine with aura, the only prospective (randomized) sham-controlled study of PFO closure for migraine with aura, the MIST trial was negative for all primary and secondary measures of migraine improvement."

Management

PFO and cryptogenic stroke or TIAs

All patients who have a paradoxical embolus in the setting of a PFO must first be evaluated for a hypercoagulable state and must avoid agents that could promote clot formation, such as cigarettes or oral contraceptives. They are also often generally advised to avoid long periods of immobility. If a PFO is thought to be implicated in a paradoxical embolus, there may also be a role for medical therapy in the prevention of clot formation. In the WARSS trial, patients were treated with either warfarin to a target INR of 1.4–2.8 or with aspirin 325 mg. In patients with a history of cryptogenic stroke, there was a 15% recurrence rate in the group treated with warfarin. The group treated with aspirin had a slightly higher recurrence rate at 16.5%. When recurrence rates were evaluated in those known to have a PFO in the PICSS substudy, a dramatic decrease was found in the group treated with warfarin (9.5% recurrence at 2 years) versus those treated with aspirin alone (17.9% recurrence at 2 years). Based on these data, many believe that warfarin is the best therapy to prevent recurrent paradoxical emboli in the setting of a PFO [16].

Until recently, closure of a PFO required surgery and cardiopulmonary bypass. However, over the past few years percutaneous closure is increasingly an option. It is important to note that there are currently no devices approved for the elective percutaneous closure of a PFO, but many devices are being tested in clinical trials investigating the use of device closure in the setting of stroke or TIAs. In situations of extreme clinical necessity, some of these devices may be obtained as part of an FDA-approved registry, or other devices, such as approved ASD devices, can be used if clinically required. The authors would emphasize that the off-label use of ASD devices to attempt closure of a PFO is not recommended. Recent editorials have addressed the pros [24] and cons [25] of percutaneous PFO closure in patients with a history of cryptogenic stroke based on the currently available data, and multiple trials are ongoing. Recently, the results of the Closure-1 trial were presented at the American Heart Association Scientific Sessions. In this study, patients were randomized to PFO closure with the STARflex device (NMT medical) versus best medical therapy consisting of warfarin or aspirin or a combination of both. At the end of 2 years, there was no difference between the groups in the composite endpoint or in the rates of stroke or TIA. The results of this trial are yet to be published in a peer reviewed journal, but the presenters called for a more conservative approach to PFO closure patient selection based on these preliminary findings [26].

PFO and hypoxemia

If a patient suffers from hypoxemia secondary to a PFO, or if a patient is not thought to be a candidate for anticoagulation, therapy is limited to closure of the defect and prevention of right-to-left shunting. No devices are currently being marketed specifically for this therapeutic approach, but studies have shown the effectiveness of PFO closure in patients with playpnea–orthodeoxia [27] and in certain congenital situations where relief of hypoxemia can improve the hemodynamic situation without compromising right heart function [28].

Tetralogy of Fallot

Tetralogy of Fallot (TOF) includes subpulmonic stenosis with right ventricular hypertrophy, a VSD, and an aorta that overrides the interventricular septum. It is the most common form of cyanotic CHD worldwide [29]. Anatomically, the key features are the anterocephalad deviation of the outflow septum and hypertrophy of the septoparietal trabeculations [30]. Because the outlet septum is a right ventricular structure, malalignment of the outlet septum results in a VSD and partially commits the aorta to the right ventricle. The VSD is large; the pulmonary valve is often unicuspid or bicuspid. Pulmonary branch stenosis and various degrees of pulmonary arterial hypoplasia may also be present, with some patients even lacking an entire main pulmonary artery (most often the left branch pulmonary artery, where it may hang onto the aorta via the ductus). A left pulmonary arch branch coarctation in the region of the ductal insertion may also be present. The biventricular aorta is usually dilated, arises from a right-sided arch in 25% of patients, and may override the septum to such a degree that more than 50% comes from the right ventricle (consistent with the definition of a double-outlet right ventricle).

Surgical repair for this complex defect includes closure of the VSD and opening of the right ventricular outflow using a Dacron or pericardial patch. This patch may or may not cross the pulmonary valve, though due to the high frequency of a rather hypoplastic pulmonary valve semilunar junction, transannular patches are common. This classic repair has been performed for over 30 years, currently leading to a substantial number of adults who require follow-up and management of late complications. Complications can include aortic regurgitation secondary to a dilated aortic root, residual right ventricular outflow obstruction, pulmonary regurgitation and a volume overloaded right ventricle, and ventricular arrhythmias leading to sudden cardiac death in some patients. In 1993, Murphy *et al.* reviewed the outcomes of patients who had undergone repair of TOF from 1955 to 1960 at the Mayo Clinic. They found that 86% of patients were still alive 32 years after surgery. Ten of 22 late deaths were secondary to sudden cardiac death (SCD) and three patients died of heart failure [29]. Therefore, the management of adult patients with TOF focuses on the prevention of these two late morbidities.

Sudden cardiac death

In 2000, Gatzoulis *et al.* set out to better define the causes and risk factors for SCD in patients who had undergone repair of TOF [31]. They identified 793 patients from six hospital databases who had a previously repaired TOF and obtained follow-up status using arrhythmia as the primary endpoint (sustained atrial fibrillation or flutter, sustained ventricular tachycardia [VT], or SCD). Reassuringly, 715 (90.2%) were arrhythmia free during the 10-year study period. Interestingly, patients who had undergone repair with a transannular patch were significantly more likely to develop sustained VT or SCD. In addition, pulmonary regurgitation irrespective of pulmonic stenosis was the main residual hemodynamic lesion in patients who had difficulty with VT or SCD [31]. Review of the electrocardiogram (EKG) and Holter data from this patient population revealed that QRS duration was greater in all three groups (atrial fibrillation, VT, SCD) than in the group of patients free from arrhythmia. In fact, a QRS duration greater than 180 ms was strongly associated with patients who suffered from VT and SCD (Figure 10.3) [31].

The findings above along with other long-term studies revealed a connection between pulmonary regurgitation and arrhythmia: patients who have undergone transannular patch repairs and more substantial infundibulectomies are left with more akinetic or aneurysmal regions of the right ventricle. This type of repair also predisposes patients to a significant amount of pulmonary regurgitation. Together, these lesions lead to progressive right ventricular dilatation and dysfunction, a widened QRS, and increased risk of ventricular arrhythmias [32]. Therefore, there is an increasing recognition that

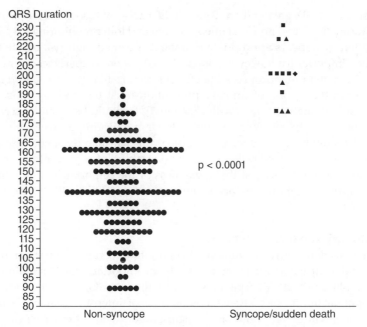

Figure 10.3 Risk of syncope or sudden death in patients following repair of tetralogy of Fallot. A QRS width of >180 ms identified the highest risk group. (Modified from Gatzoulis *et al.* [29], with permission.)

it is important to correct the pulmonary regurgitation before right ventricular dilation and QRS duration are too advanced. Other risk factors for SCD identified in this patient population include older age at the time of repair, ventricular dysfunction, and history of palliative shunt (Waterston [ascending aorta to the right pulmonary artery] or Potts [descending aorta to left pulmonary artery]) [31,33].

Despite the clearly increased risk of ventricular arrhythmia in this patient population, there are little data as to the appropriate surveillance and management of this problem. In patients who have experienced resuscitated cardiac arrest, most agree that implantable cardioverter–defibrillator (ICD) therapy is appropriate. However, indications for primary prevention are less clear. Khairy *et al.* evaluated 121 TOF patients who had ICDs placed for primary (56.2%) or secondary (43.8%) prevention. Characteristics constituting primary prevention included presyncope or syncope, non-sustained VT by Holter monitor, QRS duration 180 ms or longer, left ventricular ejection fraction (LVEF) 35% or less, and inducible VT by electrophysiology study [34]. There was a significant rate of appropriate ICD shocks in both the primary (23.5%) and the secondary prevention group (30.2%) in the 3.7 years of follow-up. The annual event rates were 7.7% in the primary prevention group and 9.8% in the secondary prevention group. Within the primary prevention group, predictors of appropriate shock included left ventricular end-diastolic pressure (LVEDP) greater than 12 mmHg (a marker of associated left ventricular dysfunction), and non-sustained VT seen on Holter monitoring [34]. Thus, ICD therapy appears appropriate in patients deemed high risk by their caregivers. Importantly, however, almost 30% of patients experienced complications other than inappropriate shocks, suggesting that the decision for ICD therapy in the setting of primary prevention must be carefully considered [34]. Asymptomatic patients with repaired TOF should be carefully screened for ventricular ectopy with periodic Holter monitoring as well as routine clinical follow-up and either echocardiograms, cardiac magnetic resonance imaging (MRI), or gated radionuclide angiography for right ventricular function. Recent trends suggest that awareness of the importance of identifying the high-risk patient has reduced sudden death in TOF by 40% from 1979 to 2005 [35].

Pulmonary valve replacement

The connection between pulmonary regurgitation, right ventricular dilatation, and ventricular arrhythmia reveals an important role for pulmonary valve replacement (PVR) in patients with repaired tetralogy of Fallot. However, the optimal timing of PVR remains an area of intense research. Certainly, in patients with severe pulmonary regurgitation who experience symptoms such as dyspnea or exercise intolerance, replacement of the pulmonary valve is beneficial. In an early study of patients undergoing PVR by Therrien *et al.*, 24% of patients were functional class III/IV prior to surgery and 0% after surgery, indicating a symptomatic benefit for some patients [36]. However, the same study discovered that there was no significant improvement in quantified exercise tolerance, right ventricular dimensions or right ventricular ejection fraction (RVEF) [36]. These data suggest that in order to prevent irreversible right ventricular dilatation and dysfunction, operative intervention should occur prior to the onset of symptoms or arrhythmia.

The increased use of cardiac MRI has shed considerable light on the timing of repair, since it is the best imaging modality to assess the size and function of the right ventricle [32]. Vliegen *et al.* studied 26 patients with repaired TOF undergoing PVR. Indication for PVR included moderate-to-severe pulmonary regurgitation with right ventricular dilatation with or without symptoms. Cardiac MRI was performed before and after surgery. The authors showed a significant decrease in both right ventricular systolic and diastolic volumes, as well as an improvement in right ventricular function when corrected for the regurgitation [37]. Oosterhof *et al.* went on to investigate if there was a preoperative threshold of right ventricular size after which right ventricular dilatation does not improve. They evaluated 71 patients with cardiac MRI before and after PVR; again, indications for surgery included severe pulmonary regurgitation with progressive right ventricular dilatation, symptoms or arrhythmias [38]. Interestingly, a decrease in right ventricular volume was seen in all patients and there was no threshold for right ventricular volume after which an improvement in right ventricular size does not occur. However, *normal* RV dimensions could only be restored in patients with a right ventricular end-diastolic volume index (RV EDVI) of less than $160 \, mL/m^2$ and a right ventricular end-systolic volume index (RV ESVI) of less than $82 \, mL/m^2$ [38]. Importantly, patients with normalization of right ventricular volumes after surgery also had a higher RVEF after surgery. Taken together, these data indicate that in order to restore normal right ventricular function and to avoid complications of arrhythmia, patients with repaired TOF and significant pulmonary regurgitation should be followed closely by cardiac MRI to evaluate right ventricular size and function. Operative intervention should occur when right ventricular dilatation is progressive but prior to an RV EDVI of $160 \, mL/m^2$ [38].

The operative mortality of PVR is low at 1–4% [39], but most young adults will require future interventions since the lifespan of prosthetic valves and conduits is limited. Therefore, a percutaneous option for PVR is desirable for many patients. In 2008, Lurz *et al.* presented their results for 155 patients undergoing percutaneous pulmonary valve implantation (Melody system, Medtronic) in Europe. The majority of these patients had a repaired TOF, mostly with a right ventricle-to-pulmonary artery conduit. Importantly, conduits have a more predictable anatomy than a native outflow tract, which makes the appropriate sizing of a percutaneous valve easier. Freedom from reoperation was 70% at 70 months and survival was 96.9% at 83 months [40]. Zahn *et al.* recently published the US experience with the Melody system in patients with a right ventricular outflow tract conduit dysfunction. Only three of 34 experienced procedural adverse events, and the criteria for procedural success were met in 93% of the attempted implantations [41]. Pulmonary regurgitant fraction as measured by cardiac MRI was reduced from an average of 27.6% to 3.35% at 6 months. Most importantly, 19% of patients had an improvement in their NYHA functional class [41]. Based on these results, the Medtronic Melody system is now approved by the FDA as a humanitarian device and other percutaneous pulmonary valves are currently under development. These technological advances promise to reduce the need for repeated surgeries in this population of young patients.

Eisenmenger syndrome

Eisenmenger syndrome is defined as pulmonary hypertension due to a high pulmonary vascular resistance with reversed or bidirectional shunting through a congenital defect [42]. Causes are generally left-to-right shunts that occur after the tricuspid valve. Pretricuspid valve shunts (i.e., ASD, partially anomalous pulmonary venous return, etc.) rarely result in pulmonary hypertension (about 15%). Most congenital causes of Eisenmenger syndrome include VSD and/or PDA. In addition to symptoms of dyspnea, palpitations, and volume retention, patients with Eisenmenger syndrome have the complications of progressive cyanosis. These include secondary erythrocytosis, hyperviscosity, iron-deficiency anemia, and hemoptysis [3]. Therapies for Eisenmenger syndrome are limited and are predominately based on observational studies. The importance of oxygen is controversial since much of the hypoxemia is related to the shunt and may not be responsive to supplemental oxygen. Sandoval *et al.* evaluated the use of nocturnal oxygen in adult patients with Eisenmenger syndrome and found no significant difference in mortality [43]. However, there are no studies of continuous oxygen therapy and home oxygen is usually prescribed for these patients as supportive care.

Many advocate the use of warfarin in patients with Eisenmenger syndrome but no RCTs demonstrate benefit for anticoagulation. In addition, the high incidence of hemoptysis in this population may make warfarin therapy difficult to tolerate. The most effective way to avoid excessive clotting in these patients is to avoid iron-deficiency anemia. In 1996, Ammash and Warnes reviewed risk factors for CVA in a population with cyanotic CHD and found the clinical variable most highly associated with CVA was iron-deficiency anemia. Other risk factors included a history of phlebotomy and not surprisingly atrial fibrillation [44]. Phlebotomy and the resultant iron-deficiency anemia lead to microcytosis, which increases the risk of CVA. Therefore, phlebotomy should only be used in the setting of *symptomatic* hyperviscosity. In addition, iron-deficiency should be immediately treated with a low dose of iron supplementation (325 mg/day) and close follow-up of hematological variables. The iron supplementation can be decreased or discontinued once normocytosis is restored [44].

The use of pulmonary vasodilators in patients with Eisenmenger syndrome has received increasing attention. In 2003, Fernandes *et al.* retrospectively reviewed records of 67 patients with Eisenmenger physiology who had been treated with epoprostenol (IV prostaglandin-I_2) and found that all patients had a significant improvement in functional class, 6-minute walking distance, and systemic oxygen saturation. In patients who underwent repeat hemodynamics after 3 months of therapy, the median PVR decreased from 41 Woods units to 21 Woods units [45]. The first randomized trial of pulmonary vasodilator therapy was published in 2006. BREATHE-5 randomized functional class III Eisenmenger patients to bosentan, an oral endothelin receptor antagonist, or placebo. Patients were evaluated after 16 weeks for changes in PVR. While PVR increased in the placebo-treated group by 5.4%, it decreased by 9.3% in the group treated with bosentan. In addition, 6-minute walk distance increased in the bosentan treated group by 43 m, while it decreased in the placebo-treated group by 9.7 m [46]. These trials suggest that pulmonary vasodilator therapy decreases PVR, improves 6-minute walk distance, and increases functional capacity. Although their effect on mortality is still unknown, the use of pulmonary vasodilator therapy in patients with Eisenmenger syndrome is an increasingly important part of the treatment arsenal and one of the few therapies for which there are randomized trials to support its benefit [47].

Pregnancy in patients with adult congenital heart disease

The major improvements in the care of pediatric patients with CHD have resulted in an increasingly large number of women who are of childbearing age who wish to become pregnant. A growing number of retrospective studies have demonstrated that, although the incidence of maternal and fetal complications is higher than in the control population, maternal death is rare [48]. However, these retrospective studies are biased by the fact that many women with severe CHD are counseled never to get pregnant. Certainly, patients with severe pulmonary hypertension or significant heart failure secondary to systemic ventricular dysfunction should avoid pregnancy since the hemodynamic changes required will be poorly tolerated. In a small study of 12 women with Eisenmenger syndrome, there were three maternal deaths (two prepartum and one 30 days after delivery) and three spontaneous abortions [49]. The seven women who reached the end of the second trimester were hospitalized; all required delivery by cesarean section in the third trimester secondary to maternal or fetal indications [49]. Women with cyanotic CHD should also avoid pregnancy secondary to a high rate of fetal complications. In a study from the Royal Brompton in 1995, the risk of maternal complications was 32% with one maternal death, and only 43% of pregnancies resulted in a live birth [50]. Thus, in women with pulmonary hypertension, cyanotic CHD or congestive heart failure, the emphasis should be on the prevention of pregnancy through contraception. If they do become pregnant, then termination should be recommended. In women with less significant CHD, successful pregnancies are possible. Individual lesions will be discussed below.

Aortic stenosis

In young women of childbearing age, the most common etiology of aortic stenosis (AS) is a congenital bicuspid aortic valve. Other causes of congenital AS include subaortic membrane and hypertrophic subaortic obstruction [51]. Early studies demonstrated a high rate of cardiac complications associated with pregnancy in women with AS secondary to the elevated LVEDP that occurs as the cardiac output increases. However, two more recent studies demonstrate acceptable outcomes for pregnant women with AS. Silversides *et al.* reviewed 39 women with 49 pregnancies in the setting of congenital AS. Ninety per cent of women had bicuspid aortic valves and 59% were classified as severe AS with peak gradients by echo/Doppler estimated as high as 67 mmHg. In the group with severe AS there were only three events (defined as pulmonary edema, arrhythmia or maternal death): two women with pulmonary edema and one with atrial arrhythmias. There were no maternal deaths [52]. In the women with mild-to-moderate AS there were no cardiac events during the antepartum and peripartum period, but four women in this group did experience a significant deterioration in their functional class [52]. There was an expected rate of obstetric and fetal complications in this study as six pregnancies (12%) resulted in premature birth, one a small for gestational age baby, or respiratory distress syndrome, but no fetal deaths [52].

Yap *et al.* reviewed 53 pregnancies in women with congenital AS and a mean aortic jet velocity of 3.3 m/s (range 1.7–5.3 m/s). Left ventricular function was normal in all women. Cardiac events including heart failure, arrhythmia, and stroke occurred in five women (9.4% of pregnancies). Two women in the severe AS group had an episode of congestive heart failure requiring medical therapy [53]. Again, there was the usual incidence of obstetric complications with 7.5% of pregnancies resulting in premature labor and 13.2% of babies born prematurely, but 11.5% of pregnancies were complicated by hypertensive disorders of pregnancy, and there was a 4% incidence of placental abruption. In summary, these data indicate that in the majority of women with AS, pregnancy is well tolerated, although the risk of obstetric and perinatal complications may be increased [53]. Improvements in both cardiac and obstetric care may account for the difference between these results and earlier studies demonstrating a high rate of both maternal and fetal mortality [54]. In pregnant patients with symptomatic AS, percutaneous balloon aortic valvuloplasty is feasible and effective [55].

Pulmonic stenosis

Pulmonic stenosis (PS) in young women can be an isolated congenital abnormality or found as part of a spectrum of congenital cardiac anomalies. Women with known doming (non-dysplastic) pulmonary valve stenosis, symptoms, and a cardiac catheterization gradient from the right ventricle to the pulmonary artery over 30 mmHg, or asymptomatic women with a gradient over 40 mmHg should undergo percutaneous balloon valvuloplasty prior to conception [56]. Those with a dysplastic pulmonary valve are generally not considered candidates for a percutaneous approach. Although there is little in the literature regarding this situation, women who conceive in the setting of known valvular PS are thought to tolerate pregnancy quite well [56]. In 2004, Hameed *et al.* reported on 17 patients with PS and compared them to controls matched in age, ethnicity, and year of delivery [57]. Only one patient had deterioration in her functional class (NYHA class I to NYHA class II). There was no statistically significant difference in obstetric or fetal complications when the patients were compared to the control group. In addition, there was no difference in outcome between the groups with severe PS and those with milder PS [57]. In the rare patient who has symptoms that are refractory to medical therapy, percutaneous valvuloplasty is feasible during the pregnancy [56].

Pulmonary regurgitation

As discussed above, pulmonary regurgitation in young women is seen most commonly after complete repair of TOF [58], though it may occur with idiopathic dilatation of the pulmonary artery or associated with valvular PS. Multiple studies have reviewed the outcome of pregnancy in patients with repaired TOF and all show favorable results, but these have included small numbers of patients not all of whom had pulmonary valve dysfunction [59,60]. Singh *et al.* evaluated 44 pregnancies in 24 women with repaired TOF and found no maternal or perinatal complications, although one infant was found to have pulmonary atresia. More recently, Meijer *et al.* evaluated 50 pregnancies in women with a history of repaired TOF [58]. Severe pulmonary regurgitation (PI) was present in 14 of the 50 pregnancies (28%) and two of the five women who experienced a cardiac event during pregnancy were from the group with severe PI. Both of these patients developed right-sided heart failure and supraventricular tachycardia late in pregnancy and were treated medically [58]. There were no maternal deaths.

In summary, the data suggest that although women with severe pulmonary regurgitation are at risk for right-sided heart failure and arrhythmia when pregnant, they respond well to medical therapy, and adverse outcomes are rare.

Aortopathies

Pregnancy requires significant changes in the musculoskeletal system and markedly increased laxity in the ligaments of the pelvic floor in order to allow the mother to carry the growing fetus as well as to prepare for delivery. This increase in laxity, governed by the hormone relaxin, is associated with the remodeling of large-diameter collagen fibers to small-diameter collagen fibers and requires activation of the collagenolytic system [61]. Elastin may also play a role in this process [61]. While the activity of these hormones is intended for the collagen of the pelvic floor, there may be ramifications for the fibrous tissue of the vascular system. For patients with a pre-existing defect in their collagen, such as women with Marfan syndrome, these changes may present a source of vascular complication. In a retrospective study of pregnancy in the setting of Marfan syndrome, five of the 38 women with Marfan syndrome experienced aortic dissection (three during pregnancy and two post-partum) as compared to no aortic dissection in the control population [62]. Three of the affected women had baseline studies indicating an aortic root diameter of over 40 mm [46]. These data, along with earlier studies of pregnancy in those with Marfan syndrome [63,64], suggest that women should be imaged prior to conception to assess the size of the aortic root, usually by computed tomography angiography (CTA) or cardiac MRI: patients with an aortic root of greater than 40 mm should avoid pregnancy as their risk of dissection is higher. Women who do become pregnant should be followed by serial echocardiograms to ensure that the aortic root size is stable.

Recent data suggest that the aortic root enlargement in Marfan syndrome is caused by excessive signaling by transforming growth factor (TGF-beta) and that angiotensin II receptor blockers (ARBs) may be effective in reducing the rate of growth of the aortic root in these patients [65]. Since ARBs are relatively contraindicated in pregnancy, this creates some dilemma in following women with Marfan syndrome and the drug should be stopped if pregnancy is contemplated. In addition, aortopathy has also been associated with bicuspid aortic valves as well as other CHDs [66,67]. Although no direct data exist, these women should also be closely monitored for ascending aortic aneurysm prior to and during pregnancy.

Ehlers-Danlos syndrome type IV, the vascular type, is known to result from mutations in the gene for type III procollagen (*COL3A1*). Complications of pregnancy include aortic aneurysm development and rupture. In one series, it led to death in 12 of the 81 women who became pregnant [68]. Even though pregnancy can be tolerated in this situation, it is ill-advised.

References

1. Marelli AJ, Mackie AS, Ionescu-Ittu R, Rahme E, Pilote L. Congenital heart disease in the general population: changing prevalence and age distribution. *Circulation* 2007;115: 163–172.
2. Warnes CA, Williams RG, Bashore TM, *et al.* ACC/AHA 2008 guidelines for the management of adults with congenital heart disease: a report of the American College of Cardiology/American Heart Association Task Force on Practice Guidelines (Writing Committee to Develop Guidelines on the Management of Adults With Congenital Heart Disease). Developed in Collaboration With the American Society of Echocardiography, Heart Rhythm Society, International Society for Adult Congenital Heart Disease, Society for Cardiovascular Angiography and Interventions, and Society of Thoracic Surgeons. *J Am Coll Cardiol* 2008;52:e1–121.
3. Gatzoulis MA, Webb GD, Daubeney PEF. *Diagnosis and Management of Adult Congenital Heart Disease.* Edinburgh: Churchill Livingstone, 2003.
4. Campbell M. Natural history of atrial septal defect. *Br Heart J* 1970;32:820–826.
5. Konstantinides S, Geibel A, Olschewski M, *et al.* A comparison of surgical and medical therapy for atrial septal defect in adults. *N Engl J Med* 1995;333:469–473.
6. Attie F, Rosas M, Granados N, Zabal C, Buendia A, Calderon J. Surgical treatment for secundum atrial septal defects in patients >40 years old. A randomized clinical trial. *J Am Coll Cardiol* 2001;38:2035–2042.
7. Mills NL, King TD. Nonoperative closure of left-to-right shunts. *J Thorac Cardiovasc Surg* 1976;72:371–378.
8. Hausdorf G, Kaulitz R, Paul T, Carminati M, Lock J. Transcatheter closure of atrial septal defect with a new flexible, self-centering device (the STARFlex Occluder). *Am J Cardiol* 1999;84:1113–1116, A10.
9. Lock JE. The adult with congenital heart disease: cardiac catheterization as a therapeutic intervention. *J Am Coll Cardiol* 1991;18:330–331.
10. Rao PS, Sideris EB. Centering-on-demand buttoned device: its role in transcatheter occlusion of atrial septal defects. *J Intervent Cardiol* 2001;14:81–89.
11. Latson LA, Zahn EM, Wilson N. Helex septal occluder for closure of atrial septal defects. *Curr Intervent Cardiol Rep* 2000;2:268–273.
12. Du ZD, Koenig P, Cao QL, Waight D, Heitschmidt M, Hijazi ZM. Comparison of transcatheter closure of secundum atrial septal defect using the Amplatzer septal occluder associated with deficient versus sufficient rims. *Am J Cardiol* 2002;90:865–869.
13. Butera G, Carminati M, Chessa M, *et al.* Percutaneous versus surgical closure of secundum atrial septal defect: comparison of early results and complications. *Am Heart J* 2006;151:228–234.
14. Khan AA, Tan JL, Li W, *et al.* The impact of transcatheter atrial septal defect closure in the older population: a prospective study. *J Am Coll Cardiol* 2010;3:276–281.
15. Mas JL, Arquizan C, Lamy C, *et al.* Recurrent cerebrovascular events associated with patent foramen ovale, atrial septal aneurysm, or both. *N Engl J Med* 2001;345:1740–1746.
16. Homma S, Sacco RL, Di Tullio MR, Sciacca RR, Mohr JP. Effect of medical treatment in stroke patients with patent foramen ovale: patent foramen ovale in Cryptogenic Stroke Study. *Circulation* 2002;105:2625–2631.
17. Kerut EK, Norfleet WT, Plotnick GD, Giles TD. Patent foramen ovale: a review of associated conditions and the impact of physiological size. *J Am Coll Cardiol* 2001;38:613–623.
18. Lamy C, Giannesini C, Zuber M, *et al.* Clinical and imaging findings in cryptogenic stroke patients with and without patent foramen ovale: the PFO-ASA Study. Atrial Septal Aneurysm. *Stroke* 2002;33:706–711.

19. Anzola GP, Morandi E, Casilli F, Onorato E. Different degrees of right-to-left shunting predict migraine and stroke: data from 420 patients. *Neurology* 2006;66:765–767.

20. Butera G, Biondi-Zoccai GG, Carminati M, *et al*. Systematic review and meta-analysis of currently available clinical evidence on migraine and patent foramen ovale percutaneous closure: much ado about nothing? *Catheter Cardiovasc Interv* 2010;75:494–504.

21. Garg P, Servoss SJ, Wu JC, *et al*. Lack of association between migraine headache and patent foramen ovale: results of a case-control study. *Circulation* 2010;121:1406–1412.

22. Dowson A, Mullen MJ, Peatfield R, *et al*. Migraine Intervention With STARFlex Technology (MIST) trial: a prospective, multicenter, double-blind, sham-controlled trial to evaluate the effectiveness of patent foramen ovale closure with STARFlex septal repair implant to resolve refractory migraine headache. *Circulation* 2008;117:1397–13404.

23. Tepper SJ, Cleves C, Taylor FR. Patent foramen ovale and migraine: association, causation, and implications of clinical trials. *Curr Pain Headache Rep* 2009;13:221–226.

24. Meier B. Catheter-based closure of the patent foramen ovale. *Circulation* 2009;120: 1837–1841.

25. McElhinney DB. Patent foramen ovale closure: let's keep the heart in mind. *Circulation* 2009;119:2967–2968.

26. Furlan A, Massaro J, Mauri L, *et al*. Closure I: a prospective, multicenter, randomized controlled trial to evaluate the safety and efficacy of the STARFlex septal closure system versus best medical therapy in patients with a stroke or transient ischemic attack due to presumed embolism through a patent foramen ovale. *Circulation* 2010;122:2218.

27. Henriksen PA, Strachan K, Selby C, Northridge DB. Percutaneous patent foramen ovale closure in a patient with platypnoea-orthodeoxia syndrome. *Heart* 2007;93:892.

28. Gelernter-Yaniv L, Khoury A, Schwartz Y, Lorber A. Transcatheter closure of right-to-left interatrial shunts to resolve hypoxemia. *Congenital Heart Dis* 2008;3:47–53.

29. Murphy JG, Gersh BJ, McGoon MD, *et al*. Long-term outcome after surgical repair of isolated atrial septal defect. Follow-up at 27 to 32 years. *N Engl J Med* 1990;323: 1645–1650.

30. Bashore TM. Adult congenital heart disease: right ventricular outflow tract lesions. *Circulation* 2007;115:1933-1947.

31. Gatzoulis MA, Balaji S, Webber SA, *et al*. Risk factors for arrhythmia and sudden cardiac death late after repair of tetralogy of Fallot: a multicentre study. *Lancet* 2000;356: 975–981.

32. Bouzas B, Kilner PJ, Gatzoulis MA. Pulmonary regurgitation: not a benign lesion. *Eur Heart J* 2005;26:433–439.

33. Pelech AN, Neish SR. Sudden death in congenital heart disease. *Pediatr Clin North Am* 2004;51:1257–1271.

34. Khairy P, Harris L, Landzberg MJ, *et al*. Implantable cardioverter-defibrillators in tetralogy of Fallot. *Circulation* 2008;117:363–370.

35. Pillutla P, Shetty KD, Foster E. Mortality associated with adult congenital heart disease: Trends in the US population from 1979 to 2005. *Am Heart J* 2009;158:874–879.

36. Therrien J, Siu SC, McLaughlin PR, Liu PP, Williams WG, Webb GD. Pulmonary valve replacement in adults late after repair of tetralogy of fallot: are we operating too late? *J Am Coll Cardiol* 2000;36:1670–1675.

37. Vliegen HW, van Straten A, de Roos A, *et al*. Magnetic resonance imaging to assess the hemodynamic effects of pulmonary valve replacement in adults late after repair of tetralogy of fallot. *Circulation* 2002;106:1703–1707.

38. Oosterhof T, Vliegen HW, Meijboom FJ, Zwinderman AH, Bouma B, Mulder BJ. Long-term effect of pulmonary valve replacement on QRS duration in patients with corrected tetralogy of Fallot. *Heart* 2007;93:506–509.

39. Yemets IM, Williams WG, Webb GD, *et al.* Pulmonary valve replacement late after repair of tetralogy of Fallot. *Ann Thorac Surg* 1997;64:526–530.
40. Lurz P, Coats L, Khambadkone S, *et al.* Percutaneous pulmonary valve implantation: impact of evolving technology and learning curve on clinical outcome. *Circulation* 2008;117:1964–1972.
41. Zahn EM, Hellenbrand WE, Lock JE, McElhinney DB. Implantation of the melody transcatheter pulmonary valve in patients with a dysfunctional right ventricular outflow tract conduit early results from the U.S. clinical trial. *J Am Coll Cardiol* 2009;54: 1722–1729.
42. Wood P. The Eisenmenger syndrome or pulmonary hypertension with reversed central shunt. *Br Med J* 1958;2:755–762.
43. Sandoval J, Aguirre JS, Pulido T, *et al.* Nocturnal oxygen therapy in patients with the Eisenmenger syndrome. *Am J Respir Critical Care Med* 2001;164:1682–1687.
44. Ammash N, Warnes CA. Cerebrovascular events in adult patients with cyanotic congenital heart disease. *J Am Coll Cardiol* 1996;28:768–772.
45. Fernandes SM, Newburger JW, Lang P, *et al.* Usefulness of epoprostenol therapy in the severely ill adolescent/adult with Eisenmenger physiology. *Am J Cardiol* 2003;91: 632–635.
46. Galie N, Beghetti M, Gatzoulis MA, *et al.* Bosentan therapy in patients with Eisenmenger syndrome: a multicenter, double-blind, randomized, placebo-controlled study. *Circulation* 2006;114:48–54.
47. Beghetti M, Galie N. Eisenmenger syndrome a clinical perspective in a new therapeutic era of pulmonary arterial hypertension. *J Am Coll Cardiol* 2009;53:733–740.
48. Khairy P, Ouyang DW, Fernandes SM, Lee-Parritz A, Economy KE, Landzberg MJ. Pregnancy outcomes in women with congenital heart disease. *Circulation* 2006;113: 517–524.
49. Avila WS, Grinberg M, Snitcowsky R, *et al.* Maternal and fetal outcome in pregnant women with Eisenmenger's syndrome. *Eur Heart J* 1995;16:460–464.
50. Presbitero P, Somerville J, Stone S, Aruta E, Spiegelhalter D, Rabajoli F. Pregnancy in cyanotic congenital heart disease. Outcome of mother and fetus. *Circulation* 1994;89: 2673–2676.
51. Yap SC, Takkenberg JJ, Witsenburg M, Meijboom FJ, Roos-Hesselink JW. Aortic stenosis at young adult age. *Expert Rev Cardiovasc Ther* 2005;3:1087–1098.
52. Silversides CK, Colman JM, Sermer M, Farine D, Siu SC. Early and intermediate-term outcomes of pregnancy with congenital aortic stenosis. *Am J Cardiol* 2003;91: 1386–1389.
53. Yap SC, Drenthen W, Pieper PG, *et al.* Risk of complications during pregnancy in women with congenital aortic stenosis. *Int J Cardiol* 2008;126:240–246.
54. Arias F, Pineda J. Aortic stenosis and pregnancy. *J Reprod Med* 1978;20:229–232.
55. McIvor RA. Percutaneous balloon aortic valvuloplasty during pregnancy. *Int J Cardiol* 1991;32:1–3.
56. Bonow RO, Carabello BA, Kanu C, *et al.* ACC/AHA 2006 guidelines for the management of patients with valvular heart disease: a report of the American College of Cardiology/ American Heart Association Task Force on Practice Guidelines (writing committee to revise the 1998 Guidelines for the Management of Patients With Valvular Heart Disease): developed in collaboration with the Society of Cardiovascular Anesthesiologists: endorsed by the Society for Cardiovascular Angiography and Interventions and the Society of Thoracic Surgeons. *Circulation* 2006;114:e84–231.
57. Hameed A. Effect of severity of pulmonic stenosis on pregnancy outcome: a case control study. *Am J Obstet Gynecol* 2004;191:93.

58. Meijer JM, Pieper PG, Drenthen W, *et al*. Pregnancy, fertility, and recurrence risk in corrected tetralogy of Fallot. *Heart* 2005;91:801–805.

59. Singh H, Bolton PJ, Oakley CM. Pregnancy after surgical correction of tetralogy of Fallot. *Br Med J (Clin Res ed)* 1982;285:168–170.

60. Lewis BS, Rogers NM, Gotsman MS. Successful pregnancy after repair of Fallot's tetralogy. *South Afr Med J* 1972;46:934-936.

61. Borg-Stein J, Dugan SA, Gruber J. Musculoskeletal aspects of pregnancy. *Am J Phys Med Rehab* 2005;84:180–192.

62. Lind J, Wallenburg HC. The Marfan syndrome and pregnancy: a retrospective study in a Dutch population. *Eur J Obstet Gynecol Reprod Biol* 2001;98:28–35.

63. Pyeritz RE. Maternal and fetal complications of pregnancy in the Marfan syndrome. *Am J Med* 1981;71:784–790.

64. Rossiter JP, Repke JT, Morales AJ, Murphy EA, Pyeritz RE. A prospective longitudinal evaluation of pregnancy in the Marfan syndrome. *Am J Obstet Gynecol* 1995;173: 1599–1606.

65. Brooke BS, Habashi JP, Judge DP, Patel N, Loeys B, Dietz HC, 3rd. Angiotensin II blockade and aortic-root dilation in Marfan's syndrome. *N Engl J Med* 2008;358:2787–2795.

66. Niwa K, Siu SC, Webb GD, Gatzoulis MA. Progressive aortic root dilatation in adults late after repair of tetralogy of Fallot. *Circulation* 2002;106:1374–1378.

67. Della Corte A, Bancone C, Quarto C, *et al*. Predictors of ascending aortic dilatation with bicuspid aortic valve: a wide spectrum of disease expression. *Eur J Cardiothorac Surg* 2007;31:397–404; discussion 405.

68. Pepin M, Schwarze U, Superti-Furga A, Byers PH. Clinical and genetic features of Ehlers-Danlos syndrome type IV, the vascular type. *N Engl J Med* 2000;342:673–680.

CHAPTER 11

Cardiac imaging

Aiden Abidov[1] and Daniel S. Berman[2,3]
[1]The University of Arizona College of Medicine, Tucson, AZ, USA
[2]Cedars-Sinai Medical Center, Los Angeles, CA, USA
[3]David Geffen School of Medicine, UCLA, Los Angeles, CA, USA

Introduction

Heart disease is one of the most common causes of death in the world. A large proportion of the morbidity and mortality is due to coronary artery disease (CAD). While effective therapies are available that can prevent CAD and its consequences, these therapies are often not effectively applied due to the following factors: (1) weak predictive power of the standard clinical risk estimators, such as the Framingham risk score, especially in those patients with asymptomatic atherosclerosis; (2) lack of tools by which to tailor the aggressiveness level of the preventive therapy in different patient populations with similar predicted risk of CAD; and (3) ambiguity of the clinical management and follow-up protocols for asymptomatic or mildly symptomatic patients with known CAD, especially after the coronary interventions. Frequently, the initial presentation of the cardiac disease is sudden death.

Non-invasive cardiac imaging with echocardiography, magnetic resonance imaging (MRI), myocardial perfusion imaging (MPI) using single photon emission computed tomography (SPECT) or positron emission tomography (PET), or coronary computed tomographic angiography (CCTA) provides an opportunity to more effectively identify cardiac disease and guide patient management. Among patients suffering sudden death from undiagnosed cardiac disease, an overwhelming majority have some form of structural heart disease, which could be identified with at least one of the these modalities.

In this chapter we attempt to analyze evidence from recent trials of the use of non-invasive cardiac imaging in the clinical management and risk stratification of the various patient populations.

Cardiovascular Clinical Trials: Putting the Evidence into Practice, First Edition.
Edited by Marcus D. Flather, Deepak L. Bhatt, and Tobias Geisler.
© 2013 Blackwell Publishing Ltd. Published 2013 by Blackwell Publishing Ltd.

Myocardial perfusion imaging with SPECT or PET

SPECT MPI

Over the last few decades, the assessment of myocardial perfusion from stress and rest SPECT MPI has become central to the management of patients with known or suspected CAD [1]. A large body of evidence supports the use of SPECT MPI for diagnosis and perhaps more importantly, for risk stratification in CAD [2]. For over a decade, electrocardiogram (EKG) gating has become part of routine SPECT MPI studies, thus providing information regarding both myocardial perfusion and function. As noted in the American College of Cardiology/American Heart Association/American Society of Nuclear Cardiology (ACC/AHA/ASNC) guidelines, "the ability of gated SPECT to provide measurement of left ventricular (LV) ejection fraction (EF), segmental wall motion, and absolute LV volumes also adds to the prognostic information that can be derived from a SPECT study" [2]. Several observational studies have defined ischemic stunning as a significant drop in stress LVEF compared to that at rest, or a new wall motion abnormality persisting long enough to be observed in post-stress SPECT MPI; this is an important non-perfusion marker of the underlying severe epicardial disease [3–6].

The ability of SPECT MPI to risk stratify patients with known or suspected CAD rests on its ability to assess the extent and severity of myocardial ischemia and infarction [7]. Several factors converge throughout non-invasive cardiac imaging to standardize interpretation and reporting of these findings. If purely qualitative terms were used for this purpose, it would be difficult to compare the results of various trials. Regarding SPECT MPI studies, three important methodological factors have provided a reasonable level of standardization of the findings and, as a result, increase the generalized applicability of the evidence from the various clinical trials.

First, qualitative visual interpretation of the perfusion defects with the simplified dichotomized approach ("normal" or "abnormal") is being replaced by the semiquantitative perfusion scores (sum of scores for each individual myocardial segment using a five-point scale: 0 = normal perfusion to 4 = absent uptake), which uniquely combine both severity and extent of the perfusion defect [8]. Extensive research data have proved an important role for summed perfusion scores in diagnosis, risk stratification, patient management, and assessment of resource utilization [8–12]. Recently, we have introduced a definition of the "% myocardium hypoperfused" at stress or rest and the "% myocardium ischemic," derived from the summed perfusion scores and normalized to the total number of the scored segments. This parameter is intuitive and provides a standardized value regardless of the number of segments in the model used for semiquantitative analysis by different centers. Both the summed segmental scoring and the % myocardium abnormal approaches have been validated in numerous studies and are now the standard for assessing all myocardial perfusion modalities.

Second, a 17-segment model of the left ventricle has been introduced for all the non-invasive cardiac imaging modalities as an optimally weighted approach for visual interpretation of regional left ventricular abnormality [13], providing further uniformity in the reporting of perfusion abnormalities, and thus further generalization of the evidence obtained in clinical trials.

Third, the development of artificial intelligence, and the intrinsically operator-independent, three-dimensional, and digital nature of the myocardial perfusion imaging are ideal for the implementation of completely automated quantitative analysis. We have introduced the total perfusion deficit (TPD) [14] as a computer-derived analog of the expert-derived semiquantitative perfusion scores, representing both defect extent and severity of perfusion defect. TPD is measured at stress and rest, and ischemic TPD is calculated from the difference (stress TPD minus rest TPD). TPD is more reproducible than the expert visual perfusion scores [15], suggesting that this type of objective, quantitative assessment of perfusion abnormalities may be more effective in assessing the effects of therapy in individual patients than visual analysis alone. Ischemic TPD was the variable used in the COURAGE (Clinical Outcomes Utilizing Revascularization and Aggressive Drug Evaluation) nuclear substudy [16] to evaluate baseline ischemia and the change in ischemia after therapy.

A variety of artifacts continue to be the principal drawback of SPECT MPI, among which variable soft tissue attenuation is the most common. In men, diaphragmatic attenuation, obscuring inferior segments, is most common, while in women it is variable breast attenuation, obscuring anterior or anterolateral segments. Two main solutions can be implemented to diminish the influence of these artifacts: radionuclide source- or CT-based attenuation correction methods [17–21] or prone imaging [22–27]. Head-to-head comparison demonstrates that both methods result in the fewest equivocal studies compared to supine acquisition [28], especially in men and mostly in inferior wall defects. Automated combined supine–prone quantification of the perfusion defects employing TPD was proven to significantly improve the diagnostic performance of the MPI studies [25].

Finally, there is an important trend in the development of both improved acquisition systems and improved image reconstruction algorithms to replace conventional SPECT approaches. Several novel camera systems have been reported with higher sensitivities compared to the traditional Anger cameras [29–31] and clinical data have been published for the high-speed MPI [31–33]. These systems, as well as new methods of image reconstruction that can be applied with conventional Anger camera systems, promise to both shorten the acquisition periods required for SPECT MPI and to substantially reduce the radiation dose associated with the procedures.

PET MPI and PET-FDG imaging

The availability of a generator-based PET radiopharmaceutical (rubidium-82 [Rb-82], half-life 75 seconds) for MPI and the wider availability of PET scanners due to their common use in cancer have recently led to the growth of

Table 11.1 Potential advantages of myocardial perfusion PET imaging compared to SPECT.

Advantage	Clinical implication
Superior image quality of PET images: • Higher spatial, temporal, and contrast resolution of PET imaging compared to that of SPECT • Routine implementation of the attenuation correction methodology (using either a CT- or radionuclide-based approach)	Fewer tissue attenuation artifacts, better image quality in obese, patients with equivocal SPECT, women, elderly, claustrophobic, patients with pacemakers, patients with multivessel CAD
PET radiotracers with higher energy and shorter half-life	Use of higher diagnostic doses with overall shorter, more convenient protocols and lower radiation exposure, compared to SPECT
Lower gastrointestinal activity	Fewer diagnostic problems with evaluation of the inferior wall
Ability to provide unique, peak stress wall motion and perfusion data	Diagnostic information comparable with first-pass RWMA (compared to delayed post-stress functional data of SPECT)
Ability to provide unique metabolic/blood flow reserve data	Important in patients with microvascular disease, diabetes, LVH, known CAD
Evaluation of the viability	Gold standard (perfusion and F18-FDG scan) before the era of CMR
Potentially better performance in serial/ sequential imaging	Important implication in the evaluation of the therapeutic effects of different treatment strategies

CAD, coronary artery disease; CMR, cardiac magnetic resonance; LVH, left ventricular hypertrophy; RWMA, regional wall motion abnormality.

PET MPI. Rb-82 MPI has all the diagnostic advantages of SPECT MPI, but is a more powerful modality (Table 11.1). PET has better spatial and temporal resolution, provides routine, robust attenuation correction, and allows quantitative assessment of regional myocardial blood flow reserve, measured from the estimation of absolute myocardial flow that is derived from the initial transit of the perfusion tracer through the left ventricle and the left ventricular myocardium. The advantage of the latter is that it may reduce the probability of serious underestimation of the extent of ischemia that can occur with relative blood flow assessment alone. Furthermore, PET metabolic imaging with F18-FDG is a well-established method for assessment of myocardial viability. The disadvantages of myocardial perfusion PET are a higher initial equipment cost and that it is currently being used only with vasodilator stress; the 75-second half-life precludes the routine use of this radiopharmaceutical with treadmill exercise due to logistics.

Non-perfusion parameters on myocardial perfusion imaging

Left ventricular systolic and diastolic parameters

EKG gating adds quantification of a wide variety of clinically pertinent parameters of function and geometry to SPECT and PET MPI including: LVEF, end-diastolic volume (EDV) and end-systolic volume (ESV) of the LV cavity, mass, LV shape indices [34], and several other variables (Table 11.2). Regional parameters of function assessed from gated MPI include LV myocardial wall motion and thickening. Diastolic function assessment is also feasible with MPI when a sufficient number of frames per cardiac cycle are acquired [35].

Assessment of regional wall motion and thickening

With gated MPI, regional ventricular function is routinely analyzed, and findings are most commonly reported in terms of abnormality of regional wall motion or thickening, either qualitatively or semiquantitatively. Stress-induced regional wall motion is a highly specific marker of significant, usually critical, stenosis in the epicardial artery supplying the segment [36].

Transient ischemic dilation ratio and lung–heart ratio

These non-perfusion markers are important in the identification of patients with severe and extensive disease. TID on images acquired after stress when compared to rest has been shown to be related to both severe and extensive ischemia [37–42]. Increased lung uptake of the perfusion tracers is considered to represent an increase in pulmonary capillary wedge pressure. When stress induced, it has prognostic significance [43]. Importantly, there is no correlation between these two parameters (meaning that their combination in the same patient is very unlikely); this makes TID and lung–heart ratio (LHR) complementary risk markers. TID ratio is considered a more specific marker of severe (multivessel or left main) CAD. Increased LHR may be related mostly to the exercise-induced LV systolic and perhaps diastolic dysfunction, independently of the underlying coronary pathology [44].

Increased right ventricular uptake

Increased right ventricular uptake of radioactivity is considered to be secondary to increased right ventricular pressure, and thus, when stress induced, to be similar in its pathophysiology to increased lung uptake of radiotracer [45].

Guidance for cardiac resynchronization therapy

Recently, the implications of nuclear imaging for the evaluation of potential candidates for cardiac resynchronization therapy (CRT) have been reviewed [46,47]. Studies have shown that an assessment of inter- and intra-ventricular dyssynchrony can be effectively performed by means of phase analysis on SPECT MPI [48–51] or gated blood pool SPECT [52]. By combining dyssynchrony assessment with the extent and location of myocardial scar, MPI has the potential to predict a favorable effect of CRT. Trials are needed to compare

Table 11.2 Functional non-perfusion parameters assessed with myocardial perfusion SPECT.

Parameter	Methodology	Clinical implications
Left ventricular ejection fraction (LVEF)	Automated quantification (volume- or count-based): • Gated stress • Gated rest	Major risk-stratification factor (all-cause, cardiac, and sudden death risk) Improves prognostic value of MPI in patients with known CAD Important for the clinical decision-making algorithms/need in revascularization Important as a sequential parameter in evaluation of the effect of therapy/revascularization
Delta EF	Rest–stress difference	Delta EF >5% is a marker of "ischemic stunning," a moderately sensitive marker of severe CAD
LV volumes	Automated quantification: • End-systolic (ESV) • End-diastolic (ESV)	Major risk-stratification factor (all-cause, cardiac, and sudden death risk)
Left ventricular enlargement at rest (LVE)	Visual	Major risk-stratification factor (all-cause, cardiac, and sudden death risk) Marker of the type of baseline cardiomyopathy (large perfusion defects + LVE = ischemic cardiomyopathy)

Transient ischemic dilation (TID) or transient cavitary dilation (TCD)	Visual comparison of stress and rest images
	Automated quantification:
	• Ungated stress/rest LV volume ratio
	• Gated:
	  – ESV-based
	  – EDV-based
		Moderately sensitive and highly specific marker of severe and extensive CAD
		Gender, protocol, and tracer specific; highly-dependent on the scan quality (edge definitions)
		Important prognostic factor: marker of possible endothelial dysfunction (syndrome X) in patients with normal epicardial disease

LHR (lung–heart ratio)	Automated quantification: • Stress • Rest	Moderately sensitive and specific marker of severe and extensive CAD Not correlated with TID (two markers are complementary)
Increased lung uptake	Visual: • Stress • Rest	Same as LHR Less specific; can be increased at rest in chronic lung disease
LV shape indices (LVSI)	Automated quantification (maximal dimension ratio): • Global • Focal	Global abnormal LVSI is a marker of remodeling of the LV Predictor of clinical CHF/CHF hospitalization in follow-up Focal abnormal LVSI is a sensitive and specific factor for severe CAD in the vessel supplying this territory/segment

(continued)

Table 11.2 (continued)

Parameter	Methodology	Clinical implications
LV mass	Automated quantification	Major factor in evaluation of the etiology and prognosis of the cardiomyopathy Sequential measurements may guide therapy
Regional wall motion abnormalities (RWMA): • Motion • Thickening	Visual qualitative: • Stress • Rest Semiquantitative scoring (using six-point scale for wall motion and four-point scale for thickening): • Stress • Rest Automated quantification: • Stress • Rest	Improves sensitivity and specificity in identification of CAD when combined with perfusion findings Associated with severe stenosis of the epicardial artery supplying the abnormal segment(s) if present on post-stress images (~30–45 min after the exercise) and resolves on rest images Improves diagnostic certainty if normal wall motion/thickening noted in the areas of perfusion abnormality (implies attenuation artifact)
Diastolic function	Automated quantification (16- or higher frame gating): • Stress • Rest	Currently underutilized Direct marker of diastolic dysfunction Important potential marker of the severity and prognosis of underlying CAD
Ventricular dyssynchrony	Automated quantification (16- or higher frame gating) Gated blood pool SPECT is preferred	Important guide marker for CRT
Coronary flow reserve	Automated quantification: Global or regional (segmental): • Stress • Rest	Currently underutilized Allows precise measurements of the direct quantification of the global and regional myocardial blood supply May play an important role in the evaluation of the effectiveness of medical therapy
Right ventricular enlargement (RVE)	Visual	Non-specific marker of pulmonary hypertension Marker of severe valvular disease or adult congenital heart disease May be observed at rest with massive pulmonary thromboembolism

CAD, coronary artery disease; CHF, congestive heart failure; CRT, cardiac resynchronization therapy; MPI, myocardial perfusion imaging.

Table 11.3 Reported sensitivity and specificity ranges of the different myocardial perfusion SPECT imaging protocols. (Reproduced from Russell and Zaret [53], with permission.)

Test type	Sensitivity (%)	Specificity (%)
Exercise treadmill test		
Thallium-201	60–82	65–82
Tc-99m sestamibi	82–97	36–90
Tc-99m tetrofosmin	80–95	77–89
Adenosine or dipyridamole		
Thallium-201	77–92	75–100
Tc-99m sestamibi	81–90	67–72
Tc-99m tetrofosmin	83–89	55–94
Dobutamine		
Thallium-201	86–100	36–100
Tc-99m sestamibi	76–100	64–100
Tc-99m tetrofosmin	80–95	72–80

this ability of MPI with echocardiography, the technique commonly being used for this purpose.

Diagnostic value of myocardial perfusion imaging

MPI has become a useful modality for diagnostic assessment of patients with either known or suspected CAD. Table 11.3 [53] gives the combined evidence for the diagnostic value of MPI. The method has proven effective in multiple clinical subsets and populations of patients: the elderly [54–57], young patients [58], women [59–61], and patients with recent [62–65] and chronic myocardial infarction (MI) [66,67], LV dysfunction [68], as a follow-up after coronary interventions (either percutaneous or surgical) [69,70] in symptomatic patients with acute chest pain [71] and asymptomatic patients with diabetes [72–74] and/or multiple risk-factors of CAD [75], even with underlying atrial fibrillation [76,77] or permanent pacemakers [78–81].

Referral bias and normalcy rate

The sensitivity and specificity of MPI used to guide referral to coronary angiography are highly influenced by post-test referral bias ("verification" bias). This bias often applies to reports of all non-invasive diagnostic modalities for establishing the diagnosis of CAD. It results in a wide variation of the reported sensitivity and specificity of SPECT MPI. If only patients with a positive test result are sent for the "gold standard" test (coronary angiography), the resultant observed sensitivity will be 100% and the specificity will be 0% [82]. The severe distortion of reported specificity prompted us to introduce the concept of the normalcy rate as a proxy for test specificity, defined as the frequency of normal MPI in patients with a low likelihood of CAD, estimated based on Bayesian analysis of age, sex, and symptom classification [83,84]. This concept was evaluated in multiple clinical studies in the field of MPI. These analyses

Table 11.4 Comparative diagnostic performance of myocardial perfusion PET and SPECT: available literature data.

Authors/population size	Year	PET tracer	Diagnostic performance			
			PET		SPECT	
			Sensitivity (%)	Specificity (%)	Sensitivity (%)	Specificity (%)
Tamaki et al. [225] n = 51	1988	N-13 ammonia	98	100	96	100
Go et al. [226] n = 202	1990	Rb-82	93	78	76	80
Stewart et al. [227] n = 81	1991	Rb-82	84	88	84	53
Marwick et al. [228] n = 50 (all-post CABG)	1991	Rb-82	91	75	73	100
Bateman et al. [229] n = 224	2006	Rb-82	86	100	81	66
Husmann et al. [230] n = 150	2008	N-13 ammonia	97	84	77	84

have repeatedly shown a normalcy rate well above 90%, supporting a high specificity of the method [2].

A few studies have compared diagnostic performance of SPECT and PET MPI. As shown in Table 11.4, studies to date have been consistent in showing that PET imaging results in improved sensitivity and specificity in the detection of obstructive CAD. Diagnostic performance of the perfusion PET is more robust in the populations considered "problematic" for perfusion SPECT, such as obese patients. Due to the multiple advantages of PET, in laboratories where both SPECT and PET MPI are available, PET MPI is increasingly favored in all patients in whom pharmacological rather than exercise stress is being used with MPI.

Role of nuclear cardiology in clinical decision-making: evidence-based approach

Whom should we scan?

This important subject is extensively covered in practice guidelines and recent appropriateness criteria [85]. The most important starting point in answering this question is the pretest likelihood of CAD, which can be estimated using either an original Diamond–Forrester approach [86] or the modified approach proposed by the ACC/AHA guidelines Table 11.5) [85,87]. For detecting CAD,

Table 11.5 Pretest likelihood* of coronary artery disease by age, gender, and symptoms. (Reproduced from Brindis *et al* [87], with permission.)

Age (years)	Gender	Typical/ Definite angina pectoris	Atypical/ probable angina pectoris	Non-anginal chest pain	Asymptomatic
30–39	Men	Intermediate	Intermediate	Low	Very low
	Women	Intermediate	Very low	Very low	Very low
40–49	Men	High	Intermediate	Intermediate	Low
	Women	Intermediate	Low	Low	Very low
50–59	Men	High	Intermediate	Intermediate	Low
	Women	Intermediate	Intermediate	Low	Very low
60–69	Men	High	Intermediate	Intermediate	Low
	Women	High	Intermediate	Intermediate	Low

*Very low likelihood, <5%; low likelihood, 5–9%; intermediate likelihood, 10–90%; high likelihood, >90%.

non-invasive testing with any of the imaging modalities has greatest benefit in patients with an intermediate pretest likelihood of CAD.

What are the estimates of risk associated with various MPI findings?

Stress-gated MPI is well documented and most commonly uses a non-invasive method for risk stratification. A new paradigm in patient management is that of a risk-based approach (as opposed to an anatomy-based approach) in patients with suspected CAD in whom symptoms are non-limiting. With a risk-based approach, the focus is on identifying patients at risk for major cardiac events. This application is summarized in the ACC/AHA/ASNC guidelines [2]. To date, there are extensive reports examining risk after a normal stress MPI, with most studies reporting rates of hard events (cardiac death or non-fatal MI) of less than 1% per year of follow-up [1,2]. Overall, when pooled data from 16 studies of over 27 000 patients followed for a mean of 26.8 months were considered, the annualized hard event rate was only 0.6%. The relative risk associated with an abnormal MPI ranges from 3% to 14% per year in these studies, indicating that SPECT MPI successfully aggregates or concentrates risk in patients with abnormal studies relative to normal studies, resulting in the former being at far greater risk than the latter.

The identification of low risk with a normal study and the reclassification of higher risk patients with abnormal studies are two of the most basic characteristics of risk stratification with tests. Based on data gathered to date from prognostic studies, risk of cardiac death is considered to be low if less than 1%, high risk if greater than 3%, and intermediate risk if 1–3%. In chronic CAD, it has been suggested that a mortality rate of greater than 3% per year can be used to identify patients with minimal symptoms whose mortality rate can be improved by myocardial revascularization. The 1–3% range for inter-mediate risk would be scaled up for patients who are very elderly or have serious comorbidities, due to increased mortality in all subgroups of these patients. Also, patients whose known or suspected CAD is seriously affecting quality of life or functional status should be considered catheterization can-didates irrespective of risk status.

Can we predict a survival benefit based on results of the baseline MPI?

Based on the evidence described above, physicians today usually do not refer patients with normal SPECT MPI for invasive coronary angiography (ICA), confident that angiographic assessment is unlikely to yield further benefit. At the other end of the spectrum, the presence of significantly limiting symptoms or a significant ischemia revealed on the MPI, commonly leads to ICA for consideration of revascularization to relieve symptoms and to improve quality of life. The need for consideration of revascularization in patients with only mild or moderate perfusion abnormalities is less clear.

The COURAGE era: new evidence supports ischemia-guided therapy

The COURAGE trial [88] was designed to assess the superiority of percutane-ous coronary intervention (PCI) coupled with optimal medical therapy in reducing the risk of death and non-fatal MI in patients with stable CAD, as compared with optimal medical therapy (OMT) alone. The population in the study was highly selected: of 35 539 screened patients, only 2287 were enrolled in the study. Inclusion criteria included stenosis of 70% or greater in one or more proximal epicardial coronary artery and objective evidence of myocar-dial ischemia (substantial resting EKG changes or inducible ischemia with either exercise or pharmacological vasodilator stress) or at least one coronary stenosis of at least 80% and classic angina without provocative testing. Exclu-sion criteria included persistent class IV angina, a markedly positive stress test (substantial ST-segment depression or hypotensive response during stage 1 of the Bruce protocol), refractory heart failure or cardiogenic shock, an ejec-tion fraction of less than 30%, revascularization within the previous 6 months, and coronary anatomy not suitable for PCI. The patients were randomized to undergo PCI with OMT (PCI group, n = 1149 patients) or to receive OMT alone (OMT group, n = 1138 patients). Patients were followed for an average of 4.5 years. OMT patients were allowed to cross-over to revascularization if they had progressive or refractory symptoms. The main results of the trial demonstrated that as an initial management strategy in patients with stable CAD, PCI did not reduce the risk of death, MI, or other major cardiovascular events when added to OMT [87]. The authors concluded that "as an initial management approach, optimal medical therapy without routine PCI can be implemented safely in the majority of patients with stable coronary artery disease. However, approximately one third of these patients may subse-quently require revascularization for symptom control or for subsequent development of an acute coronary syndrome."

Since this large randomized trial showed no survival advantage with the addition of PCI, the question must be raised as to whether stress imaging has a role in guiding selection of patients for revascularization. If patients with stable symptoms do not benefit from revascularization, catheterization is not needed, and, thus, no stress imaging is needed to identify the potential catheterization candidate.

As a part of the COURAGE study, an important nuclear substudy addressed how SPECT MPI testing may shape clinical outcomes. In this substudy of 314 patients in whom both pre- and 6–18-month post-randomization SPECT MPI was performed, patients assigned to PCI + OMT (n = 159) demonstrated significantly greater ischemia reduction when compared to patients receiving OMT alone (n = 155) (33% vs 19%; p = 0.0004]. Importantly, among the relatively smaller subset of patients with "moderate-to-severe pretreatment ischemia," a significantly greater proportion showed significant ischemia reduction (≥5% reduction in ischemic myocardium) with a strategy of PCI + OMT as opposed to OMT (78% vs 52%; p = 0.007). Despite the lack of improved survival with PCI + OMT versus OMT alone in the main COURAGE study, the substudy suggests that the former may be a superior approach to reduce ischemic burden, particularly in patients with extensive ischemia [16]. The study was, however, insufficiently powered to examine this question, and the results must be considered hypothesis generating. Nonetheless, the substudy provides evidence suggesting that imaging of myocardial ischemia could affect patient outcomes through guiding decisions for revascularization. Of note, the post-therapy residual ischemia was strongly predictive of outcomes in both the PCI and the OMT alone groups (Figure 11.1).

Since the COURAGE nuclear substudy was only hypothesis generating, a "COURAGE II" trial is being proposed, incorporating the results of ischemia testing—either as an inclusion criterion or a stratification factor—and this may further clarify the initially reported results and allow us to better understand what constitutes optimal patient management. Future study should also differentiate distinct cohorts for PCI and coronary artery bypass grafting (CABG), characterize the type and completeness of medical therapy, and assess whether the ejection fraction and/or the amount of ischemia needed to observe patient benefits vary according to the population studied. In other words, assessment of the clinical effectiveness of an imaging modality (in this case, SPECT MPI) must be coupled with detailed evaluation of the numerous factors studied in both clinical and test results. Only in this way can an imaging test be studied relative to its ability to shape clinical outcomes among patients who are subject to common medical decisions.

More recently, the results of the FAME (Fractional Flow Reserve Versus Angiography for Multivessel Evaluation) study [89] provide further support to the concept that assessment of the amount of inducible myocardial ischemia may be of benefit in predicting benefit from revascularization. This study revealed that guiding PCI by means of physiological data (fractional flow reserve; FFR) was associated with a significantly lower incidence of major adverse cardiac events (MACE) compared with routine angiography-guided

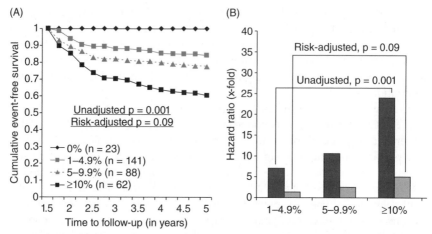

Figure 11.1 Results of the COURAGE nuclear substudy. (A) Kaplan–Meier survival for patients according to residual ischemia (0%, 1–4.9%, 5–9.9%, and ≥10% ischemic myocardium) after 6–18 months of percutaneous coronary intervention (PCI) + medical therapy (MT) or MT. Overall event-free survival was 100%, 84.4%, 77.7%, and 60.7%, respectively, for 0%, 1–4.9%, 5–9.9%, and ≥10% ischemic myocardium (p < 0.001). In a risk-adjusted Cox model (controlling for randomized treatment), this difference was not significant (p = 0.09). (B) Unadjusted (dark gray bars) and risk-adjusted (light gray bars) hazard ratios for the extent and severity of residual ischemia at 6–18 months of follow-up. (Reproduced from Shaw *et al.* [16], with permission from Wolters Kluwer Health.)

PCI in patients with multivessel disease, without a significant increase in the procedure time. Since the findings of FFR and MPI are strongly related [90], the FAME study provides indirect support for guiding revascularization decisions based on non-invasive assessment of ischemia.

Summary

The above discussion suggests that SPECT MPI is an effective diagnostic, prognostic, and clinical management tool based on robust evidence from multiple high-quality trials; however, nearly all of the data are from observational series and the vast majority of the available data on outcomes is with SPECT rather than PET. There is far less written about the prognostic implications of PET MPI than SPECT MPI. However, given the overall higher accuracy of PET MPI for detecting obstructive CAD, it is considered likely that the relationships between PET MPI and subsequent patient outcomes will be at least as strong as those observed with SPECT MPI. Randomized clinical trials, with both SPECT and PET, are needed to test the hypothesis that ischemia detected by SPECT or PET MPI is predictive of outcome benefit from revascularization.

Echocardiography

Over the last five decades, there has been remarkable and continuous development in the technology and methodology of echocardiography, with fast implementation of the novel techniques and protocols into daily clinical practice after accumulation of evidence reflecting clinical benefits of this modality [91]. The armamentarium of modern echocardiography includes a wide variety of echo techniques, allowing detailed characterization of cardiac anatomy and geometry, function, central hemodynamics, coronary circulation, and myocardial viability [92].

While technological development has led to invasive ultrasound techniques, including intravascular ultrasound (IVUS) and intracardiac echocardiography (ICE), coverage of these techniques is beyond the scope of this overview.

Recent technical advances in echocardiography: evolution of the methodology and clinical implications

The most important technical advances in the field of clinical echocardiography have been recently presented in several excellent reviews [93–96]; below is an abbreviated list of the most important developments:

• Two-dimensional echocardiography, which has almost completely eliminated use of M-mode echo.
• Doppler imaging technology and tissue Doppler imaging (TDI), which opened a new diagnostic horizon in the evaluation of central hemodynamics, valvular heart disease, and mechanisms of systolic and diastolic congestive heart failure using cardiac ultrasound [94–98].
• Computer technologies and systems for digital storage, processing, and review [92].
• Transducer technologies both for detailed clinical echocardiography exams and "quick-look" portable and handheld devices; "harmonic" imaging; introduction of the multilane transesophageal echocardiography (TEE) methodology compared to monoplane/biplane imaging.
• Three-dimensional echocardiography methodology [92,99].
• Echocardiography contrast agents for improving assessment of LV function and with potential for assessment of myocardial perfusion [100].
• Speckle tracking imaging (STI) for the assessment of cardiac mechanics and strain imaging [93].
• Evaluation of mechanical dyssynchrony using either triplane tissue synchronization imaging, color-coded TDI, or STI.

We present only a brief review of important clinical applications of echocardiography. As noted below, there is abundant evidence supporting the wide use of this modality for the three major goals of any cardiac imaging: precise diagnosis, effective prognostication, and active role in the clinical decision-making process. Echocardiography has many strengths, including no radiation, no contrast (for most applications), comprehensive cardiac assessment, and broad clinical experience and data. Its principal weaknesses are its dependence on the patient's cooperation and body habitus, the experience of the technician, and, given the largely subjective nature of the interpretation, the experience of the interpreter. Perhaps most importantly, current echocardiography is not truly three dimensional, such that parts of the myocardium may not be visualized, and this lack of compete visualization may not be recognized by the interpreter.

Role of echocardiography in the clinical decision-making process and guidance of the therapy in various clinical settings: existing evidence and future implications

Critically ill and hemodynamically unstable patients

In critically ill patients, assessment of cardiac volumes and function is often of paramount importance in guiding management. Thus, assessment of left and right ventricular function has become one of the most frequent indications for the echocardiography exam both in cardiac and medical intensive care unit (ICU) patients [101]. Trials consistently demonstrate strong performance of both transthoracic echocardiography (TTE) and TEE in this complicated patient population [102,103].

Based on existing evidence and expert guidelines, biventricular systolic function should be evaluated with echocardiography in all ICU patients with unexplained hemodynamic instability; this information is vital for guiding further clinical management or resuscitation. Diastolic function in the ICU setting should be evaluated in cases of increased filling pressures (elevated pulmonary capillary wedge pressure) with normal or subnormal LVEF. Evaluation of right ventricular function can assist in understanding of the underlying pathological process in patients with hemodynamic instability. This evaluation is especially important in patients with known or suspected pulmonary embolism, since a severely dilated and hypokinetic right ventricle is predictive of massive clot, and is an indication to alter medical management (initiation of vasopressors, thrombolytic therapy, surgical consult for possible embolectomy) [104,105]. An exceptionally important application for the bedside evaluation of patients is pericardial effusion/cardiac tamponade, both of which are relatively frequent in the ICU; bedside echocardiography-guided pericardiocentesis is an effective tool in resolving tamponade in a majority of circumferential effusions. While prospective, large-scale randomized controlled studies focusing on endpoints like cost-effectiveness, morbidity or mortality are not available regarding the use of TTE or TEE in the ICU, practice experience clearly supports the necessity of having echocardiography readily available in these settings [106].

Detection of coronary artery disease

Echocardiography is an important tool of modern cardiology practice in the evaluation of obstructive CAD. An echocardiography "hallmark" of CAD is the presence of either rest or stress-induced wall motion abnormalities (WMA) matching well-defined vascular territories [107]. Inducible WMA is, in general, a presentation of the ischemia, whereas resting WMA, especially with myocardial thinning, is considered "indicative" of the scar [108]. Pooled data from multiple studies demonstrate good diagnostic performance of non-contrast stress echocardiography regardless of the stressor type [107]. With ICA applied as a gold standard, meta-analysis of pooled data (17 trials, n = 1405 patients) has demonstrated a similarly high diagnostic accuracy for stress echocardiography and MPI [109]. Adding digital imaging processing (background subtraction and color coding) has been shown to further improve diagnostic image quality of the stress echocardiogram [110]. There is growing evidence of the excellent diagnostic potential of myocardial contrast echocardiography for the assessment of the myocardial perfusion [111].

Prognostic assessment of patients with known or suspected coronary artery disease

Stress echocardiography with either exercise or pharmacological stress has been shown to have prognostic value in various clinical populations [90]. Stress echocardiography has a high negative predictive value, similar to that of MPI (Table 11.6) [112]. Of interest, in the recently published CECaT trial (Cost-effectiveness of functional cardiac testing in the diagnosis and management of CAD: a randomised controlled trial) [113], 898 patients were randomized to angiography, stress SPECT, cardiac magnetic resonance (CMR), or stress echocardiography. The main outcome measures were exercise time (modified Bruce protocol) and cost-effectiveness compared with angiography (diagnosis, treatment, and follow-up costs). Stress echocardiography patients had a 10% test failure rate, significantly shorter total exercise time and time to angina at 6 months post-treatment, and a greater number of adverse events, leading to significantly higher costs compared to MPI. Given the level of skill required for stress echocardiography, the authors considered that it may be best to reserve this test for those who have a contraindication to SPECT and are unable or unwilling to have CMR.

Appropriateness criteria for echocardiography have recently been published [114]. There is considerable overlap in the uses of stress echocardiography and stress MPI (see above). In general, a pattern appears to be emerging in the US in which echocardiography is more often used in patients with low–intermediate pretest likelihood of CAD (related to the higher specificity of the method), whereas those with high–intermediate and high likelihood of the disease, or established CAD are more commonly referred to stress MPI. Presence of valvular pathology or functional valvular lesions (ischemic mitral regurgitation) favors the choice of stress echocardiography.

With respect to selection of the modality for stress imaging in a given patient, factors such as availability of equipment, technical expertise, and clinical expertise found at an individual testing site are considered more important than differences in the capabilities of the modalities in selecting a test for a given patient. This consideration applies to echocardiography, SPECT or PET MPI, or stress CMR.

Assessment of myocardial viability

The hallmark of viability on dobutamine echocardiography is the improvement of wall motion during the infusion of low-dose dobutamine (5–10 μg/kg/min) [108]. Dobutamine echocardiography demonstrates a high accuracy in prediction of functional recovery of the dysfunctional segments after revascularization, and the results are comparable to those obtained with MPI [108] and CMR [115] (Figure 11.2). Moreover, prediction of the global LVEF

Table 11.6 Summary estimates of rates after a negative test and negative predictive value for myocardial infarction or cardiac death for women and men in exercise myocardial perfusion imaging and exercise echocardiography. (Reproduced from Metz et al. [112], with permission.)

Exercise imaging modality and events	n	Mean follow-up (months)	Mean age (years)	Women (%)	Summary event rate after a negative test (%) (95% CI)	Negative predictive value (%) (95 CI)	Annualized event rate (%)
MI and cardiac death							
MPI	8008	36	54	34	1.21 (0.98–1.48)	98.8 (98.5–99.0)	0.45
Thallium	868	45	57	32	3.11 (2.05–4.53)	96.9 (95.5–97.9)	0.70
Sestamibi	1802	32	58	35	1.28 (0.81–1.92)	98.7 (98.1–99.2)	0.34
Thallium/sestamibi	4938	23	61	39	0.83 (0.60–1.13)	99.2 (98.9–99.4)	0.45
Tetrofosmin	400	43	57	28	1.5 (0.55–3.25)	98.5 (96.8–99.4)	0.42
Echo	3021	33	56	46	1.56 (1.14–2.07)	98.4 (97.9–98.9)	0.54
Revascularization and unstable angina							
MPI	1756	36	52	36	3.42 (2.61–4.40)	96.6 (95.6–97.4)	1.25
Echo	380	32	54	45	2.63 (1.26–4.84)	97.4 (95.2–98.7)	0.95

MI, myocardial infarction; MPI, myocardial perfusion imaging.

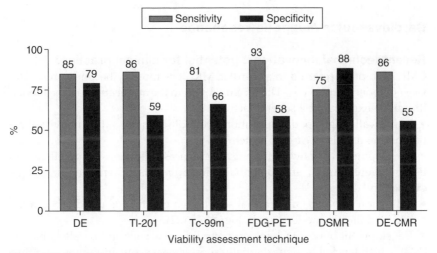

Figure 11.2 Sensitivity and specificity of different imaging methods for assessing myocardial viability. CMR, cardiac magnetic resonance; DE, delayed enhancement; DSMR, dobutamine-stress magnetic resonance; PET, positron emission tomography. (Data from Tomlinson *et al.* [115] and Bax *et al.* [116].)

improvement is also feasible [116]. However, due to the current lack of specific information regarding tissue characterization, echocardiography may not be as effective in identifying scar as CMR or in identifying jeopardized but viable myocardium as FDG metabolism with PET. Whether novel techniques (TDI), STI, or novel perfusion echocardiography contrast agents will change this requires further investigation. Comparing echocardiography and SPECT for viability, an interesting observation was made several years ago by Bax *et al.* Either test can be effective as a first test. A normal or severely abnormal result with either is usually definitive for viability and non-viability, respectively. However, when intermediate results are seen on initial testing, improvement in viability assessment is provided by using the complementary examination [117].

Cardiac resynchronization therapy

CRT represents one of the most recent advances in heart failure management; utilization of biventricular pacing, allowing correction of atrioventricular, interventricular, and intraventricular conduction delays, resulting in improved left ventricular contractility in selected patients [118]. Novel echocardiography-guided protocols, utilizing TDI and STI, can accurately predict positive response to CRT in the form of reverse remodeling (reduction in LV volumes, improved EF, and reduced mitral regurgitation), and improved survival [96,116,119]. Further study would appear to be warranted to determine the relative effectiveness and cost-effectiveness of assessment of dyssynchrony and scar with echocardiography compared with CMR, SPECT, and PET.

Cardiovascular magnetic resonance

Recent technical innovations: potential for clinical practice

CMR (also often referred to as cardiac MRI) has recently become a powerful tool of modern cardiology. The recent growth in the applications of the modality can be explained by several factors:

• Intrinsically high spatial resolution of the CMR images, allowing visualization of fine details of cardiac structures.

• Development of new CMR pulse sequences, allowing an excellent soft tissue differentiation, and potentially including an atherosclerotic plaque evaluation [120].

• Validation of *in vivo* myocardial scar imaging, which is rapidly becoming a gold standard in modern cardiology [121,122].

• Development of new technology, including new coils and parallel imaging [123], which has led to a substantially shorter scan acquisition time, and thus improved patient comfort and decreased motion artifacts.

• Incorporation of the steady-state free precession (SSFP) sequences (otherwise known as True FISP, FIESTA, or balanced FFE), providing substantially higher quality of the ciné images and single shots compared to the images obtained by conventional gradient-echo techniques; this sequence has rapidly become a "gold standard" approach to LV volumes, mass, and function measurements [118].

• Validation of clinical protocols for the CMR perfusion [124], especially involving semiquantitative visual or computer-based approaches, which makes the methodology more useful in daily practice.

Limitations of CMR are its operator-dependent acquisition (experienced technician needed) and the cost of the equipment. Another limitation relates to nephrogenic systemic fibrosis, a fortunately extremely rare but often fatal disorder [125,126], which has been linked to the use gadolinium contrast agents for MRI in patients with impaired renal function, resulting in contraindication of contrast CMR studies in patients with renal failure. Safety concerns currently make CMR generally contraindicated in patients with implanted pacemakers and cardioverter defibrillators (ICSs). CMR is generally not an appropriate methodology for unstable patients (those with significant arrhythmias, acute ischemia or heart failure) and cannot be used without anesthesia in some patients with claustrophobia.

Assessment of myocardial scar/fibrosis

The high diagnostic specificity of delayed enhancement (DE) using gadolinium contrast in CMR, coupled with the high spatial resolution of MRI, allows MRI to assess the presence, transmural extent, location, and precise size of a myocardial scar [119.127]. The understanding of the mechanisms of infarct healing and ventricular remodeling has been advanced through the ability of CMR to distinguish transmural and subendocardial infarction. The presence and location of DE evidence of myocardial fibrosis also is useful for the diagnosis and management of patients with a variety of non-ischemic cardiomyopathic processes. Among these conditions, the most commonly cited have been hypertrophic cardiomyopathy, cardiac amyloidosis [128,129], sarcoidosis [130–132], and myocarditis [130,133].

DE on CMR allows differentiation of even small infarcts, not identified on MPI or echocardiography images. In this regard, in a relatively small (n = 83) but elegant study, comparing the ability of CMR with MPI to detect small infarcts [134], the diagnostic value of CMR was found to be superior to SPECT in detecting myocardial necrosis early after acute MI. The finding was explained by the ability of CMR to detect small subendocardial infarcts missed by SPECT MPI. The authors further noted that due to the definite technical advantages of CMR, it may help to accurately assess MI size and to serve as a surrogate endpoint instead of early mortality in clinical trials evaluating the efficacy of reperfusion therapies during the acute setting of infarction.

Several studies demonstrating a potential advantage of the high spatial resolution of CMR in the evaluation of myocardial scar in different clinical settings are presented in Table 11.7 [135]. An interesting and important clinical application of scar imaging by CMR is determination of tachycardia in attempts to refine the selection of patients for ICD placement. In this regard, Bello *et al.* [136] have shown in a small group of patients referred for electrophysiological testing that the size of the scar determined by DE-CMR was a more powerful predictor for the risk of inducible ventricular tachycardia than LVEF.

Assessment of myocardial viability

Previously published data based on MPI and dobutamine-stress echocardiography have confirmed that presence and extent of the functional recovery (both global and regional) carries not only symptomatic but also a clear prognostic benefit [137]. CMR defines not only the location and function of the involved myocardial segments but also a transmurality of the lesion, revealing areas with completely destroyed cell integrity, presented as a DE on post-contrast images; it shows excellent diagnostic performance in predicting recovery of the infarcted myocardium (Figure 11.3) [138]. Accuracy of the CMR for viability assessment may be enhanced by adding a low-dose dobutamine stress to the standard cardiac protocol [139], especially in the segments with non-transmural (25–50%) delayed hyperenhancement on contrast CMR [140].

Overall, many of the functional and structural parameters obtained by CMR can also be acquired with dobutamine stress echocardiography, when all myocardial segments are available for the analysis. Dobutamine challenge results with MRI, added on top of rest imaging, provide information regarding the presence of stunned or hibernating myocardium, and are predictive of both recovery of the function and future adverse events [141]. A recently published review [113] has suggested the following diagnostic approach when myocardial viability is concerned: initial two-dimensional echocardiography exam in order to assess quality of the image and visualization of all the

Table 11.7 Studies of spatial extent of infarcts using CMR delayed-enhancement imaging. (Reproduced from Gibbons *et al.* [135], with permission.)

Author	Patients	Number of patients	Use of CMR	Infarct imaging results
Porto *et al.* [231]	<30-mm stent	52	Detect new small MI after PCI	23% of vessels showed new MI Change in plaque volume correlated with MI mass (r = 0.58; P < 0.001).
Cino *et al.* [232]	Remote STEMI	48	Reference standard to test EKG localization of MI	EKG sensitivity low in lateral and limited anteroapical infarcts, high (>80%) for others. EKG specificity high (>98%) for all locations
Valeti *et al.* [233]	HOCM, septal alcohol ablation or myectomy	24	For each procedure: size, extent, and location of defects	Septal myectomy—discrete resection in anteroseptal alcohol ablation—variable; usually transmural MI; sparing of basal septum in 25%
Harris *et al.* [234]	Congenital heart disease	73	Localize fibrosis	31 of 34 patients with previous patch repair of RVOT had fibrosis in the RVOT, 14 of 34 had fibrosis in the ventricular septal defect patch (P < 0.001). Patients with RVOT patch repairs were more likely to have fibrosis of the aortic valve (P = 0.002) and ascending aorta (P = 0.05)

EKG, electrocardiogram; HOCM, hypertrophic obstructive cardiomyopathy; IVUS, intravascular ultrasound; MI, myocardial infarction; MRI, magnetic resonance imaging; PCI, percutaneous coronary intervention; RV, right ventricular; RVOT, right ventricular outflow tract; STEMI, ST-segment elevation myocardial infarction.

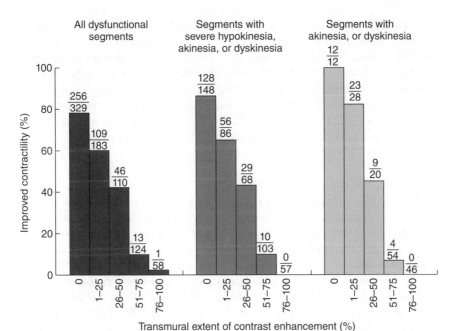

Figure 11.3 Relationship between the transmural extent of contrast enhancement before revascularization and the likelihood of increased contractility after revascularization. (Reproduced from Kim *et al.* [138], with kind permission from Springer Science+Business Media.)

segments; if the image is not adequate, proceed with CMR (adding low-dose dobutamine if needed); otherwise, if the echocardiography images are adequate, proceed with a dobutamine stress echocardiography. However, there is no evidence from randomized clinical trials supporting this approach in terms of the outcomes or cost-effectiveness. A similar sequential approach could also begin with SPECT or PET.

Based on current evidence, CMR, SPECT, PET, and echocardiography are all accurate methods for assessment of myocardial viability and/or scarring. According to the pooled data for all modalities from multiple trials, the presence of viable/non-viable myocardium is a powerful predictor of outcome after the revascularization [142]. So far, there are no large-scale clinical trials prospectively evaluating prognostic benefits of CMR in patients undergoing revascularization and there are no trials comparing the effectiveness of CMR to the other non-invasive imaging modalities for this purpose. Although CMR was part of the STITCH (Surgical Treatment for Ischemic Heart Failure) trial, it was not applied in all patients and few patients had delayed enhancement CMR for assessment of viability. A subset of the STITCH population did have dobutamine echocardiography and nuclear stress and MPI procedures. Surprisingly, while patients with viability had greater survival than patients without viability, no treatment interaction was noted; there was no observed surgical advantage over OMT in heart failure patients with low EFs who had viability. While these data cast some doubt on the clinical utility of viability imaging, several aspects of the STITCH trial remain problematic in drawing these conclusions. These include the selection of the patient population (patients with extensive viability may have been selectively excluded from randomization in the trial); the fact that only half of the patients underwent either of these tests and that the echocardiography and nuclear data were combined to evaluate treatment benefit; PET scanning was not used; and the extent of viability as a variable could not be evaluated in a small sample size [143].

Assessment of myocardial ischemia

CMR can assess myocardial perfusion in several different ways. Stress-induced wall motion abnormalities in patients with stable chest pain syndromes or rest wall-motion abnormalities in those with acute presentation allow a diagnostic approach similar to that employed by stress echocardiography. In addition, contrast-enhanced CMR can be used at rest and under vasodilator stress, providing evaluation of rest and stress perfusion abnormalities, similar to MPI. Finally, evaluation of the global and segmental coronary flow reserve, analogous to that in PET, offers the potential to add diagnostic value. The presence of DE has been reported to improve the specificity of CMR. The superior spatial resolution of MRI offers the potential of detecting subendocardial ischemia. Indeed, many published reports have been favorable for perfusion CMR [144–147]. Reported sensitivities and specificities of the stress CMR are within the ranges 74–84% and 58–66%, respectively. Increasing the contrast dose (0.05 mmol/kg) has been reported to improve sensitivity (91%) [148]; the specificity of stress perfusion defects by CMR, however, remains challenging. This specificity may be improved by incorporating the DE results into the interpretation of the rest/stress perfusion studies [121,149,150].

Prediction of prognosis

Since CMR has become available in clinical practice only relatively recently, the body of evidence supporting its prognostic value compared to the more mature imaging modalities (such as stress echocardiography and MPI) is more limited. Nonetheless, recently several important studies have utilized CMR for the prediction of prognosis not only in patients with coronary pathology but also in patients with other cardiac disorders. Based on data from 461 patients who had undergone stress CMR (assessment of both adenosine-stress myocardial perfusion reserve and dobutamine-stress wall motion), both abnormal myocardial reserve or stress wall motion abnormality were predictive of both cardiac death and non-fatal MI (HR, 10.57; $p < 0.001$; HR, 4.72; $p < 0.002$, respectively) [151].

Several studies have demonstrated that the amount of myocardial scar or fibrosis as defined by DE-CMR is an independent and incremental predictor of adverse cardiac outcome. This was shown in different clinical subsets, including patients with CAD [152,153] and non-ischemic cardiomyopathy

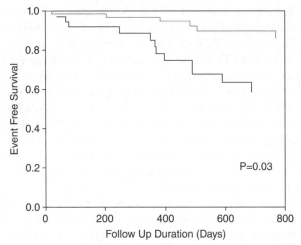

Figure 11.4 Prognostic value of delayed-enhancement cardiac magnetic resonance (DE-CMR) in patients with dilated cardiomyopathy. Kaplan–Meier survival estimates for the primary endpoint of all-cause mortality. Data are adjusted for baseline differences in age, left ventricular (LV) end-systolic volume, LV end-diastolic volume, LV ejection fraction, right ventricular ejection fraction, and treatment with digoxin. Lower line indicates patients with late gadolinium enhancement; upper line indicates patients without late gadolinium enhancement. (Reproduced from Assomull *et al.* [154] with permission.)

(Figure 11.4) [154]. Unique information carried by the CMR provides prognostic input beyond the standard predictors of survival, such as LVEF and volumes. For instance, in patients with clinical indications for an ICD, a significant association of inducible sustained monomorphic ventricular tachycardia during electrophysiological testing and infarcted tissue heterogeneity as defined by DE-CMR was recently demonstrated [155]. In patients with ischemic cardiomyopathy, the extent of DE was found to predict clinical response to CRT therapy [156,157].

Summary

In summary, CMR is a unique and rapidly evolving tool of modern cardiac imaging, providing unique diagnostic and prognostic information in multiple clinical settings and patient populations. The versatility of the method and absence of radiation exposure add to the value of the test; thus many cardiac imaging experts predict a great future for this modality with substantial expansion of CMR application in the years to come [158].

Coronary CT angiography

Technological advances and development of the methodology

Coronary CT angiography (CCTA) is a rapidly growing area in modern cardiac imaging. In the first description of CT, Sir Godfrey Hounsfield recognized that the potential of CCTA could one day become a reality [159]. Since the earliest days of CT, accurate, non-invasive coronary angiography has been a major goal. While CCTA was performed in the late 1990s with electron beam CT (EBCT), the development of multislice spiral CT (MSCT) paved the way for the method to become a reality. As soon as 16-slice MSCT scanners were available, it became clear that the modality would have an important clinical role. However, it was not until the 64-slice scanner was developed, with rotation times of 400 ms or less, that the method reached a plateau, resulting in broad dissemination of the approach. While there are still many questions that must be answered regarding specific applications, it would appear that CCTA is a methodology that will have a dramatic effect on the practice of clinical cardiology.

The principal dramatic change brought about by CCTA has been its ability to reveal fine details of coronary anatomy [160]. Contrast cardiac CT also provides high resolution three-dimensional images of the structural anatomy of the ventricles [161,162], atria and left atrial appendage [163,164], pericardium [165] and large vessels [166–168], and functional performance of the cardiac chambers [169]. Importantly, non-contrast EKG-gated cardiac CT has enabled the accurate measurement of coronary artery calcification, opening up the opportunity for improved assessment of patients with subclinical coronary atherosclerosis.

Future applications of cardiac CT include the possibility of assessment of rest and post-stress myocardial perfusion, and evaluation of the myocardial scar and fibrosis based on contrast enhancement patterns [158,170,171]. With further improvement in CCTA technology, it has become feasible to visualize not only the presence but also the fine details of the morphology of the coronary atherosclerotic plaque (Figure 11.5) [172–174], demonstrating the potential to recognize high-risk features associated with particular findings. Recently, based on these new advances, many researchers have expressed their hope in redefining the stratification of patients based not only on overall extent and severity of atherosclerosis, but also on the vulnerability of the individually assessed coronary plaques [175].

Chronologically, one the most important initial milestones in the development of CCTA was the expansion of knowledge based on the evaluation of coronary artery calcium (CAC) EBCT and the methodology of the CAC quantification, with further evidence confirming the important prognostic value of this parameter [176]. Despite a significant correlation between the overall atherosclerotic burden (as defined by the total CAC score) and prevalence of obstructive CAD, there was no good correlation found between the severity of the calcification and severity of the lumen obstruction in individual lesions [177]; early in the development of CAC scanning it was reported that the area of calcium on CT is roughly only one-fifth that of the total area of histologically identified plaque [178], and thus, a considerable number of patients with CAD may have non-calcified ("soft," lipid-rich) plaque, which would not be flow limiting.

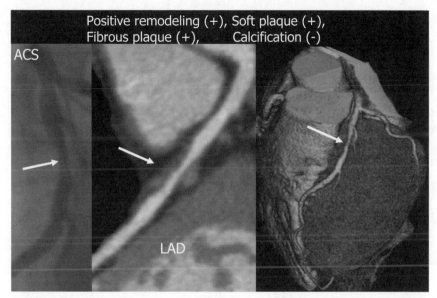

Positive remodeling (+), Soft plaque (+), Fibrous plaque (+), Calcification (-)

ACS

LAD

Figure 11.5 The CT characteristics of a culprit lesion in a patient presenting with acute coronary syndrome as compared to invasive coronary angiogram. The white arrows show the site of luminal obstruction or culprit lesion. (Modified from Motoyama S, *et al*. [172], with permission.)

Table 11.8 Sensitivity and specificity of coronary CT angiography for the detection of coronary artery stenoses in comparison to invasive coronary angiography. (Reproduced from Achenbach [179], with kind permission from Springer Science + Business Media.)

Scanner type	Number of studies	Per-segment analysis		Per-patient analysis	
		Sensitivity (%)	Specificity (%)	Sensitivity (%)	Specificity (%)
4-slice CT	22	84	93	91	83
16-slice CT	26	83	96	97	81
64-slice CT	6	93	96	99	93

Regarding contrast coronary CT studies, EBCT was highly limited. Despite a high temporal resolution and low radiation dose to the patient, it is a "single slice" approach that does not allow isotropic voxel sizing; due to this limitation the data cannot be evaluated as a true three-dimensional dataset in a manner that would allow sufficiently clear visualization of the coronary lumen from many perspectives—a feature upon which CCTA relies heavily. This was an important consideration when the research interest in this field switched to the MSCT. Rapid technical improvement within just a decade led to the development of the powerful 64-slice MSCT scanners by all major CT vendors, providing significantly better spatial resolution compared to both EBCT and 16-slice MSCT systems; these 64-slice systems are considered a current industry standard for CCTA [179] (Table 11.8).

An "Achilles heel" of CCTA is a need for a low heart rate and regular rhythm in order to avoid artifact due to coronary artery motion. With most systems heart rate reduction to 60 beats per minute (bpm) or below is considered optimal. While one manufacturer has developed a scanner with 83-ms temporal resolution, even this scanner reveals improved CCTA scan quality at lower heart rates [180]. With most scanners available in 2012, there is still dependence on a slow heart rate (near 60bpm) and a regular rhythm for consistent reliable results, especially when low radiation exposure protocols are utilized. Although a multicenter trial with dual-source CT without beta-blockers is currently being performed, in most centers beta-blockers are routinely employed to achieve an adequately low heart rate.

The technology for CCTA continues to change rapidly, with most recently faster scanners (temporal resolution approaching 60ms), scanners with higher resolution (reported to be 0.2mm vs. as low as 0.5mm with 64-slice systems), and increased coverage (up to 16cm with a single rotation with a 320-slice scanner), the latter providing one-beat CCTA. Finally, improvements in the technology are also related to the important issue of radiation dose reduction; recently, concern has been widely expressed about the increased radiation exposure of the population due to the high number of the diagnostic radiology procedures in general, and CT scans in particular [181,182]. With the development of simple acquisition algorithms with tube current modulation and energy reduction [183,184], and implementation of "best practice" methodology in accord with the ALARA ("as low as reasonably achievable") principle, the radiation dose during CCTA has been reduced significantly [185]. With the use of dose modulation and other approaches such as prospective gating, the routine dose with CCTA in many centers is now less than 10mSv, and in some centers is in the range of 2mSv [180]. If these dose levels become the community standard, CCTA will be associated with lower radiation doses than with the standard SPECT or PET MPI procedures in use today [181].

Prognostic value

CAC is thought to develop when the body attempts to contain and stabilize inflamed coronary plaque [186]. In general, evidence of CAC reflects a more advanced stage of plaque development. CAC is considered pathognomomic of coronary atherosclerosis. A quantitative relationship has been demonstrated between CAC and histopathological evidence of coronary plaque area. Moreover, calcified plaque assessment correlates with pathological assessment of the total amount of calcified plus non-calcified plaque [174]. As such, CAC serves as an indirect but proportional marker for global atherosclerotic burden.

The majority of studies in this field have concentrated on the prognostic value of CAC. Pooled data demonstrate the excellent potential of CAC in risk stratification of patients above and beyond clinical and historical data [172]. In the development of the estimators of risk considerable attention has been given to consideration of CAC distribution by age, gender, and other clinical variables in order to further "fine-tune" the prediction of cardiac risk

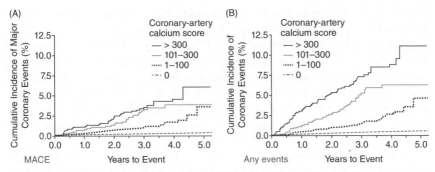

Figure 11.6 Unadjusted Kaplan–Meier cumulative-event curves for coronary events among participants with coronary-artery calcium scores of 0, 1–100, 101–300, and >300. (A) Rates for major adverse cardiac events (MACE) and (B) rates for any coronary event. The differences between all curves are statistically significant (p < 0.001). (Reproduced from Detrano *et al.* [189], Copyright © 2008 Massachusetts Medical Society. All rights reserved.)

[172,187,188]. A highly regarded recent study reported distribution of the follow-up cardiac events by CAC score in four ethnic groups in the MESA (Multi-Ethnic Study of Atherosclerosis) trial, a population-based study of 6722 patients from a registry [189]. CAC was a significant predictor of both major cardiac events (cardiac death or MI) and any coronary events in the overall population (Figure 11.6), as well as separately in the four ethnic groups during a median follow-up of 3.9 years [188].

Moreover, analysis of the data from the same registry [190] demonstrated that risk stratification based on standard absolute cut-off points of CAC (<100, 100–400 and >400 Agatston units) performed much better than age–sex–race/ethnicity-specific percentiles in terms of model fit and discrimination. Importantly, consideration of CAC significantly improves the classification of risk compared to a prediction model based on traditional risk factors [191]. Furthermore, while carotid intima-media thickness (CIMT) has been shown to be predictive of cardiac events in many studies, the MESA trial demonstrated that CAC score was a far stronger predictor of events than CIMT [192]. In one recent observation [193], only the presence of CAC itself, rather than other "traditional" CAD predictors, was predictive of CAC progression.

That CAC and SPECT MPI measurements provide highly complementary information in assessing patients with suspected CAD has been shown in a large study from our lab comparing the frequency of ischemia on MPI with the magnitude of CAC abnormality in a total of 1195 patients without known coronary disease, who underwent both stress MPI and CAC tomography within 7.2 ± 44.8 days [194]. Among the patients with a CAC of less than 100 Agatston units, MPI ischemia was rare, occurring in less than 2% of such patients. This low frequency of ischemia with a CAC score of less than 100 Agatston units was seen in patients with and without clinical symptoms. As the CAC score increased in magnitude above 100 Agatston units, the frequency of myocardial ischemia on MPI increased progressively.

This study has raised several important clinical considerations. First, it helped to define indications for stress MPI referral after CAC imaging. According to the results, referral for MPI is generally not needed when the CAC score is less than 100 Agatston units due to the very low likelihood of observing inducible MI in such patients. Conversely, when the CAC score is greater than 400 Agatston units, stress MPI (or another stress imaging modality) would appear to be generally beneficial, because the frequency of inducible ischemia is substantial within this CAC range, even in asymptomatic patients.

Of note, the wide range of CAC scores (CCSs) in the patients with normal MPI studies exposes an important limitation relevant to all forms of so-called "physiological" stress imaging testing: they do not effectively screen for subclinical atherosclerosis. Our study was also important in documenting the insensitivity of MPS for detecting coronary atherosclerosis (in contrast to detecting patients with hemodynamically significant CAD). Of 1119 patients with normal MPS studies, a large proportion had a high enough CCS that there would be consensus that aggressive medical management is warranted: 56% had a CCS of greater than 100 and 31% of greater than 400. These findings suggest that if testing begins with MPI in a given patient, further assessment of atherosclerotic burden by CAC testing may be useful in assessment of the need for aggressive attempts to prevent coronary events.

To date few data indicate that aggressive treatment of patients with subclinical atherosclerosis defined by CAC reduces subsequent cardiac events. In a randomized clinical trial, a part of the St Francis Heart Study, showed a trend toward less progression of the CCS in patients treated with statins versus a control group, but this failed to reach statistical significance [195]. However, given the clearly strong relationship between CAC measurements and events, a randomized trial withholding aggressive treatment in the control arm might be ethically problematic. It appears that there is a recent trend toward recommendation of CAC testing for asymptomatic patients, at least those at intermediate clinical risk, and for aggressive treatment of those with prognostically important amounts of CAC.

As previously noted, when the CCS is greater than 400, stress imaging for silent myocardial ischemia is now accepted practice [85]. A recent study supported this approach by showing that when such testing for ischemia is negative, the short-term cardiac event rates are low [196]. In an analysis of 1089 patients who had non-ischemic exercise MPI after CAC testing, during a mean follow-up of 32 ± 16 months, less than 1% underwent early revascularization, and the annualized cardiac event rate was less than 1% in all the CAC subgroups, including those with CCS greater than 1000.

Finally, in a recent subanalysis of more than 10000 patients from the CONFIRM multinational registry, among patients with a CCS of 0, 13% had non-obstructive CAD and 3.5% had obstructive disease. Of note, 3.9% of patients with a CAC score of 0 and 50% stenosis experienced a cardiac event (HR, 5.7; 95% CI, 2.5–13.1; p < 0.001) compared with 0.8% of patients with a CCS of 0 and no obstructive CAD [197].

In summary, CAC measurements appear useful in asymptomatic patients with risk factors and an intermediate clinical risk, i.e., when the need for aggressive preventive measures is not already clear. Currently there is widespread agreement that a CCS of greater than 100 defines a patient population deserving aggressive therapy, and a score of greater than 400 defines a sufficiently high risk that patients deserve prevention according to secondary prevention guidelines, and that this score also defines a threshold above which further testing for ischemia is considered appropriate.

Diagnostic and prognostic impact in different clinical populations

CCTA allows visualization of the vascular wall and lumen, thus significantly improving the diagnosis of non-obstructive plaque and eliminating a diagnostic problem well-known to clinicians who have to deal with "lumenograms" acquired on ICA.

Numerous studies of the diagnostic accuracy of CCTA compared with CTA have been performed. These studies have limitations such as referral bias, as discussed above for MPI, as well as limitations related to the use of ICA as a gold standard per se. The issues of referral bias are less prominent with CCTA than with MPI since nearly all of the correlative studies have been performed on patients already determined as needing ICA, in contrast to the MPI correlative studies in which the decision to perform ICA was frequently governed by the MPI test result itself. Nonetheless, this modality has been subjected to more assessments of sensitivity and specificity in patient groups being sent for ICA than any of the other non-invasive cardiac imaging modalities. On the basis of a large body of evidence, CCTA is considered the most accurate non-invasive test for the detection of CAD as defined by ICA.

With regard to the clinical selection of patients and their referral for either ICA or CCTA, in a large multinational study of patients referred for CCTA (CONFIRM Registry), determination of pretest likelihood of angiographically significant CAD using ICA-based guideline probabilities (based on age, gender, and typicality of the chest pain) greatly overestimated the actual prevalence of disease [198].

A meta-analyses of the sensitivity and specificity of CCTA pooled data from 28 CCTA studies [199]; the diagnostic performance of CCTA was found to be excellent (Figure 11.7).

Recently, several large multicenter trials regarding the accuracy of CCTA for detecting CAD compared with ICA have been published. A recent prospective, multicenter, multivendor study conducted with "real-world" analysis (no patients or segments were excluded because of impaired image quality attributable to either coronary motion or calcifications), involved 360 symptomatic patients with acute and stable anginal syndromes who were between 50 and 70 years of age and were referred for diagnostic conventional ICA, which was compared with CCTA [200]. In this population of patients with intermediate-to-high and high pre-test likelihood of CAD, CCTA was reliable in ruling out significant CAD (Table 11.9). CCTA specificity in this study was lower than in most other reports, probably due to the inclusion of all the

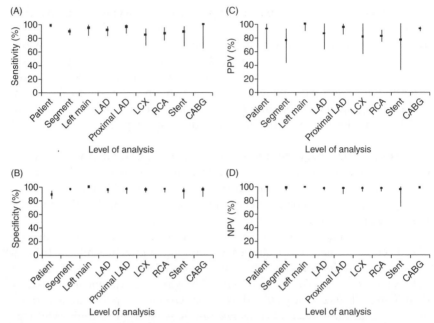

Figure 11.7 Left panel: Pooled estimates (18 studies; n = 1286; 95% CI) for different levels of analysis. Left main artery: owing to numerical difficulties with the hierarchical summary receiver operating characteristic symmetric model, sensitivity (A) and specificity (B) were pooled using the weighted average method and confidence intervals rather than credible intervals were reported. Right panel: Median (C) positive and (D) negative predictive values (PPV and NPV) across studies (range). CABG, coronary artery bypass graft; LAD, left anterior descending; LCX, left circumflex; RCA, right coronary artery. (Reproduced from Mowatt *et al* [199], with permission from BMJ Publishing Group Ltd.)

Table 11.9 Appropriate indications for CT coronary angiography. (Adapted from Achenbach [179], with kind permission from Springer Science + Business Media.)

Detection of CAD with prior test results: evaluation of chest pain syndromes
Uninterpretable or equivocal stress test result (exercise, perfusion, or stress echocardiography)

Detection of CAD (symptomatic): evaluation of chest pain syndrome
Intermediate pretest probability of CAD, EKG uninterpretable or unable to exercise

Detection of CAD (symptomatic): acute chest pain
Intermediate pretest probability of CAD, no EKG changes, and serial enzymes are negative

Evaluation of coronary arteries in patients with new-onset heart failure to assess etiology

Evaluation of suspected coronary anomalies

CAD, coronary artery disease; EKG, electrocardiogram.

segments and patients despite observed artifacts. An important observation from this study is that the majority of the false-positive and false-negative studies were clustered around the cut-off of 50% luminal stenosis.

Another important recently published prospective multicenter trial (ACCU-RACY; Assessment by Coronary Computed Tomographic Angiography of Individuals Undergoing Invasive Coronary Angiography) [201] investigated 230 symptomatic patients with intermediate-to-high and high likelihood of CAD who were referred for ICA; in this study, 64-slice CCTA showed high diagnostic accuracy for detection of obstructive coronary stenosis at both 50% and 70% stenosis thresholds. The authors also concluded that the 99% negative predictive value at the patient and vessel level observed in this study establishes CCTA as an effective non-invasive alternative to ICA to rule out obstructive coronary artery stenosis. In this study, the prevalence of obstructive CAD was 12.5%. Similar high diagnostic accuracy of CCTA compared to ICA was demonstrated in the CACTUS (Coronary Angiography by Computed Tomography with the use of a Submillimeter resolution) trial [202] that included 243 patients with an intermediate pre-test probability for CAD.

In a subsequent multicenter trial, the CORE 64 (Coronary Artery Evaluation using 64-Row Multidetector Computed Tomography Angiography) study, the overall accuracy was similar, but with somewhat lower negative predictive value [203]. However, this difference is most likely attributed to the manner in which lesions were assessed in the presence of coronary artery calcification, which may have obscured the coronary lumen, as well as to differences in prevalence of obstructive CAD in the various studies.

Particularly in patients with an intermediate likelihood of CAD, the clinical implications of a normal CCTA study are generally clear: the high negative predictive value implies that the symptoms leading to testing are very unlikely to be due to obstructive CAD. The clinical implications of the abnormal CCTA study are often, however, less clear. While the coronary angiographic correlations have been excellent, the correlations between CCTA and functional measures of ischemia have been much lower. In the studies to date in which both SPECT MPI and CCTA have been performed, less than 50% of the patients with CCTA studies showing greater than 50% stenosis demonstrated ischemia on SPECT MPI [204–207] (Figure 11.8). Since a stenosis of greater than 70% is now more widely required as an angiographic criterion for the need for revascularization, it would be of interest to observe the relationship between CCTA and ischemia using this angiographic cut-off. However, given the lack of excellent correlation between angiographic stenosis and coronary flow reserve, the current "gold standard" for hemodynamic significance [88], it is likely that 50% of such lesions, even those meeting the greater than 70% stenosis criterion, will not demonstrate ischemia.

Evidence from several observational series suggests that CCTA is the most effective imaging modality for the evaluation of coronary anomalies [208–210]. Another documented area in which CCTA is highly accurate is in the evaluation of the bypass patency in symptomatic patients with either venous or arterial coronary bypasses [211]. While simultaneous assessment

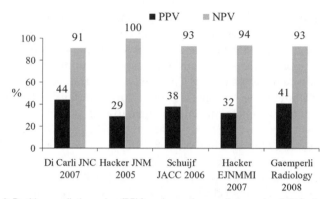

Figure 11.8 Positive predictive value (PPV) and negative predictive value (NPV) of coronary computed tomographic angiography (>50% stenosis) with respect to myocardial perfusion imaging. (Based on data from references [204–207, 215].)

of the native coronary anatomy in the post-bypass population is challenging due to the high frequency of artifacts related to heavy calcifications, distorted anatomy, and surgical clips, the accuracy for detection of graft patency approaches 100%.

Some recently published data suggest the usefulness of CCTA for the evaluation of coronary stent patency [212,213]; in a small population (100 patients/128 stents) the reported sensitivity, specificity, and positive and negative predictive value of the dual-source CCTA, calculated in all stents, were 94%, 92%, 77%, and 98%, respectively. Due to the limited spatial resolution of CT and artifacts associated with the metal in coronary stents, CCTA is more accurate for in-stent stenosis in large stents (over 3 mm). Overall, more clinical evidence is needed in support of this application.

CCTA is a new modality in the armamentarium of advanced cardiac imaging. Thus, available prognostic data only cover either relatively small populations or provide a limited (either short- or mid-term) follow-up. Nevertheless, initial publications in this field demonstrate the powerful predictive value of CCTA, with excellent prognosis in those patients who have no evidence of atherosclerosis on their index scan [214,215].

More detailed analysis of a large population (n = 1127) has shown that in patients with chest pain, CCTA identifies increased risk for all-cause death [216]. In this population, a negative CCTA was associated with extremely low all-cause mortality. Notably, the CCTA predictors of death included proximal left anterior descending artery (LAD) stenosis and number of vessels with greater than 50% and greater than 70% stenosis. Of importance, there was an appropriate increase in the death rate associated with each step of increased jeopardy when the CCTA was assessed by the Duke Jeopardy score (Figure 11.9) [209].

Regarding the cost-effectiveness of CCTA, interesting data have emerged from the analysis of the Medicare claims in a large population of patients

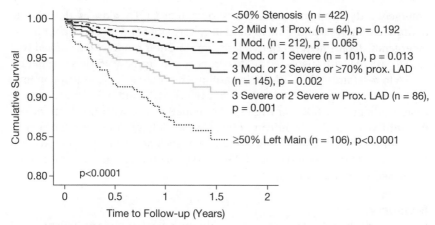

R-A p<0.0001 (adjusting for risk factors, chest pain, + dyspnea), Mild (30-49%), Mod. (50-69%), & Severe (≥70%).

Figure 11.9 Cumulative survival in patients exhibiting plaque by the Duke prognostic coronary artery disease index. Risk-adjusted p < 0.001 (controlling for age, family history, and dyslipidemia). LAD, left anterior descending artery; Mod, moderate; Prox, proximal. (Reproduced from Min *et al.* [216], with permission.)

without known CAD who underwent CCTA (n = 1938) or stress MPI (n = 7752) [217]. Patients who underwent CCTA, compared with matched patients who underwent SPECT, incurred lower overall healthcare and CAD expenditures while experiencing similarly low rates of CAD hospitalization, outpatient visits, MI, and angina. These data suggest that CCTA may be a cost-effective alternative to SPECT for the initial coronary evaluation of patients without known CAD. In the same study, the SPECT MPI approach was seen to be more cost-effective than CCTA in patients with known CAD.

The recent multicenter randomized CT-STAT (Coronary Computed Tomographic Angiography for Systematic Triage of Acute Chest Pain Patients to Treatment) trial tested performance of CCTA compared to standard of care (stress MPI) in patients with acute low risk chest pain. The study demonstrated a 54% reduction in time to diagnosis and a 38% reduction in cost of care in the CCTA arm as compared with the MPI arm [218].Whether CCTA is equal to or superior to MPI for assessment of patients with suspected CAD remains an unanswered question. A large randomized clinical trial comparing CCTA to functional testing (MPI, stress echo, stress EKG), PROMISE (PROspective Imaging Study for Evaluation of Chest Pain) study, is currently being conducted. Several observational studies have demonstrated the usefulness of CCTA in patients with acute chest pain and low clinical risk (TIMI risk score 3 or less) [219–222]. In these trials, CCTA has been shown as a safe, accurate, and fast methodology, performing better in terms of time-to-diagnosis and cost-effectiveness, compared to the standard of care [212]. A pilot single-center randomized trial comparing CCTA to rest/stress MPI in the emergency department setting has shown that CCTA reduces the time to definitive diagnosis and time to discharge for patients with chest pain in the emergency department [212]. In a large, multicenter randomized clinical trial of 750 patients with suspected acute coronary syndrome at 15 sites comparing CCTA to rest/stress SPECT MPI, the authors reported a 53% reduction in time to diagnosis using CCTA compared to SPECT MPI, and a 38% reduction in costs to diagnosis. Both strategies were equally safe, with no difference in 6-month MACEs. The American College of Cardiology along with the Society of Cardiovascular CT and other professional societies developed initial clinical appropriateness criteria for CCTA in 2006, with revisions of these criteria published in mid 2010 [223].

Summary

In summary, the role of CCTA in the evaluation of symptomatic patients with intermediate likelihood of CAD is currently supported by the significant body of evidence, acquired from multiple studies (including several large multicenter trials). How useful CCTA is as a tool for the assessment of the coronary anatomy in asymptomatic patients still remains unclear. A large randomized clinical trial comparing CCTA to different stress perfusion modalities in patients without known CAD and at least intermediate pretest likelihood of CAD is underway. Trials like this are considered highly important in answering the question currently being raised as a prerequisite to uniform coverage of this procedure by various insurance entities; namely, does CCTA improve health outcomes [224]. Indeed, this important question has not been well answered for any of the non-invasive cardiac imaging modalities. It is anticipated that randomized clinical trials addressing these issues will be forthcoming.

Acknowledgement

The authors thank Xingping Kang MD for her expert assistance in preparation of the manuscript and illustrative materials for this chapter.

References

1. Berman DS, Hachamovitch R, Shaw L, Hayes SW, Germano G. Nuclear cardiology. In: Fuster V, Alexander RW, O'Rourke RA, et al., eds. *Hurst's The Heart*. 11 ed. McGraw-Hill, 2004.
2. Klocke FJ, Baird MG, Lorell BH, *et al*. ACC/AHA/ASNC guidelines for the clinical use of cardiac radionuclide imaging–executive summary: a report of the American College of Cardiology/American Heart Association Task Force on Practice Guidelines (ACC/AHA/ASNC Committee to Revise the 1995 Guidelines for the Clinical Use of Cardiac Radionuclide Imaging). *J Am Coll Cardiol* 2003;42:1318–1333.
3. Germano G, Erel J, Kiat H, Kavanagh PB, Berman DS. Quantitative LVEF and qualitative regional function from gated thallium-201 perfusion SPECT. *J Nucl Med* 1997; 38:749–754.

4. Germano G, Kiat H, Kavanagh PB, *et al*. Automatic quantification of ejection fraction from gated myocardial perfusion SPECT. *J Nucl Med* 1995;36:2138–2147.
5. Germano G, Berman DS. *Clinical Gated Cardiac SPECT*. Armonk, New York: Futura Publishing, 1999.
6. Faber TL, Stokely EM, Peshock RM, Corbett JR. A model-based four-dimensional left ventricular surface detector. *IEEE Trans Med Imaging* 1991;10:321–329.
7. Ladenheim ML, Pollock BH, Rozanski A, *et al*. Extent and severity of myocardial hypoperfusion as predictors of prognosis in patients with suspected coronary artery disease. *J Am Coll Cardiol* 1986;7:464–471.
8. Berman DS, Kiat H, Friedman JD, *et al*. Separate acquisition rest thallium-201/stress technetium-99m sestamibi dual-isotope myocardial perfusion single-photon emission computed tomography: a clinical validation study. *J Am Coll Cardiol* 1993;22: 1455–1464.
9. Iskandrian AS, Chae SC, Heo J, Stanberry CD, Wasserleben V, Cave V. Independent and incremental prognostic value of exercise single-photon emission computed tomographic (SPECT) thallium imaging in coronary artery disease. *J Am Coll Cardiol* 1993;22: 665–670.
10. Iskandrian AS, Chae SC, Heo J, Stanberry CD, Wasserleben V, Cave V. Independent and incremental prognostic value of exercise single-photon emission computed tomographic (SPECT) thallium imaging in coronary artery disease. *J Am Coll Cardiol* 1993;22: 665–670.
11. Hachamovitch R, Berman DS, Kiat H, Cohen I, Friedman JD, Shaw LJ. Value of stress myocardial perfusion single photon emission computed tomography in patients with normal resting electrocardiograms: an evaluation of incremental prognostic value and cost-effectiveness. *Circulation* 2002;105:823–829.
12. Sharir T, Germano G, Kang X, *et al*. Prediction of myocardial infarction versus cardiac death by gated myocardial perfusion SPECT: risk stratification by the amount of stress-induced ischemia and the poststress ejection fraction. *J Nucl Med* 2001;42:831–837.
13. Cerqueira MD, Weissman NJ, Dilsizian V, *et al*. Standardized myocardial segmentation and nomenclature for tomographic imaging of the heart: a statement for healthcare professionals from the Cardiac Imaging Committee of the Council on Clinical Cardiology of the American Heart Association. *Circulation* 2002;105:539–542.
14. Slomka PJ, Nishina H, Berman DS, *et al*. Automated quantification of myocardial perfusion SPECT using simplified normal limits. *J Nucl Cardiol* 2005;12:66–77.
15. Berman DS, Kang X, Gransar H, *et al*. Quantitative assessment of myocardial perfusion abnormality on SPECT myocardial perfusion imaging is more reproducible than expert visual analysis. *J Nucl Cardiol* 2009;16:45–53.
16. Shaw LJ, Berman DS, Maron DJ, *et al*. Optimal medical therapy with or without percutaneous coronary intervention to reduce ischemic burden: results from the Clinical Outcomes Utilizing Revascularization and Aggressive Drug Evaluation (COURAGE) trial nuclear substudy. *Circulation* 2008;117:1283–1291.
17. Heller GV, Links J, Bateman TM, *et al*. American Society of Nuclear Cardiology and Society of Nuclear Medicine joint position statement: attenuation correction of myocardial perfusion SPECT scintigraphy. *J Nucl Cardiol* 2004;11:229–230.
18. Hendel RC, Corbett JR, Cullom SJ, DePuey EG, Garcia EV, Bateman TM. The value and practice of attenuation correction for myocardial perfusion SPECT imaging: a joint position statement from the American Society of Nuclear Cardiology and the Society of Nuclear Medicine. *J Nucl Cardiol* 2002;9:135–143.
19. Bateman TM, Cullom SJ. Attenuation correction single-photon emission computed tomography myocardial perfusion imaging. *Semin Nucl Med* 2005;35:37–51.

20. Thompson RC, Heller GV, Johnson LL, *et al*. Value of attenuation correction on ECG-gated SPECT myocardial perfusion imaging related to body mass index. *J Nucl Cardiol* 2005;12:195–202.

21. Singh B, Bateman TM, Case JA, Heller G. Attenuation artifact, attenuation correction, and the future of myocardial perfusion SPECT. *J Nucl Cardiol* 2007;14:153–164.

22. Kiat H, Van Train KF, Friedman JD, *et al*. Quantitative stress-redistribution thallium-201 SPECT using prone imaging: methodologic development and validation. *J Nucl Med* 1992;33:1509–1515.

23. Lisbona R, Dinh L, Derbekyan V, Novales-Diaz JA. Supine and prone SPECT Tc-99m MIBI myocardial perfusion imaging for dipyridamole studies. *Clin Nucl Med* 1995; 20:674–677.

24. O'Connor MK, Bothun ED. Effects of tomographic table attenuation on prone and supine cardiac imaging. *J Nucl Med* 1995;36:1102–1106.

25. Nishina H, Slomka PJ, Abidov A, *et al*. Combined supine and prone quantitative myocardial perfusion SPECT: Method development and clinical validation in patients with no known coronary artery disease. *J Nucl Med* 2006;47:51–58.

26. Perault C, Loboguerrero A, Liehn JC, *et al*. Quantitative comparison of prone and supine myocardial SPECT MIBI images. *Clin Nucl Med* 1995;20:678–684.

27. Segall GM, Davis MJ. Prone versus supine thallium myocardial SPECT: a method to decrease artifactual inferior wall defects. *J Nucl Med* 1989;30:548–555.

28. Malkerneker D, Brenner R, Martin WH, *et al*. CT-based attenuation correction versus prone imaging to decrease equivocal interpretations of rest/stress Tc-99m tetrofosmin SPECT MPI. *J Nucl Cardiol* 2007;14:314–323.

29. Funk T, Kirch DL, Koss JE, Botvinick E, Hasegawa BH. A novel approach to multipinhole SPECT for myocardial perfusion imaging. *J Nucl Med* 2006;47:595–602.

30. Madsen MT. Recent advances in SPECT imaging. *J Nucl Med* 2007;48:661–673.

31. Sharir T, Ben-Haim S, Merzon K, *et al*. High-speed myocardial perfusion imaging: initial clinical comparison with conventional dual detector Anger camera imaging. *J Am Coll Cardiol Imaging* 2008;1:156–163.

32. Berman DS, Kang X, Tamarappoo B, *et al*. Stress thallium-201/rest technetium-99m sequential dual isotope high-speed myocardial perfusion imaging. *J Am Coll Cardiol Cardiovasc Imaging* 2009;2:273–282.

33. Gambhir SS, Berman DS, Ziffer Z, *et al*. A novel high sensitivity rapid acquisition Single-Photon cardiac imaging camera. *J Nucl Med* 2009;50:635–643.

34. Germano G, Berman DS. *Clinical Gated Cardiac SPEC*, 2nd ed. New York: Blackwell Futura, 2006.

35. Akincioglu C, Berman DS, Nishina H, *et al*. Assessment of diastolic function using 16-frame 99mTc-sestamibi gated myocardial perfusion SPECT: normal values. *J Nucl Med* 2005;46:1102–1108.

36. Sharir T, Bacher-Stier C, Dhar S, *et al*. Post exercise regional wall motion abnormalities detected by Tc-99m sestamibi gated SPECT: a marker of severe coronary artery disease. *J Nucl Med* 1998;39:87P–88P.

37. Abidov A, Bax JJ, Hayes SW, *et al*. Integration of automatically measured transient ischemic dilation ratio into interpretation of adenosine stress myocardial perfusion SPECT for detection of severe and extensive CAD. *J Nucl Med* 2004;45:1999–2007.

38. Abidov A, Bax JJ, Hayes SW, *et al*. Transient ischemic dilation ratio of the left ventricle is a significant predictor of future cardiac events in patients with otherwise normal myocardial perfusion SPECT. *J Am Coll Cardiol* 2003;42:1818–1825.

39. Mazzanti M, Germano G, Kiat H, *et al*. Identification of severe and extensive coronary artery disease by automatic measurement of transient ischemic dilation of the left

ventricle in dual-isotope myocardial perfusion SPECT. *J Am Coll Cardiol* 1996;27: 1612–1620.

40. Weiss AT, Berman DS, Lew AS, *et al.* Transient ischemic dilation of the left ventricle on stress thallium-201 scintigraphy: a marker of severe and extensive coronary artery disease. *J Am Coll Cardiol* 1987;9:752–759.

41. Villanueva FS, Kaul S, Smith WH, Watson DD, Varma SK, Beller GA. Prevalence and correlates of increased lung/heart ratio of thallium-201 during dipyridamole stress imaging for suspected coronary artery disease. *Am J Cardiol* 1990;66:1324–1328.

42. Romanens M, Gradel C, Saner H, Pfisterer M. Comparison of 99mTc-sestamibi lung/ heart ratio, transient ischaemic dilation and perfusion defect size for the identification of severe and extensive coronary artery disease. *Eur J Nucl Med* 2001;28:907–910.

43. Gill JB, Ruddy TD, Newell JB, Finkelstein DM, Strauss HW, Boucher CA. Prognostic importance of thallium uptake by the lungs during exercise in coronary artery disease. *N Engl J Med* 1987;317:1486–1489.

44. Morel O, Pezard P, Furber A, *et al.* Thallium-201 right lung/heart ratio during exercise in patients with coronary artery disease: relation to thallium-201 myocardial single-photon emission tomography, rest and exercise left ventricular function and coronary angiography. *Eur J Nucl Med* 1999;26:640–646.

45. Williams KA, Hill KA, Sheridan CM. Noncardiac findings on dual-isotope myocardial perfusion SPECT. *J Nucl Cardiol* 2003;10:395–402.

46. Henneman MM, van der Wall EE, Ypenburg C, *et al.* Nuclear imaging in cardiac resynchronization therapy. *J Nucl Med* 2007;48:2001–2010.

47. Ypenburg C, Westenberg JJ, Bleeker GB, *et al.* Noninvasive imaging in cardiac resynchronization therapy–part 1: selection of patients. *Pacing Clin Electrophysiol* 2008;31: 1475–1499.

48. Chen J, Garcia EV, Folks RD, *et al.* Onset of left ventricular mechanical contraction as determined by phase analysis of ECG-gated myocardial perfusion SPECT imaging: development of a diagnostic tool for assessment of cardiac mechanical dyssynchrony. *J Nucl Cardiol* 2005;12:687–695.

49. Chen J, Faber TL, Cooke CD, Garcia EV. Temporal resolution of multiharmonic phase analysis of ECG-gated myocardial perfusion SPECT studies. *J Nucl Cardiol* 2008; 15:383–391.

50. Trimble MA, Velazquez EJ, Adams GL, *et al.* Repeatability and reproducibility of phase analysis of gated single-photon emission computed tomography myocardial perfusion imaging used to quantify cardiac dyssynchrony. *Nucl Med Commun* 2008;29: 374–381.

51. Henneman MM, Chen J, Dibbets-Schneider P, *et al.* Can LV dyssynchrony as assessed with phase analysis on gated myocardial perfusion SPECT predict response to CRT? *J Nucl Med* 2007;48:1104–1111.

52. Van Kriekinge SD, Nishina H, Ohba M, Berman DS, Germano G. Automatic global and regional phase analysis from gated myocardial perfusion SPECT imaging: application to the characterization of ventricular contraction in patients with left bundle branch block. *J Nucl Med* 2008;49:1790–1797.

53. Russell RR, 3rd, Zaret BL. Nuclear cardiology: present and future. *Curr Probl Cardiol* 2006;31:557–629.

54. Iskandrian AS, Heo J, Decoskey D, Askenase A, Segal BL. Use of exercise thallium-201 imaging for risk stratification of elderly patients with coronary artery disease. *Am J Cardiol* 1988;61:269–272.

55. Amanullah AM, Kiat H, Hachamovitch R, *et al.* Impact of myocardial perfusion single-photon emission computed tomography on referral to catheterization of the very

elderly. Is there evidence of gender-related referral bias? *J Am Coll Cardiol* 1996;28: 680–686.

56. Lima RS, De Lorenzo A, Pantoja MR, Siqueira A. Incremental prognostic value of myocardial perfusion 99m-technetium-sestamibi SPECT in the elderly. *Int J Cardiol* 2004;93:137–143.

57. Hachamovitch R, Kang X, Amanullah AM, *et al*. Prognostic implications of myocardial perfusion single-photon emission computed tomography in the elderly. *Circulation* 2009;120:2197–2206.

58. Rocci R, de Ambroggi L, Radice M, *et al*. Thallium-201 myocardial imaging in young asymptomatic subjects with "ischaemic" changes in exercise electrocardiogram. *Acta Cardiol* 1979;34:217–232.

59. Hachamovitch R, Berman DS, Kiat H, *et al*. Effective risk stratification using exercise myocardial perfusion SPECT in women: gender-related differences in prognostic nuclear testing. *J Am Coll Cardiol* 1996;28:34–44.

60. Shaw LJ, Hachamovitch R, Redberg RF. Current evidence on diagnostic testing in women with suspected coronary artery disease: choosing the appropriate test. *Cardiol Rev* 2000;8:65–74.

61. Hachamovitch R, Berman DS, Kiat H, *et al*. Gender-related differences in clinical management after exercise nuclear testing. *J Am Coll Cardiol* 1995;26:1457–1464.

62. Dakik HA, Mahmarian JJ, Kimball KT, Koutelou MG, Medrano R, Verani MS. Prognostic value of exercise 201Tl tomography in patients treated with thrombolytic therapy during acute myocardial infarction. *Circulation* 1996;94:2735–2742.

63. Mahmarian JJ, Pratt CM, Nishimura S, Abreu A, Verani MS. Quantitative adenosine 201Tl single-photon emission computed tomography for the early assessment of patients surviving acute myocardial infarction. *Circulation* 1993;87:1197–1210.

64. Mahmarian JJ, Mahmarian AC, Marks GF, Pratt CM, Verani MS. Role of adenosine thallium-201 tomography for defining long-term risk in patients after acute myocardial infarction. *J Am Coll Cardiol* 1995;25:1333–1340.

65. Mahmarian J. Management decisions in survivors of acute myocardial infarction using radionuclide imaging. *ACC Curr J Rev* 1999;8:50–56.

66. Pratt CM, Mahmarian JJ, Morales-Ballejo H, Casareto R, Moye LA. Design of a randomized, placebo-controlled multicenter trial on the long-term effects of intermittent transdermal nitroglycerin on left ventricular remodeling after acute myocardial infarction. Transdermal Nitroglycerin Investigators Group. *Am J Cardiol* 1998;81: 719–724.

67. Mahmarian JJ, Shaw LJ, Olszewski GH, Pounds BK, Frias ME, Pratt CM. Adenosine sestamibi SPECT post-infarction evaluation (INSPIRE) trial: A randomized, prospective multicenter trial evaluating the role of adenosine Tc-99m sestamibi SPECT for assessing risk and therapeutic outcomes in survivors of acute myocardial infarction. *J Nucl Cardiol* 2004;11:458–469.

68. Abidov A, Hachamovitch R, Berman DS. Modern nuclear cardiac imaging in diagnosis and clinical management of patients with left ventricular dysfunction. *Minerva Cardioangiol* 2004;52:505–519.

69. Giedd KN, Bergmann SR. Myocardial perfusion imaging following percutaneous coronary intervention: the importance of restenosis, disease progression, and directed reintervention. *J Am Coll Cardiol* 2004;43:328–336.

70. Zellweger MJ, Lewin HC, Lai S, *et al*. When to stress patients after coronary artery bypass surgery? Risk stratification in patients early and late post-CABG using stress myocardial perfusion SPECT: implications of appropriate clinical strategies. *J Am Coll Cardiol* 2001;37:144–152.

71. Heller GV, Stowers SA, Hendel RC, *et al.*, eds. Clinical value of acute rest technetium-99m tetrofosmin tomographic myocardial perfusion imaging in patients with acute chest pain and nondiagnostic electrocardiograms. *J Am Coll Cardiol* 1998;31:1101–1107.

72. De Lorenzo A, Lima RS, Siqueira-Filho AG, Pantoja MR. Prevalence and prognostic value of perfusion defects detected by stress technetium-99m sestamibi myocardial perfusion single-photon emission computed tomography in asymptomatic patients with diabetes mellitus and no known coronary artery disease. *Am J Cardiol* 2002;90: 827–832.

73. Wackers FJ, Young LH, Inzucchi SE, *et al.* Detection of silent myocardial ischemia in asymptomatic diabetic subjects: the DIAD study. *Diabetes Care* 2004;27:1954–1961.

74. Wackers FJ, Young LH, Inzucchi SE, *et al.* Detection of silent myocardial ischemia in asymptomatic diabetic subjects: the DIAD study. *Diabetes Care* 2004;27:1954-61.

75. Hachamovitch R, Berman DS, Shaw LJ, *et al.* Incremental prognostic value of myocardial perfusion single photon emission computed tomography for the prediction of cardiac death: differential stratification for risk of cardiac death and myocardial infarction. *Circulation* 1998;97:535–543.

76. Abidov A, Hachamovitch R, Rozanski A, Hayes SW, Santos MM, Sciammarella MG, et al. Prognostic implications of atrial fibrillation in patients undergoing myocardial perfusion single-photon emission computed tomography. *J Am Coll Cardiol* 2004;44: 1062–1070.

77. Askew JW, Miller TD, Hodge DO, Gibbons RJ. The value of myocardial perfusion single-photon emission computed tomography in screening asymptomatic patients with atrial fibrillation for coronary artery disease. *J Am Coll Cardiol* 2007;50:1080–1085.

78. Lapeyre AC, 3rd, Poornima IG, Miller TD, Hodge DO, Christian TF, Gibbons RJ. The prognostic value of pharmacologic stress myocardial perfusion imaging in patients with permanent pacemakers. *J Nucl Cardiol* 2005;12:37–42.

79. ten Cate TJ, Visser FC, Panhuyzen-Goedkoop NM, Verzijlbergen JF, van Hemel NM. Pacemaker-related myocardial perfusion defects worsen during higher pacing rate and coronary flow augmentation. *Heart Rhythm* 2005;2:1058–1063.

80. Posma JL, Blanksma PK, Van Der Wall EE, Vaalburg W, Crijns HJ, Lie KI. Effects of permanent dual chamber pacing on myocardial perfusion in symptomatic hypertrophic cardiomyopathy. *Heart* 1996;76:358–362.

81. Lakkis NM, He ZX, Verani MS. Diagnosis of coronary artery disease by exercise thallium-201 tomography in patients with a right ventricular pacemaker. *J Am Coll Cardiol* 1997;29:1221–1225.

82. Rozanski A, Berman D, Gray R, *et al.* Preoperative prediction of reversible myocardial asynergy by postexercise radionuclide ventriculography. *N Engl J Med* 1982;307: 212–216.

83. Maddahi J, Garcia EV, Berman DS, Waxman A, Swan HJ, Forrester J. Improved noninvasive assessment of coronary artery disease by quantitative analysis of regional stress myocardial distribution and washout of thallium-201. *Circulation* 1981;64:924–935.

84. Van Train KF, Berman DS, Garcia EV, *et al.* Quantitative analysis of stress thallium-201 myocardial scintigrams: a multicenter trial. *J Nucl Med* 1986;27:17–25.

85. Hendel RC, Budoff MJ, Cardella JF, *et al.* ACC/AHA/ACR/ASE/ASNC/HRS/ NASCI/RSNA/SAIP/SCAI/ SCCT/SCMR/SIR 2008 Key Data Elements and Definitions for Cardiac Imaging: A Report of the American College of Cardiology/ American Heart Association Task Force on Clinical Data Standards (Writing Committee to Develop Clinical Data Standards for Cardiac Imaging). *Circulation* 2009;119: 154–186.

86. Diamond GA, Forrester JS. Analysis of probability as an aid in the clinical diagnosis of coronary-artery disease. *N Engl J Med* 1979;300:1350–1358.

87. Brindis RG, Douglas PS, Hendel RC, *et al.* ACCF/ASNC appropriateness criteria for single-photon emission computed tomography myocardial perfusion imaging (SPECT MPI): a report of the American College of Cardiology Foundation Quality Strategic Directions Committee Appropriateness Criteria Working Group and the American Society of Nuclear Cardiology endorsed by the American Heart Association. *J Am Coll Cardiol* 2005;46:1587–1605.

88. Boden WE, O'Rourke RA, Teo KK, *et al.* Optimal medical therapy with or without PCI for stable coronary disease. *N Engl J Med* 2007;356:1503–1516.

89. Tonino PA, De Bruyne B, Pijls NH, *et al.* Fractional flow reserve versus angiography for guiding percutaneous coronary intervention. *N Engl J Med* 2009;360:213–224.

90. Samady H, Lepper W, Powers ER, *et al.* Fractional flow reserve of infarct-related arteries identifies reversible defects on noninvasive myocardial perfusion imaging early after myocardial infarction. *J Am Coll Cardiol* 2006;47:2187–2193.

91. Cheitlin MD, Armstrong WF, Aurigemma GP, *et al.* ACC/AHA/ASE 2003 guideline update for the clinical application of echocardiography–summary article: a report of the American College of Cardiology/American Heart Association Task Force on Practice Guidelines (ACC/AHA/ASE Committee to Update the 1997 Guidelines for the Clinical Application of Echocardiography). *J Am Coll Cardiol* 2003;42:954–970.

92. Feigenbaum H, Armstrong WF, Ryan T, eds. *Feigenbaum's Echocardiography*, 6th ed. Lippincott Williams & Wilkins, 2005.

93. Liao SL, Garcia MJ. New advances in quantitative echocardiography. *J Nucl Cardiol* 2008;15:255–265.

94. Burns AT, McDonald IG, Thomas JD, Macisaac A, Prior D. Doin' the twist: new tools for an old concept of myocardial function. *Heart* 2008;94:978–983.

95. Yu CM, Sanderson JE, Marwick TH, Oh JK. Tissue Doppler imaging a new prognosticator for cardiovascular diseases. *J Am Coll Cardiol* 2007;49:1903–1914.

96. Van de Veire NR, De Sutter J, Bax JJ, Roelandt JR. Technological advances in tissue Doppler imaging echocardiography. *Heart* 2008;94:1065–1074.

97. Kirkpatrick JN, Vannan MA, Narula J, Lang RM. Echocardiography in heart failure: applications, utility, and new horizons. *J Am Coll Cardiol* 2007;50:381–396.

98. Lester SJ, Tajik AJ, Nishimura RA, Oh JK, Khandheria BK, Seward JB. Unlocking the mysteries of diastolic function: deciphering the Rosetta Stone 10 years later. *J Am Coll Cardiol* 2008;51:679–689.

99. Soliman OI, Kirschbaum SW, van Dalen BM, *et al.* Accuracy and reproducibility of quantitation of left ventricular function by real-time three-dimensional echocardiography versus cardiac magnetic resonance. *Am J Cardiol* 2008;102:778–783.

100. Dolan MS, Gala SS, Dodla S, *et al.* Safety and efficacy of commercially available ultrasound contrast agents for rest and stress echocardiography a multicenter experience. *J Am Coll Cardiol* 2009;53:32–38.

101. Beaulieu Y. Bedside echocardiography in the assessment of the critically ill. *Crit Care Med* 2007;35 (5 Suppl):S235–249.

102. Joseph MX, Disney PJ, Da Costa R, Hutchison SJ. Transthoracic echocardiography to identify or exclude cardiac cause of shock. *Chest* 2004;126:1592–1597.

103. Bruch C, Comber M, Schmermund A, Eggebrecht H, Bartel T, Erbel R. Diagnostic usefulness and impact on management of transesophageal echocardiography in surgical intensive care units. *Am J Cardiol* 2003;91:510–513.

104. Vieillard-Baron A, Page B, Augarde R, *et al.* Acute cor pulmonale in massive pulmonary embolism: incidence, echocardiographic pattern, clinical implications and recovery rate. *Intensive Care Med* 2001;27:1481–1486.

105. Vieillard-Baron A, Prin S, Chergui K, Dubourg O, Jardin F. Echo-Doppler demonstration of acute cor pulmonale at the bedside in the medical intensive care unit. *Am J Respir Crit Care Med* 2002;166:1310–1319.

106. Huttemann E. Transoesophageal echocardiography in critical care. *Minerva Anesthesiol* 2006;72:891–913.

107. Cerqueira MD, Weissman NJ, Dilsizian V, *et al*. Standardized myocardial segmentation and nomenclature for tomographic imaging of the heart: a statement for healthcare professionals from the Cardiac Imaging Committee of the Council on Clinical Cardiology of the American Heart Association. *Circulation* 2002;105:539–542.

108. Schuijf JD, Shaw LJ, Wijns W, *et al*. Cardiac imaging in coronary artery disease: differing modalities. *Heart* 2005;91:1110–1117.

109. Schinkel AF, Bax JJ, Geleijnse ML, *et al*. Noninvasive evaluation of ischaemic heart disease: myocardial perfusion imaging or stress echocardiography? *Eur Heart J* 2003; 24:789–800.

110. Kaufmann BA, Wei K, Lindner JR. Contrast echocardiography. *Curr Probl Cardiol* 2007; 32:51–96.

111. Weyman AE. The year in echocardiography. *J Am Coll Cardiol* 2007;49:1212–1219.

112. Metz LD, Beattie M, Hom R, Redberg RF, Grady D, Fleischmann KE. The prognostic value of normal exercise myocardial perfusion imaging and exercise echocardiography: a meta-analysis. *J Am Coll Cardiol* 2007;49:227–237.

113. Sharples L, Hughes V, Crean A, *et al*. Cost-effectiveness of functional cardiac testing in the diagnosis and management of coronary artery disease: a randomised controlled trial. The CECaT trial. *Health Technol Assess* 2007;11:iii–iv, ix–115.

114. ACCF/ASE/AHA/ASNC/HFSA/HRS/SCAI/SCCM/SCCT/SCMR 2011 Appropriate use criteria for echocardiography. *J Am Coll Cardiol* 2011;57;1126–1166.

115. Tomlinson DR, Becher H, Selvanayagam JB. Assessment of myocardial viability: comparison of echocardiography versus cardiac magnetic resonance imaging in the current era. *Heart Lung Circ* 2008;17:173–185.

116. Bax JJ, Poldermans D, Elhendy A, Boersma E, Rahimtoola SH. Sensitivity, specificity, and predictive accuracies of various noninvasive techniques for detecting hibernating myocardium. *Curr Probl Cardiol* 2001;26:147–186.

117. Bax JJ, Maddahi J, Poldermans D, *et al*. Sequential (201)Tl imaging and dobutamine echocardiography to enhance accuracy of predicting improved left ventricular ejection fraction after revascularization. *J Nucl Med* 2002;43:795–802.

118. Albouaini K, Egred M, Rao A, Alahmar A, Wright DJ. Cardiac resynchronisation therapy: evidence based benefits and patient selection. *Eur J Intern Med* 2008;19:165–172.

119. Delgado V, Ypenburg C, van Bommel RJ, *et al*. Assessment of left ventricular dyssynchrony by speckle tracking strain imaging comparison between longitudinal, circumferential, and radial strain in cardiac resynchronization therapy. *J Am Coll Cardiol* 2008;51:1944–1952.

120. Fuster V, Kim RJ. Frontiers in cardiovascular magnetic resonance. *Circulation* 2005;112: 135–144.

121. Kim RJ, Albert TS, Wible JH, *et al*. Performance of delayed-enhancement magnetic resonance imaging with gadoversetamide contrast for the detection and assessment of myocardial infarction: an international, multicenter, double-blinded, randomized trial. *Circulation* 2008;117:629–637.

122. Mahrholdt H, Wagner A, Judd RM, Sechtem U, Kim RJ. Delayed enhancement cardiovascular magnetic resonance assessment of non-ischaemic cardiomyopathies. *Eur Heart J* 2005;26:1461–1474.

123. Niendorf T, Sodickson DK. Parallel imaging in cardiovascular MRI: methods and applications. *NMR Biomed* 2006;19:325–341.

124. Klem I, Heitner JF, Shah DJ, *et al.* Improved detection of coronary artery disease by stress perfusion cardiovascular magnetic resonance with the use of delayed enhancement infarction imaging. *J Am Coll Cardiol* 2006;47:1630–1638.

125. Swaminathan S, High WA, Ranville J, *et al.* Cardiac and vascular metal deposition with high mortality in nephrogenic systemic fibrosis. *Kidney Int* 2008;73:1413–1418.

126. Saxena SK, Sharma M, Patel M, Oreopoulos D. Nephrogenic systemic fibrosis: an emerging entity. *Int Urol Nephrol* 2008;40:715–724.

127. Judd RM, Wagner A, Rehwald WG, Albert T, Kim RJ. Technology insight: assessment of myocardial viability by delayed-enhancement magnetic resonance imaging. *Nat Clin Pract Cardiovasc Med* 2005;2:150–158.

128. Thomson LE. Cardiovascular magnetic resonance in clinically suspected cardiac amyloidosis: diagnostic value of a typical pattern of late gadolinium enhancement. *J Am Coll Cardiol* 2008;51:1031–1032.

129. Maceira AM, Prasad SK, Hawkins PN, Roughton M, Pennell DJ. Cardiovascular magnetic resonance and prognosis in cardiac amyloidosis. *J Cardiovasc Magn Reson* 2008; 10:54.

130. Matoh F, Satoh H, Shiraki K, *et al.* The usefulness of delayed enhancement magnetic resonance imaging for diagnosis and evaluation of cardiac function in patients with cardiac sarcoidosis. *J Cardiol* 2008;51:179–188.

131. Steel KE, Kwong RY. Application of cardiac magnetic resonance imaging in cardiomyopathy. *Curr Heart Fail Rep* 2008;5:128–135.

132. Bohl S, Wassmuth R, Abdel-Aty H, *et al.* Delayed enhancement cardiac magnetic resonance imaging reveals typical patterns of myocardial injury in patients with various forms of non-ischemic heart disease. *Int J Cardiovasc Imaging* 2008;24:597–607.

133. Zagrosek A, Wassmuth R, Abdel-Aty H, Rudolph A, Dietz R, Schulz-Menger J. Relation between myocardial edema and myocardial mass during the acute and convalescent phase of myocarditis—a CMR study. *J Cardiovasc Magn Reson* 2008;10:19.

134. Ibrahim T, Bulow HP, Hackl T, *et al.* Diagnostic value of contrast-enhanced magnetic resonance imaging and single-photon emission computed tomography for detection of myocardial necrosis early after acute myocardial infarction. *J Am Coll Cardiol* 2007;49: 208–216.

135. Gibbons RJ, Araoz PA, Williamson EE. The year in cardiac imaging. *J Am Coll Cardiol* 2007;50:988–1003.

136. Bello D, Fieno DS, Kim RJ, *et al.* Infarct morphology identifies patients with substrate for sustained ventricular tachycardia. *J Am Coll Cardiol* 2005;45:1104–1108.

137. Bax JJ, van der Wall EE, Harbinson M. Radionuclide techniques for the assessment of myocardial viability and hibernation. *Heart* 2004;90 (Suppl 5):v26–33.

138. Kim RJ, Hillenbrand HB, Judd RM. Evaluation of myocardial viability by MRI. *Herz* 2000;25:417–430.

139. Wellnhofer E, Olariu A, Klein C, *et al.* Magnetic resonance low-dose dobutamine test is superior to SCAR quantification for the prediction of functional recovery. *Circulation* 2004;109:2172–2174.

140. Isbell DC, Kramer CM. Magnetic resonance for the assessment of myocardial viability. *Curr Opin Cardiol* 2006;21:469–472.

141. Cigarroa CG, deFilippi CR, Brickner ME, Alvarez LG, Wait MA, Grayburn PA. Dobutamine stress echocardiography identifies hibernating myocardium and predicts recovery of left ventricular function after coronary revascularization. *Circulation* 1993;88:430–436.

142. Allman KC, Shaw LJ, Hachamovitch R, Udelson JE. Myocardial viability testing and impact of revascularization on prognosis in patients with coronary artery disease and left ventricular dysfunction: a meta-analysis. *J Am Coll Cardiol* 2002;39:1151–1158.

143. Bonow RB, Maurer G, Lee KL *et al.*, for the STICH Trial Investigators. Myocardial viability and survival in ischemic left ventricular dysfunction. *N Engl J Med* 2011;364:1617–1625.

144. Wilke N, Jerosch-Herold M, Wang Y, *et al.* Myocardial perfusion reserve: assessment with multisection, quantitative, first-pass MR imaging. *Radiology* 1997;204:373–384.

145. Al-Saadi N, Nagel E, Gross M, *et al.* Noninvasive detection of myocardial ischemia from perfusion reserve based on cardiovascular magnetic resonance. *Circulation* 2000;101: 1379–1383.

146. Al-Saadi N, Nagel E, Gross M, *et al.* Improvement of myocardial perfusion reserve early after coronary intervention: assessment with cardiac magnetic resonance imaging. *J Am Coll Cardiol* 2000;36:1557–1564.

147. Schwitter J, Nanz D, Kneifel S, *et al.* Assessment of myocardial perfusion in coronary artery disease by magnetic resonance: a comparison with positron emission tomography and coronary angiography. *Circulation* 2001;103:2230–2235.

148. Paetsch I, Jahnke C, Wahl A, *et al.* Comparison of dobutamine stress magnetic resonance, adenosine stress magnetic resonance, and adenosine stress magnetic resonance perfusion. *Circulation* 2004;110:835–842.

149. Schwitter J, Wacker CM, van Rossum AC, *et al.* MR-IMPACT: comparison of perfusion-cardiac magnetic resonance with single-photon emission computed tomography for the detection of coronary artery disease in a multicentre, multivendor, randomized trial. *Eur Heart J* 2008;29:480–489.

150. Thomson LE, Fieno DS, Abidov A, *et al.* Added value of rest to stress study for recognition of artifacts in perfusion cardiovascular magnetic resonance. *J Cardiovasc Magn Reson* 2007;9:733–740.

151. Jahnke C, Nagel E, Gebker R, *et al.* Prognostic value of cardiac magnetic resonance stress tests: adenosine stress perfusion and dobutamine stress wall motion imaging. *Circulation* 2007;115:1769–1776.

152. Barclay JL, Egred M, Kruszewski K, *et al.* The relationship between transmural extent of infarction on contrast enhanced magnetic resonance imaging and recovery of contractile function in patients with first myocardial infarction treated with thrombolysis. *Cardiology* 2007;108:217–222.

153. Tarantini G, Razzolini R, Cacciavillani L, *et al.* Influence of transmurality, infarct size, and severe microvascular obstruction on left ventricular remodeling and function after primary coronary angioplasty. *Am J Cardiol* 2006;98:1033–1040.

154. Assomull RG, Prasad SK, Lyne J, *et al.* Cardiovascular magnetic resonance, fibrosis, and prognosis in dilated cardiomyopathy. *J Am Coll Cardiol* 2006;48:1977–1985.

155. Schmidt A, Azevedo CF, Cheng A, *et al.* Infarct tissue heterogeneity by magnetic resonance imaging identifies enhanced cardiac arrhythmia susceptibility in patients with left ventricular dysfunction. *Circulation* 2007;115:2006–2014.

156. White JA, Yee R, Yuan X, *et al.* Delayed enhancement magnetic resonance imaging predicts response to cardiac resynchronization therapy in patients with intraventricular dyssynchrony. *J Am Coll Cardiol* 2006;48:1953–1960.

157. Ypenburg C, Roes SD, Bleeker GB, *et al.* Effect of total scar burden on contrast-enhanced magnetic resonance imaging on response to cardiac resynchronization therapy. *Am J Cardiol* 2007;99:657–660.

158. Fraser AG, Buser PT, Bax JJ, *et al.* The future of cardiovascular imaging and non-invasive diagnosis: a joint statement from the European Association of Echocardiography, the Working Groups on Cardiovascular Magnetic Resonance, Computers in Cardiology, and Nuclear Cardiology, of the European Society of Cardiology, the European Association of Nuclear Medicine, and the Association for European Paediatric Cardiology. *Eur Heart J* 2006;27:1750–1753.

159. Hounsfield GN. Computerized transverse axial scanning (tomography). 1. Description of system. *Br J Radiol* 1973;46:1016–1022.

160. Bluemke DA, Achenbach S, Budoff M, *et al*. Noninvasive coronary artery imaging: magnetic resonance angiography and multidetector computed tomography angiography: a scientific statement from the American Heart Association Committee on cardiovascular imaging and intervention of the Council on cardiovascular radiology and intervention, and the Councils on clinical cardiology and cardiovascular disease in the young. *Circulation* 2008;118:586–606.

161. Leschka S, Oechslin E, Husmann L, *et al*. Pre- and postoperative evaluation of congenital heart disease in children and adults with 64-section CT. *Radiographics* 2007;27: 829–846.

162. Krombach GA, Niendorf T, Gunther RW, Mahnken AH. Characterization of myocardial viability using MR and CT imaging. *Eur Radiol* 2007;17:1433–1444.

163. Sra J. Cardiac image integration implications for atrial fibrillation ablation. *J Interv Card Electrophysiol* 2008;22:145–154.

164. Sra J, Narayan G, Krum D, *et al*. Computed tomography-fluoroscopy image integration-guided catheter ablation of atrial fibrillation. *J Cardiovasc Electrophysiol* 2007;18:409–414.

165. Broderick LS, Brooks GN, Kuhlman JE. Anatomic pitfalls of the heart and pericardium. *Radiographics* 2005;25:441–453.

166. Mao SS, Ahmadi N, Shah B, *et al*. Normal thoracic aorta diameter on cardiac computed tomography in healthy asymptomatic adults: impact of age and gender. *Acad Radiol* 2008;15:827–834.

167. Alkadhi H, Desbiolles L, Husmann L, *et al*. Aortic regurgitation: assessment with 64-section CT. *Radiology* 2007;245:111–121.

168. Lin FY, Devereux RB, Roman MJ, *et al*. Assessment of the thoracic aorta by multidetector computed tomography: age- and sex-specific reference values in adults without evident cardiovascular disease. *J Cardiovasc Comput Tomogr* 2008;2:298–308.

169. Lin FY, Devereux RB, Roman MJ, *et al*. Cardiac chamber volumes, function, and mass as determined by 64-multidetector row computed tomography: mean values among healthy adults free of hypertension and obesity. *J Am Coll Cardiol Imaging* 2008;1: 782–786.

170. Mahnken AH, Koos R, Katoh M, et al. Assessment of myocardial viability in reperfused acute myocardial infarction using 16-slice computed tomography in comparison to magnetic resonance imaging. *J Am Coll Cardiol* 2005;45:2042–2047.

171. Gerber BL, Belge B, Legros GJ, *et al*. Characterization of acute and chronic myocardial infarcts by multidetector computed tomography: comparison with contrast-enhanced magnetic resonance. *Circulation* 2006;113:823–833.

172. Motoyama S, Kondo T, Sarai M, *et al*. Multislice computed tomographic characteristics of coronary lesions in acute coronary syndromes. *J Am Coll Cardiol* 2007;50:319–326.

173. Schaar JA, Mastik F, Regar E, *et al*. Current diagnostic modalities for vulnerable plaque detection. *Curr Pharm Des* 2007;13:995–1001.

174. Goldstein JA, Dixon S, Safian RD, Hanzel G, Grines CL, Raff GL. Computed tomographic angiographic morphology of invasively proven complex coronary plaques. *J Am Coll Cardiol Imaging* 2008;1:249–251.

175. Lin FY, Saba S, Weinsaft JW, *et al*. Relation of plaque characteristics defined by coronary computed tomographic angiography to ST-segment depression and impaired functional capacity during exercise treadmill testing in patients suspected of having coronary heart disease. *Am J Cardiol* 2009;103:50–58.

176. Greenland P, Bonow RO, Brundage BH, *et al*. ACCF/AHA 2007 clinical expert consensus document on coronary artery calcium scoring by computed tomography in global

cardiovascular risk assessment and in evaluation of patients with chest pain: a report of the American College of Cardiology Foundation Clinical Expert Consensus Task Force (ACCF/AHA Writing Committee to Update the 2000 Expert Consensus Document on Electron Beam Computed Tomography). *Circulation* 2007;115:402–426.

177. Rumberger JA, Sheedy PF, 2nd, Breen JF, Fitzpatrick LA, Schwartz RS. Electron beam computed tomography and coronary artery disease: scanning for coronary artery calcification. *Mayo Clin Proc* 1996;71:369–377.

178. Rumberger JA, Simons DB, Fitzpatrick LA, Sheedy PF, Schwartz RS. Coronary artery calcium area by electron-beam computed tomography and coronary atherosclerotic plaque area. A histopathologic correlative study. *Circulation* 1995;92:2157–2162.

179. Achenbach S. Developments in coronary CT angiography. *Curr Cardiol Rep* 2008; 10:51–59.

180. Achenbach S. Calcification, heart rate, and diagnostic accuracy of coronary computed tomography angiography. *J Cardiovasc Comput Tomogr* 2007;1:152–154.

181. Einstein AJ, Moser KW, Thompson RC, Cerqueira MD, Henzlova MJ. Radiation dose to patients from cardiac diagnostic imaging. *Circulation* 2007;116:1290–1305.

182. Einstein AJ, Henzlova MJ, Rajagopalan S. Estimating risk of cancer associated with radiation exposure from 64-slice computed tomography coronary angiography. *JAMA* 2007;298:317–323.

183. Hausleiter J, Meyer T, Hadamitzky M, *et al*. Radiation dose estimates from cardiac multislice computed tomography in daily practice: impact of different scanning protocols on effective dose estimates. *Circulation* 2006;113:1305–1310.

184. Gutstein A, Dey D, Cheng V, *et al*. Algorithm for radiation dose reduction with helical dual source coronary computed tomography angiography in clinical practice. *J Cardiovasc Comput Tomogr* 2008;2:311–322.

185. Hausleiter J, Meyer T, Hermann F, *et al*. Estimated radiation dose associated with cardiac CT angiography. *JAMA* 2009;301:500–507.

186. Greenland P, Bonow RO, Brundage BH, *et al*. ACCF/AHA 2007 clinical expert consensus document on coronary artery calcium scoring by computed tomography in global cardiovascular risk assessment and in evaluation of patients with chest pain: a report of the American College of Cardiology Foundation Clinical Expert Consensus Task Force (ACCF/AHA Writing Committee to Update the 2000 Expert Consensus Document on Electron Beam Computed Tomography) developed in collaboration with the Society of Atherosclerosis Imaging and Prevention and the Society of Cardiovascular Computed Tomography. *J Am Coll Cardiol* 2007;49:378–402.

187. Hoff JA, Chomka EV, Krainik AJ, Daviglus M, Rich S, Kondos GT. Age and gender distributions of coronary artery calcium detected by electron beam tomography in 35,246 adults. *Am J Cardiol* 2001;87:1335–1339.

188. McClelland RL, Chung H, Detrano R, Post W, Kronmal RA. Distribution of coronary artery calcium by race, gender, and age: results from the Multi-Ethnic Study of Atherosclerosis (MESA). *Circulation* 2006;113:30–37.

189. Detrano R, Guerci AD, Carr JJ, *et al*. Coronary calcium as a predictor of coronary events in four racial or ethnic groups. *N Engl J Med* 2008;358:1336–1345.

190. Budoff MJ, Nasir K, McClelland RL, *et al*. Coronary calcium predicts events better with absolute calcium scores than age-sex-race/ethnicity percentiles: MESA (Multi-Ethnic Study of Atherosclerosis). *J Am Coll Cardiol* 2009;53:345–352.

191. Polonsky TS, McClelland RL, Jorgensen NW, *et al*. Coronary artery calcium score and risk classification for coronary heart disease prediction. *JAMA* 2010;303:1610–1616.

192. Folsom AR, Kronmal RA, Detrano RC, *et al*. Coronary artery calcification compared with carotid intima-media thickness in the prediction of cardiovascular disease

incidence: the Multi-Ethnic Study of Atherosclerosis (MESA). *Arch Intern Med* 2008;168: 1333–1339.

193. Min JK, Lin FY, Gidseg DS, *et al.* Determinants of coronary calcium conversion among patients with a normal coronary calcium scan: what is the "warranty period" for remaining normal? *J Am Coll Cardiol* 2010;55:1110–1117.

194. Berman DS, Wong ND, Gransar H, *et al.* Relationship between stress-induced myocardial ischemia and atherosclerosis measured by coronary calcium tomography. *J Am Coll Cardiol* 2004;44:923–930.

195. Arad Y, Goodman KJ, Roth M, Newstein D, Guerci AD. Coronary calcification, coronary disease risk factors, C-reactive protein, and atherosclerotic cardiovascular disease events: the St. Francis Heart Study. *J Am Coll Cardiol* 2005;46:158–165.

196. Rozanski A, Gransar H, Wong ND, *et al.* Clinical outcomes after both coronary calcium scanning and exercise myocardial perfusion scintigraphy. *J Am Coll Cardiol* 2007;49: 1352–1361.

197. Villines TC, Hulten EA, Shaw LJ, *et al.* Prevalence and severity of coronary artery disease and adverse events among symptomatic patients with coronary artery calcification scores of zero undergoing coronary computed tomography angiography. Results from the CONFIRM (Coronary CT Angiography Evaluation for Clinical Outcomes: An International Multicenter) Registry. *J Am Coll Cardiol* 2011;58: 2533–2540.

198. Cheng VY et al. Performance of the traditional age, sex, and angina typicality-based approach for estimating pretest probability of angiographically significant coronary artery disease in patients undergoing coronary computed tomographic angiography. *Circulation* 2011;124:2423–2432.

199. Mowatt G, Cook JA, Hillis GS, *et al.* 64-Slice computed tomography angiography in the diagnosis and assessment of coronary artery disease: systematic review and meta-analysis. *Heart* 2008;94:1386–1193.

200. Meijboom WB, Meijs MF, Schuijf JD, *et al.* Diagnostic accuracy of 64-slice computed tomography coronary angiography: a prospective, multicenter, multivendor study. *J Am Coll Cardiol* 2008;52:2135–2144.

201. Budoff MJ, Dowe D, Jollis JG, *et al.* Diagnostic performance of 64-multidetector row coronary computed tomographic angiography for evaluation of coronary artery stenosis in individuals without known coronary artery disease: results from the prospective multicenter ACCURACY (Assessment by Coronary Computed Tomographic Angiography of Individuals Undergoing Invasive Coronary Angiography) trial. *J Am Coll Cardiol* 2008;52:1724–1732.

202. Hausleiter J, Meyer T, Hadamitzky M, *et al.* Non-invasive coronary computed tomographic angiography for patients with suspected coronary artery disease: the Coronary Angiography by Computed Tomography with the Use of a Submillimeter resolution (CACTUS) trial. *Eur Heart J* 2007;28:3034–3041.

203. Miller JM, Rochitte CE, Dewey M, *et al.* Diagnostic performance of coronary angiography by 64-row CT. *N Engl J Med* 2008;359:2324–2336.

204. Di Carli MF, Dorbala S, Curillova Z, *et al.* Relationship between CT coronary angiography and stress perfusion imaging in patients with suspected ischemic heart disease assessed by integrated PET-CT imaging. *J Nucl Cardiol* 2007;14:799–809.

205. Hacker M, Jakobs T, Matthiesen F, *et al.* Comparison of spiral multidetector CT angiography and myocardial perfusion imaging in the noninvasive detection of functionally relevant coronary artery lesions: first clinical experiences. *J Nucl Med* 2005;46: 1294–1300.

206. Schuijf JD, Wijns W, Jukema JW, *et al*. Relationship between noninvasive coronary angiography with multi-slice computed tomography and myocardial perfusion imaging. *J Am Coll Cardiol* 2006;48:2508–2514.

207. Hacker M, Jakobs T, Hack N, *et al*. Sixty-four slice spiral CT angiography does not predict the functional relevance of coronary artery stenoses in patients with stable angina. *Eur J Nucl Med Mol Imaging* 2007;34:4–10.

208. Cademartiri F, La Grutta L, Malago R, *et al*. Prevalence of anatomical variants and coronary anomalies in 543 consecutive patients studied with 64-slice CT coronary angiography. *Eur Radiol* 2008;18:781–791.

209. Wang XM, Wu LB, Sun C, *et al*. Clinical application of 64-slice spiral CT in the diagnosis of the Tetralogy of Fallot. *Eur J Radiol* 2007;64:296–301.

210. Budoff MJ, Ahmed V, Gul KM, Mao SS, Gopal A. Coronary anomalies by cardiac computed tomographic angiography. *Clin Cardiol* 2006;29:489–493.

211. Meyer TS, Martinoff S, Hadamitzky M, *et al*. Improved noninvasive assessment of coronary artery bypass grafts with 64-slice computed tomographic angiography in an unselected patient population. *J Am Coll Cardiol* 2007;49:946–950.

212. Maintz D, Seifarth H, Raupach R, *et al*. 64-slice multidetector coronary CT angiography: in vitro evaluation of 68 different stents. *Eur Radiol* 2006;16:818–826.

213. Hecht HS, Zaric M, Jelnin V, Lubarsky L, Prakash M, Roubin G. Usefulness of 64-detector computed tomographic angiography for diagnosing in-stent restenosis in native coronary arteries. *Am J Cardiol* 2008;101:820–824.

214. Pundziute G, Schuijf JD, Jukema JW, *et al*. Prognostic value of multislice computed tomography coronary angiography in patients with known or suspected coronary artery disease. *J Am Coll Cardiol* 2007;49:62–70.

215. Gaemperli O, Valenta I, Schepis T, *et al*. Coronary 64-slice CT angiography predicts outcome in patients with known or suspected coronary artery disease. *Eur Radiol* 2008;18:1162–1173.

216. Min JK, Shaw LJ, Devereux RB, *et al*. Prognostic value of multidetector coronary computed tomographic angiography for prediction of all-cause mortality. *J Am Coll Cardiol* 2007;50:1161–1170.

217. Min JK, Shaw LJ, Berman DS, Gilmore A, Kang N. Costs and clinical outcomes in individuals without known coronary artery disease undergoing coronary computed tomographic angiography from an analysis of Medicare category III transaction codes. *Am J Cardiol* 2008;102:672–678.

218. Goldstein JA, Chinnaiyan KM, Abidov A, *et al*. The CT-STAT (Coronary Computed Tomographic Angiography for Systematic Triage of Acute Chest Pain Patients to Treatment) trial. *J Am Coll Cardiol* 2011;58:1414–1422.

219. Stillman AE, Oudkerk M, Ackerman M, *et al*. Use of multidetector computed tomography for the assessment of acute chest pain: a consensus statement of the North American Society of Cardiac Imaging and the European Society of Cardiac Radiology. *Eur Radiol* 2007;17:2196–2207.

220. Goldstein JA, Gallagher MJ, O'Neill WW, Ross MA, O'Neil BJ, Raff GL. A randomized controlled trial of multi-slice coronary computed tomography for evaluation of acute chest pain. *J Am Coll Cardiol* 2007;49:863–871.

221. Hoffmann U, Nagurney JT, Moselewski F, *et al*. Coronary multidetector computed tomography in the assessment of patients with acute chest pain. *Circulation* 2006; 114:2251–2260.

222. Hoffmann U, Pena AJ, Moselewski F, *et al*. MDCT in early triage of patients with acute chest pain. *AJR Am J Roentgenol* 2006;187:1240–1247.

223. Taylor AJ, Cerqueira M, Hodgson JM, *et al.* ACCF/SCCT/ACR/AHA/ASE/ASNC/ NASCI/SCAI/SCMR 2010 appropriate use criteria for cardiac computed tomography. A report of the American College of Cardiology Foundation Appropriate Use Criteria Task Force, the Society of Cardiovascular Computed Tomography, the American College of Radiology, the American Heart Association, the American Society of Echocardiography, the American Society of Nuclear Cardiology, the North American Society for Cardiovascular Imaging, the Society for Cardiovascular Angiography and Interventions, and the Society for Cardiovascular Magnetic Resonance. *J Am Coll Cardiol* 2010;56:1864–1894.

224. Berman DS. From the Desk of the President. President's page: Clearing the higher bar. *J Cardiovasc CT* 2009;3:63–64.

225. Tamaki N, Yonekura Y, Yamashita K, *et al.* Relation of left ventricular perfusion and wall motion with metabolic activity in persistent defects on thallium-201 tomography in healed myocardial infarction. *Am J Cardiol* 1988;62:202–208.

226. Go RT, Marwick TH, MacIntyre WJ, *et al.* A prospective comparison of rubidium-82 PET and thallium-201 SPECT myocardial perfusion imaging utilizing a single dipyridamole stress in the diagnosis of coronary artery disease. *J Nucl Med* 1990;31: 1899–1905.

227. Stewart RE, Heyl B, O'Rourke RA, Blumhardt R, Miller DD. Demonstration of differential post-stenotic myocardial technetium-99m-teboroxime clearance kinetics after experimental ischemia and hyperemic stress [see comments]. *J Nucl Med* 1991;32: 2000–2008.

228. Marwick TH, Go RT, MacIntyre WJ, Saha GB, Underwood DA. Myocardial perfusion imaging with positron emission tomography and single photon emission computed tomography: frequency and causes of disparate results. *Eur Heart J* 1991;12:1064–1069.

229. Bateman TM, Heller GV, McGhie AI, *et al.* Diagnostic accuracy of rest/stress ECG-gated Rb-82 myocardial perfusion PET: comparison with ECG-gated Tc-99m sestamibi SPECT. *J Nucl Cardiol* 2006;13:24–33.

230. Husmann L, Wiegand M, Valenta I, *et al.* Diagnostic accuracy of myocardial perfusion imaging with single photon emission computed tomography and positron emission tomography: a comparison with coronary angiography. *Int J Cardiovasc Imaging* 2008; 24:511–518.

231. Porto I, Selvanayagam JB, Van Gaal WJ, *et al.* Plaque volume and occurrence and location of periprocedural myocardial necrosis after percutaneous coronary intervention: insights from delayed enhancement magnetic resonance imaging, thrombolysis in myocardial infarction myocardial perfusion grade analysis, and intravascular ultrasound. *Circulation* 2006;114:662–669.

232. Cino JM, Pujadas S, Carreras F, *et al.* Utility of contrast-enhanced cardiovascular magnetic resonance (CE-CMR) to assess how likely is an infarct to produce a typical ECG pattern. *J Cardiovasc Magn Reson* 2006;8:335–344.

233. Valeti US, Nishimura RA, Holmes DR, *et al.* Comparison of surgical septal myectomy and alcohol septal ablation with cardiac magnetic resonance imaging in patients with hypertrophic obstructive cardiomyopathy. *J Am Coll Cardiol* 2007;49:350–357.

234. Harris MA, Johnson TR, Weinberg PM, Fogel MA. Delayed enhancement cardiovascular magnetic resonance identifies fibrous tissue in children after surgery for congenital heart disease. *J Thorac Cardiovasc Surg* 2007;133:676–681.

CHAPTER 12

Prevention of cardiovascular disease

Alice J. Owen and Christopher M. Reid
Monash University, Melbourne, VIC, Australia

Introduction

The substantial economic and social costs of cardiovascular disease (CVD) make prevention an imperative worldwide. In the USA alone, the total direct and indirect costs (including health expenditure and lost productivity) of CVD and stroke for 2010 were estimated to be US$503 billion, compared to US$228 billion for cancer [1]. In both developed and developing countries, CVD is a major cause of death. In many developing countries, where nutritional deficiencies and communicable diseases have been prominent causes of mortality, there has been a shift toward an increasing burden of mortality and morbidity associated with CVD [2]. Between 1988 and 1998 a decrease in coronary heart disease (CHD) death rates in those aged 35–74 years was noted in countries such as Australia, Sweden, and the US, associated with improved prevention and treatment, whilst countries such as Kazakhstan and Ukraine experienced substantial increases in cardiovascular mortality (Figure 12.1) [3,4]. However, it has been suggested that the gains made in CVD prevention may be undone by the looming epidemics of obesity and diabetes.

Strategies for prevention of CVD have a number of foci:
• Preventing or slowing the development of atherosclerosis through population-wide prevention strategies, e.g., smoking cessation, promotion of physical activity, healthy eating, which are less likely to have an immediately discernible/tangible effect on CVD as measured by morbidity/mortality rates.
• Preventing a first cardiovascular event or the signs or symptoms of advanced CVD in persons at high risk, e.g., those with known risk factors such as hypertension, dyslipidemia or diabetes. As this group is more likely to have a cardiovascular event in the near future, implementation of prevention strategies is more likely to have measurable effectiveness in terms of reducing CVD morbidity and mortality in the medium term.

Cardiovascular Clinical Trials: Putting the Evidence into Practice, First Edition.
Edited by Marcus D. Flather, Deepak L. Bhatt, and Tobias Geisler.
© 2013 Blackwell Publishing Ltd. Published 2013 by Blackwell Publishing Ltd.

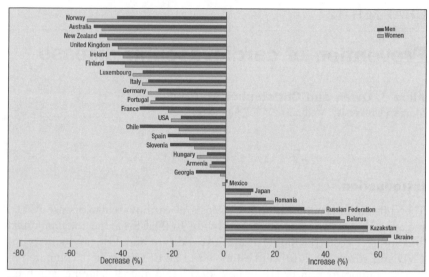

Figure 12.1 Changes in death rates from CAD, aged 35–74, 1990-2000. (Reproduced from Allender *et al.* [4].)

• Preventing subsequent cardiovascular events in those with established/ advanced CVD. This group is at greatest risk of having a cardiovascular event and is a priority for CVD prevention activities.

The first two strategies above describe *primary* prevention, while the last describes *secondary* CVD prevention. As CVD is a disease which develops over a lifetime, the greatest benefit would clearly be achieved by effective early primary prevention; however, for cost and feasibility reasons, the majority of placebo-controlled clinical trials focusing upon CVD prevention have been aimed at either those at high risk of a primary event or in the secondary prevention setting.

The goals of CVD prevention in clinical practice according to the European Fourth Joint Task Force for CVD are listed in Table 12.1.

Cardiovascular disease: etiology and assessment

Although CVD can be a consequence of congenital cardiac dysfunction, in the majority of cases, atherosclerosis is thought to be the underlying pathology leading to CVD. The critical pathways governing the initiation of an atherosclerotic lesion remain an area of ongoing discovery; however, it is currently accepted that disruption of endothelial function through inflammation and/ or injury to the vessel wall leads to the accumulation of cholesterol esters, other lipids, calcium, and cellular debris within the intima of the vessel wall. Suggested causative agents of endothelial injury include oxidized low-density lipoprotein (LDL) cholesterol, infectious agents, toxic chemicals derived from cigarette smoking, chronic inflammatory system activity, and high concentrations of blood glucose and homocysteine [5].

Table 12.1 Goals of cardiovascular disease (CVD) prevention in clinical practice.

The European Fourth Joint Task Force for CVD prevention gives the following as objectives of CVD prevention in clinical practice [7]:

1. Assist those at low risk of CVD to maintain this state lifelong and to help those at increased total CVD risk to reduce it.
2. To achieve the characteristics of people who tend to stay healthy:
No smoking
Healthy food choices
Physically active: at least 30 min of moderate activity each day
BMI <25 kg/m^2 and avoidance of central obesity
BP <140/90 mmHg
Total cholesterol <5 mmol/L (~190 mg/dL)
LDL-cholesterol <3 mmol/L (~115 mg/dL)
Blood glucose <6 mmol/L (110 mg/dL)
3. To achieve more rigorous risk factor control in high-risk subjects, especially those with CVD or diabetes:
Blood pressure under 130/80 mmHg under 130/80 mmHg if feasible
Total cholesterol <4.5 mmol/L (~175 mg/dL) with an option of <4 mmol/L (~155 mg/dL) if feasible
LDL cholesterol <2.5 mmol/L (~100 mg/dL) with an option of <2 mmol/L (~80 mg/dL) if feasible; Fasting blood glucose <6.0 mmol/L (~110 mg/dL) and glycosylated hemoglobin (HbA1c) <6.5% if feasible
4. To consider cardioprotective drug therapy in these high-risk subjects, especially for those with established atherosclerotic CVD

The effect of an intervention on CVD in large-scale prevention trials is often determined by survival analysis of "hard" outcome measures, examining the numbers of coronary (e.g., myocardial infarction [MI]) or cerebrovascular (e.g., stroke) events, or disease-specific and/or all-cause mortality in the trial population over time. Extent or progression of CVD can be assessed using measures such as carotid artery intimal–medial thickness (IMT), arterial stiffness, echocardiography, carotid artery ultrasound, magnetic resonance imaging (MRI) of the heart, and computed tomography (CT) scans of the heart and major vessels. IMT, measured by B-mode ultrasound, is a non-invasive method that has been found to be a good predictor of cardiovascular events [6]. Arterial stiffness is another widely used surrogate endpoint for CVD, and has been shown to predict risk of CVD events and mortality [7]. It can be measured either invasively or non-invasively, with European Society of Cardiology guidelines recommending aortic pulse wave velocity as the "gold standard" measure of regional aortic stiffness and a useful tool for assessment of subclinical target organ damage [8].

Landmark studies of cardiovascular disease risk

Mortality from atherosclerotic CVD grew rapidly in industrialized nations after World War II. During this time, a number of key studies in ambulant populations have been central to establishing the major factors driving this risk.

The Framingham Study is one of the earliest and best-known epidemiological studies in the field, and remains a source of data used to derive algorithms for estimating CVD risk in populations the world over. Baseline data collection commenced in 1950, and the original population sample consisted of 5127 male and female residents of the small town of Framingham, Massachusetts, USA, aged 30–59 years and free of CHD [9]. The Framingham Study subsequently extended its follow-up and evolved to include new cohorts (the children and grandchildren of the original participants) and new outcome measures and risk markers, including genetic markers of risk. The Framingham Study has provided key information about the epidemiology of CVD, particularly the relationship between blood pressure and risk of developing CVD, and age and tobacco smoking as risk factors for CVD.

Another major epidemiological study of risk of the same era was the Seven Countries Study which examined risk of heart attack and stroke in contrasting populations from Europe, Japan, and the US; it played a key role in elucidating the impact of serum cholesterol on the risk of CHD and the influence of cultural and lifestyle factors upon CVD risk [10]. The intercohort differences in CHD mortality noted in the Seven Countries Study (highest age-adjusted death rate being 288 in 1000 over 25 years in East Finland, compared to the lowest in the farming community of Tanushimaru, Japan of 45 in 1000 over 25 years [11]) were one of a number of findings which informed the development of the World Health Organization (WHO) MONICA (Multinational MONItoring of trends and determinants in CArdiovascular disease) Project. MONICA was established in the early 1980s to examine worldwide trends in CVD, monitoring a population of 10 million men and women aged 25–64 years over a decade. MONICA made an important contribution to international standardization of cardiovascular mortality, morbidity and risk factor measurement [12].

In the 1970s the MRFIT (Multiple Risk Factor Intervention Trial) screened 356 222 US males aged 35–57 years, without previous MI, for suitability for inclusion in a clinical trial to examine the effectiveness of smoking cessation, blood pressure lowering, and dietary modification interventions to reduce cardiovascular risk as compared with "usual care." The intervention trial enrolled 12 866 participants and has achieved notoriety as a classic example of confounding, as it appeared that the control "usual care" group voluntarily adopted the lifestyle changes [13]. However, the MRFIT Group also utilized the screening data to form a powerful cohort with standardized serum cholesterol measurements and long-term mortality follow-up. In 1986 it reported a continuous, graded, and strong relationship between serum cholesterol and 6-year risk of CHD death, which held for all risk groups [14]. Of all CHD deaths, 46% were estimated by MRFIT to be excess deaths attributable to serum cholesterol of 4.65 mmol/L (180 mg/dL) or greater.

A number of large-scale clinical trials and registries have informed our understanding of the risk and prevention of secondary CVD. These include the EUROASPIRE survey which aimed to describe clinical practice in Europe in relation to secondary prevention of CHD following the 1994 publication of joint recommendations for prevention of CHD in clinical practice [15]. The Euro Heart Survey pooled a number of CVD surveys and registries including those examining acute coronary syndromes, diabetes, heart failure, stable angina, adult CHD, atrial fibrillation and percutaneous coronary interventions to assess CVD clinical guideline adherence and compare clinical practice across Europe. The multinational REACH and GRACE registries have examined treatment and outcomes in those with atherothrombosis and acute coronary events, respectively [16].

Key risk factors

Major epidemiological studies of CVD, including the selection described above, have elucidated key risk factors for CVD and allowed us to estimate the proportion of risk attributable to individual risk factors. International studies have shown that the contributions of these risk factors may vary slightly between populations, but the major CVD risk factors remain largely consistent across populations and over time. This is well demonstrated by the INTERHEART case–control study which found that over 90% of the age-standardized risk of an initial acute MI could be attributed to nine key modifiable risk factors; smoking, hypertension, diabetes, abdominal obesity, high ApoB/ApoA1 ratio, diet, exercise, fruit and vegetable intake, and psychosocial factors. The odds ratios for these risk factors were directionally similar across all countries and ethnic groups in INTERHEART; however, some quantitative differences were apparent [17].

Lipids
Elevated LDL-cholesterol is a major risk factor for CVD, with the majority of blood cholesterol usually carried in the LDL fraction. LDL-cholesterol lowering treatment, in particular with statin therapy, is one of the most widely demonstrated CVD preventive strategies, supported by a large number of high-quality, randomized, placebo-controlled clinical trials. A meta-analysis of more than 90000 participants in 14 statin trials found that for every 1 mmol/L reduction in LDL-cholesterol there was a 21% reduction in major vascular events [18]. Reduction of LDL-cholesterol is now a central component of CVD risk reduction programs.

High-density lipoprotein (HDL) is considered cardioprotective due to its ability to facilitate reverse cholesterol transport, but it has also been shown to have anti-inflammatory and antioxidant activity, and to inhibit smooth muscle proliferation. These functions are important in preventing or slowing development of atherosclerotic lesions, and low levels of HDL are a significant risk factor for CVD [19]. The presence of low HDL combined with elevated levels of fasting plasma triglyceride commonly occurs in groups at elevated risk of CVD, such as those with diabetes or renal disease, and these dyslipidemias are important risk factors in these patient groups.

Lipoprotein(a) [Lp(a)] is an LDL-like lipoprotein associated with significant, although modest, increases in vascular disease risk [20]. The amounts of Lp(a) are regulated substantially by genetics rather than the dietary factors commonly associated with increased LDL. Lp(a) contains a unique protein component called apolipoprotein(a), comprised of a variable number of kringle IV-type 2 repeats, giving apolipoprotein(a) homology with plasminogen, which is thought to confer enhanced atherogenicity to the lipoprotein. Copy number variation within the LPA gene determines the size of the apolipoprotein(a) isoform and influences plasma levels of Lp(a); however, regulation of Lp(a) remains incompletely understood. The PROCARDIS Consortium recently utilized single-nucleotide polymorphism arrays to examine the associations between LPA gene variants and CVD. It found two genetic variants in the LPA gene associated with both increased Lp(a) levels and increased risk of coronary disease, with these two common variants explaining 36% of the variation in Lp(a) levels [21].

Each LDL, intermediate-density lipoprotein (IDL), very low-density lipoprotein (VLDL), and Lp(a) carries one copy of apolipoprotein B_{100} (commonly abbreviated to ApoB), whilst HDL contains the unique apolipoprotein A1 (apoA1). The ratio of blood levels of these apolipoproteins (ApoB/ApoA1) is sometimes used as a marker of cholesterol-associated CVD risk, and has been found to account for more than 50% of the attributable risk of MI in INTER-HEART [17]. In an analysis combining 68 long-term prospective studies, it was shown that measurement of the apolipoproteins as opposed to cholesterol levels does not offer any additional discrimination for vascular disease risk [22], which is also supported by analysis of CHD risk in the Framingham cohort [23].

The major lipid clinical guidelines, including the National Cholesterol Education Panel (NCEP) Adult Treatment Panel III (ATPIII) guidelines [24], have a strong focus on targeting LDL-cholesterol levels. There has been a shift toward tailoring of LDL-cholesterol goals for specific CVD risk groups, with overall CVD risk level and presence of certain risk factors driving both the LDL target goal and the suggested treatment modalities. Both the strength of the relationship between LDL-cholesterol and CVD mortality and the efficacy of LDL-cholesterol–lowering therapies are driving this focus. Whilst low HDL-cholesterol is also a strong and independent risk factor, therapeutic options for raising HDL are limited if behavioral and lifestyle changes fail to address the low HDL levels, with convincing long-term mortality outcome data for pharmacological HDL-raising therapies yet to be obtained.

Blood pressure

Worldwide, half of the burden of ischemic heart disease and stroke is attributable to high blood pressure [25]. The incidence of hypertension has been growing steadily, and those in the US who are normotensive at age 55 years now have a 90% lifetime risk of developing hypertension [26]. It should be noted that the threshold levels used to classify hypertension (≥140/90 mmHg) are an artificial construct used mostly to assist clinicians, patients, and healthcare funders with treatment decisions. It has become apparent that the relationship between cardiovascular risk and blood pressure is a continuum, at least down to levels of 115/75 mmHg [27].

A meta-analysis of more than 460 000 participants in 147 randomized blood pressure-lowering drug trials found a 22% reduction in risk of CHD and 41% reduction in risk of stroke with a lowering of 10 mmHg systolic or 5 mmHg diastolic [28]. In practice there remains a significant degree of lost therapeutic benefit in antihypertensive treatment. Even amongst those who are treated for hypertension, the proportion reaching their target blood pressure goals is often less than 50% [29]. In those with comorbidities such as renal disease, diabetes, and heart failure, achievement of blood pressure targets is particularly important to limit target-organ damage, and aggressive antihypertensive treatment using two or more antihypertensive agents is often required. Consideration of 24-hour control of blood pressure may be necessary, particularly in those with blunted nocturnal dipping, requiring careful attention to time and type of antihypertensive agent administration.

Smoking

Smoking is clearly associated with adverse health outcomes, in those who smoke and also in those exposed to second-hand smoke. Smoking is a well-defined, strong, independent risk factor for CVD. The INTERHEART study found that the risk of MI increased by 5.6% for every additional cigarette smoked per day [30]. Smoking cessation is an effective CVD prevention strategy; within 3 years of quitting, risk of MI in INTERHEART had almost halved [30]. Even in those with established coronary disease, smoking cessation has been shown to confer a 36% relative risk reduction in mortality [31].

As can be seen in Table 12.2 [32], smoking cessation is a tremendously cost-effective intervention for reducing CVD burden. This population modeling suggests that smoking cessation is the only intervention that will save money in the long term, with the savings achieved through reductions in cardiovascular events offsetting the costs of the intervention program (Table 12.1). Low-dose aspirin use by individuals at high risk of developing CVD is the next most cost-effective intervention at a population level. The arbitrary, but often accepted, level at which an intervention is considered cost-effective is around US$50 000. This will clearly vary with the ability of the healthcare decision-maker to fund the cost of the intervention.

Diabetes and metabolic syndrome

The worldwide prevalence of diabetes is increasing, with estimates suggesting that it may affect up to 300 million people by the year 2030 [33]. CVD is the major cause of mortality in diabetes, and diabetes has been shown to be associated with a two- to four-fold increase in risk of fatal CVD [34]. The impaired postprandial response in diabetes results in elevated levels of glucose and triglycerides, associated with increased oxidative stress, inflammation, and endothelial dysfunction [35]. The majority of the day is spent in

Table 12.2 Modeling effects of interventions over 30 years on outcomes and costs in the US population. (Data from Kahn *et al.* [32].)

Cost/benefit over 30-year period of CVD prevention activities in model US population, assuming maximum feasible performance of intervention*	Cost (US$)/QALY[a]
Provide aspirin if 10-year MI risk ≥10%	2779
Lower LDL-cholesterol to <160 mg/dL (4.1 mmol/L) in low-risk individuals	272061
Lower LDL-cholesterol to <130 mg/dL (3.3 mmol/L) in high-risk individuals	83327
Lower LDL-cholesterol to <100 mg/dL (2.6 mmol/L) in those with coronary artery disease	39130
Lower blood pressure to ≤140/90 mmHg in individuals without diabetes	52983
Lower HbA1C to <7.0% in individuals with diabetes	48759
Lower blood pressure to ≤130/80 mmHg in individuals with diabetes	25317
Lower LDL-cholesterol to <100 mg/dL (2.6 mmol/L) in individuals with diabetes	67199
Reduce fasting plasma glucose to <110 mg/dL (6.1 mmol/L) in those with impaired fasting glucose	17478
Smoking cessation	−1755
Reduce weight to body mass index (BMI) <30 kg/m²	18941

[a]QALY refers to quality-adjusted life year and is used to measure the effect of a treatment/ intervention on both quantity and quality of life. A QALY of 1 denotes 1 year of life in perfect health, while 1 year of life with a reduced quality of life is calculated as a fraction of 1.

a postprandial state for most persons in developed countries, and a number of studies have shown that postprandial blood glucose is a better predictor of cardiovascular events than fasting blood glucose in diabetes [36], although most CVD risk assessment tools still use fasting glucose. Individuals with diabetes are also at greater risk of developing hypertension due to sympathetic overactivity, with salt retention and stimulation of renin–angiotensin–aldosterone system activity.

Metabolic syndrome is a risk factor for both CVD and diabetes, but it should be noted that historically, depending upon the criteria used to classify metabolic syndrome, it can be either inclusive or exclusive of diabetes itself. The ATP III and the International Diabetes Federation definitions use the clustering of three or more cardiometabolic risk factors, which include central obesity, elevated plasma triglycerides, low HDL, hypertension, and insulin resistance [37]. In contrast, the WHO definition of metabolic syndrome uses diabetes as a core criterion with the additional clustering of two or three other cardiometabolic risk factors.

In a cohort of US men in whom diabetes and metabolic syndrome status was assessed using ATP III criteria, metabolic syndrome was associated with a two-fold increase in CVD mortality risk, while diabetes (either with or without metabolic syndrome) was associated with a three-fold increase in risk [38], highlighting the need to aggressively address CVD risk in patients with diabetes, regardless of their metabolic syndrome status. In INTERHEART, metabolic syndrome defined by WHO and IDF criteria was associated with increased risk of MI (OR, 2.69 and 2.20, respectively), compared to MI risks for diabetes (OR, 2.72), hypertension (OR, 2.60), central obesity (OR, 1.32), and low HDL (OR, 1.30) [39].

Obesity

Obesity, defined as a body mass index (BMI) of greater than $30 \, kg/m^2$, has been shown to be associated with a variety of adverse health outcomes, including cardiovascular health outcomes. The increasing prevalence of obesity is of concern, with rates of around 30% for Australia and the UK, 40% in the US, and up to 70% in some Pacific island nations in 2005 [40]. Obesity is associated with increased blood pressure, reduced arterial compliance, impaired glucose handling, and heightened inflammation. BMI has been the most commonly reported measure of obesity in clinical trials; however, it has been suggested that central or abdominal obesity may be more atherogenic, in particular visceral (intra-abdominal) obesity [41]. Whilst waist circumference does not have the ability to distinguish between visceral and subcutaneous abdominal fat, it is the most readily accessible measure for central obesity in clinical practice and large-scale clinical trials.

Weight loss is generally associated with improvements in risk factors, such as glucose handling, arterial compliance, blood pressure, and lipids [42]; however, whether this translates to reductions in cardiovascular mortality has yet to be firmly established. Long-term prospective studies have been complicated by the difficulties in distinguishing whether or not weight loss was intentional (i.e., whether related to illness or a personal choice independent of ill-health), and long-term follow-up of weight-loss intervention trials is hampered by the considerable difficulties in maintaining weight stability following weight-loss interventions.

Psychosocial factors

Depression, hostility, and anxiety have all been found to be associated with increased risk of CHD and cardiovascular mortality, with INTERHEART finding that almost 30% of the attributable risk of MI could be accounted for by psychosocial factors [17]. In a Scottish population-based study, socioeconomic deprivation was shown to be associated with increased risk of presence of an atherosclerotic plaque and elevated IMT, even after accounting for traditional and emerging CVD risk factors [43].

Non-modifiable risk factors

Sex and age are strong predictors of risk of CVD. Lifetime risk of developing CHD at age 40 years is almost 50% for men and just over 30% for women [44]. Family history of CVD (particularly CVD occurring in first-degree relatives below the age of 60 years) is an independent predictor of CVD [45]. In some cases there are clearly defined gene variants which show association with CVD. One of the most common and earliest described was the LDL-receptor (*LDL-R*) gene variant associated with familial hypercholesterolemia (FH), which results in plasma cholesterol levels more than twice that of normal. Associations between apolipoprotein E gene (*APOE*) polymorphisms and atherosclerotic disease have been found [46]; however, whether *APOE* gene variants are a predictor independent of other risk factors such as cholesterol remains to be firmly established. At the time of writing, genome-wide association screening approaches have been used to identify more than a dozen loci associated with MI or CAD, with about half of these associated with LDL or Lp(a) [47]. The Coronary Artery Disease Genome-wide Replication and Meta-analysis (CARDIoGRAM) Collaboration unifies the major genome-wide association studies to bring together more than 22 000 cases and more than 60 000 controls, and should make a substantial contribution to our understanding of common genetic variations and risk of MI and CAD [48]. At present, there is no convincing randomized trial evidence to support the cost-effectiveness of genome-wide screening of genetic markers for cardiovascular risk prediction, although companies offering such services have begun to proliferate. Furthering our understanding of the complex interactions between genes and environment is likely to be important in advancing the utility of genetic risk markers.

New biomarkers

Emerging biomarkers for CVD risk, including those relating to inflammation (e.g., C-reactive protein [CRP], interleukin-6), hemostasis (fibrinogen, von Willebrand factor), oxidative stress (oxidized LDL, advanced glycation end-products), renal function (cystatin-C), and myocardial dysfunction (B-type natriuretic peptide, BNP) are being evaluated for their potential to assist clinicians with prevention and treatment of CVD.

CRP is an acute-phase inflammatory marker produced by hepatic and adipose tissue in response to inflammatory stress. In contrast to other acute-phase inflammatory markers it is more stable (with a half-life of ~18 hours), and the development of highly sensitive immunoassays has enabled quantification of CRP levels across the normal range (i.e., high-sensitivity CRP or hs-CRP), making random sampling of CRP feasible. A number of observational studies have noted relationships between elevated hs-CRP and adverse cardiovascular events [49,50], although the pathophysiology of CRP has yet to be defined. A meta-analysis of CRP in the secondary CVD prevention setting suggested its value as a prognostic biomarker in those with stable coronary disease was inconclusive [51]. As it currently stands, the available evidence would suggest that whilst CRP has associations with risk of CVD, these are not causal [52].

Lipoprotein-associated phospholipase A_2 (Lp-PLA$_2$) is a subtype of the phospholipase A_2 enzyme family which hydrolyze phospholipids and oxidized phospholipids into potent proinflammatory and proatherogenic mediators. Associated with LDL, Lp(a), and HDL, Lp-PLA$_2$ has been suggested to play a critical role in atherogenesis and its clinical sequelae. A meta-analysis of a number of prospective studies examining Lp-PLA$_2$ and risk of CVD has found that both Lp-PLA$_2$ activity and mass have continuous associations with risk of CHD and vascular mortality [53].

BNP is a polypeptide secreted by ventricular myocytes in response to increased ventricular stretch and wall tension. Active BNP or the more stable N-terminal proBNP (NT-proBNP) have proven useful for guiding pharmacological therapy in chronic heart failure, associated with improvement in the proportions of patients reaching medication dose targets and reductions in all-cause mortality in patients younger than 75 years [54]. The usefulness of BNP to predict CVD risk outside the heart failure setting remains to be established, with a recent meta-analysis suggesting that measurement of BNP afforded only modest improvement in discrimination of CVD risk above that of traditional risk factors [55].

Elevated levels of the amino acid metabolite homocysteine may be caused by aging, renal function impairment, nutritional deficiencies, genetics, and some drugs, and can be reduced by folic acid and vitamin B_{12} supplementation. A meta-analysis of 20 prospective studies found that a 5 µmol/L increase in plasma homocysteine level was associated with a 32% increase in risk of ischemic heart disease and a 59% increase in risk of stroke [56]. As renal disease is associated with both substantially increased risk of CVD and risk of hyperhomocysteinemia, this population has been a focus of clinical trials of folate/vitamin B supplementation, which have had mostly unremarkable results. The increasingly widespread practice in many developed countries of supplementing grain and other food products with folate (primarily for prevention of neural tube defects in pregnancy), has been suggested as a possible reason that the results of clinical trials of vitamin B/folate supplementation for CVD prevention have been equivocal.

Risk assessment

Concept of risk assessment

The aim of cardiovascular risk assessment is to be more effective in identifying those at risk and to facilitate more efficient use of treatment and prevention resources, as opposed to the traditional approach of addressing individual risk factors through separate clinical guidelines for each individual factor.

The tools used for assessment of an individual's future risk of developing CVD are derived from multifactorial probabilistic causal models of CVD arising from the substantial volume of cardiovascular epidemiological data collected over the past few decades. Key cardiovascular risk factors are imputed into multiple variable risk prediction equations to estimate the numerical probability that the individual will develop CVD within a defined time-frame (*absolute risk*).

The *relative risk* is the ratio of the *absolute risk* of the individual (or group) to that of a low-risk group. The denominator in the relative risk calculation could be either the whole population or a group with low levels of the risk factors contributing to the risk algorithm. Whilst relative risk has been suggested to be a useful tool for clinicians and patients to gauge the level of risk relative to healthy peers, many clinical guidelines worldwide have moved toward the use of *absolute* CVD risk assessment in clinical practice. Absolute risk assessment has the ability to provide a clearer assessment of overall risk than that achieved by examining single risk factors, and is particularly useful in identifying those at greatest risk for targeting of treatment and prevention strategies which might be cost-effective only when applied to those at highest risk of disease.

Risk scores and quantitative assessment

Although derived from a cohort who were primarily Caucasian residents of a small town in a specific area of the US in the middle of the last century, the series of risk scores developed from the Framingham cohort continues to form the basis of risk calculators used around the world. A large number of risk calculators built upon the Framingham risk algorithm are derived from those published by Anderson *et al.* in 1991 [57]. The most recently released Framingham equation [58] uses slightly different endpoints and no longer distinguishes between fatal and non-fatal cardiovascular events.

There are a number of important considerations and limitations to these (and all other) risk equations which ought to be considered:

• The populations from which the algorithms are derived and how comparable/relevant they are to the individual/group under consideration in the risk assessment

• The outcomes/endpoints collected by the study, which form the basis of the risk equation, and how these are defined: Does the equation distinguish fatal and non-fatal events? What types of cardiovascular diseases/events have been used in calculating the risk score?

• Necessity/potential for application of population-specific disease-free survival rates within the equation

• How the changing population environment in terms of contemporary clinical management and CVD epidemiology might impact upon the mathematical model underpinning the equation.

With wider application of these risk scores, it has become evident that Framingham may overpredict risk in some populations [59] and underpredict it in others [60]. In light of this, the Systematic Coronary Risk Estimation (SCORE) Project aimed to develop a European primary prevention risk estimation tool for use in clinical practice, assembled from existing cohorts across Europe. The individual cohorts contributing data to SCORE did not uniformly collect information on diabetes, so this was not included in the algorithm. As diabetes imposes a three-fold increase in risk of fatal CHD [34], and the impact of risk factors such as blood pressure might be magnified in diabetes [61], this omission was a significant limitation, which was addressed by the United Kingdom Prospective Diabetes Study (UKPDS) group. The UKPDS risk score is designed for estimation of absolute risk of CHD and stroke in type II diabetes, and it has been shown to be a better predictor of risk than Framingham or SCORE [62].

Emerging biomarkers of CVD risk are yet to show improvements in CVD risk prediction of a magnitude sufficient to include them in the most commonly used CVD risk prediction scores. Obesity and metabolic syndrome are strongly related to a number of CVD risk factors such as dyslipidemia, hypertension, and inflammation, but modeling of large-scale studies and risk equations have suggested that the risk imposed by obesity is already largely covered in other aspects of risk assessment, and that addition of obesity to risk equations does not add substantially to CVD risk assessment [63,64].

Risk assessment in the clinic

Some patients will be at high risk because they have established CVD, comorbidities associated with a high CVD risk (e.g., chronic kidney disease or diabetes), or very high-risk levels of an individual risk factor (e.g., diagnosed with a familial dyslipidemia). In these cases, risk stratification using risk assessment charts may be less useful in guiding treatment or preventive strategies, but it is these patients who are of highest priority for clinic-based CVD prevention activities and absolute risk assessment may be useful as a patient educational tool.

The American College of Cardiology Foundation/American Heart Association 2009 performance measures for primary prevention of CVD in adults recommend global risk assessment for all male patients 35 years and over, and all female patients 45 years and over at an interval of at least every 5 years. In those at increased risk, CVD risk assessment should be undertaken more frequently [65]. A 2006 survey of use of CVD risk assessment scores by physicians in Europe and North, South, and Central America found that almost 50% reported regular use of CVD risk scores, with the time taken for assessment being the major reason for non-use of risk scores [66].

Population-based prevention

Tobacco

Tobacco use is one of the most important avoidable causes of CVD worldwide. The WHO Framework Convention on Tobacco Control seeks parties to the convention to address tobacco use through a number of strategies which include: development of a national infrastructure for tobacco control (government units either stand-alone or within health ministries) which is protected from commercial or other vested interests of the tobacco industry; price and tax measures to reduce tobacco consumption; protection from tobacco smoke in enclosed spaces; packaging and labeling of tobacco products; bans on tobacco advertising and sponsorship; educational public health campaigns; and accessibility of smoking cessation programs. Some strategies, such as plain labeling of tobacco products have not been tested, and a proposal in Australia to implement this measure is being vehemently resisted by the tobacco industry [67]. Increasing cigarette cost and exposure to tobacco control media campaigns have been shown to reduce population smoking prevalence, whilst in that study nicotine replacement therapies had no impact on population smoking prevalence [68]. Workplace smoking bans are effective tools to reduce both smoking prevalence and the number of cigarettes consumed by smokers [69], and are associated with reduced rates of acute MI [70]. Concerns have been raised that the rapidly evolving information technology environment may undermine the effectiveness of tobacco advertising bans, e.g., through social networking media [71].

Lifestyle
Physical inactivity, diet, and obesity are important modifiable issues for CVD prevention, and addressing these issues should be part of first-line therapy for CVD prevention.

A number of dietary interventions have been extensively examined under clinical trial conditions for their medium-term impact on CVD risk factor levels; these include the DASH (Dietary Approaches to Stop Hypertension) diet, Mediterranean-style diets, and high protein diets. The DASH diet (rich in fruit, vegetables, and low-fat dairy, and relatively low in saturated and total fat) was shown to significantly reduce blood pressure: by (systolic/diastolic) 5.5/3.0 mmHg overall and 11.4/5.5 mmHg in those with hypertension [72]. A 2006 study comparing examples of these three diet types found all were able to reduce blood pressure, LDL-cholesterol, and estimated 10-year risk of CHD [73]. Individualized, intensive lifestyle modification programs are effective in reducing CVD risk factors, but across an entire population the costs of supporting such interventions in the long-term are prohibitive.

The effect of dietary saturated fat on plasma cholesterol is well described, and clinical guidelines for lowering CVD risk universally advocate lowering of dietary saturated fat intake by individuals. Evidence has shown that *trans*-fatty acids also powerfully raise LDL-cholesterol, in addition to lowering HDL-cholesterol [74]. *Trans*-fats are formed in substantial quantities during partial hydrogenation of liquid vegetable oils for use in margarines, commercial cooking, and food processing. Mandatory restrictions on commercial use of *trans*-fats appears to be a more effective method for reducing their intake than voluntary reductions, food labeling, and education [75], and modeling of data from prospective studies suggests that in the US between 6% and 19% of CHD events could be avoided with a substantial reduction of *trans*-fats in the food supply [74].

Conversely, intake of very long chain omega-3 polyunsaturated fats (eicosapentaenoic acid [EPA] and docosahexaenoic acid [DHA] found in significant quantities in fish) has been shown to be associated with a reduced CVD risk [76]. American Heart Association (AHA) guidelines suggest that in those with established CVD, 1000 mg/day EPA + DHA should be consumed (through diet and/or supplements), whereas for primary prevention at least 500 mg/day EPA + DHA is recommended (which can generally be achieved through consumption of two meals of fatty fish per week) [77]. The landmark GISSI studies have provided randomized controlled trial evidence of the effectiveness of very long chain omega-3 fatty acids in reducing cardiovascular mortality, with a 36% reduction in cardiovascular mortality seen post MI (GISSI-P) [78], and a 9% reduction in all-cause mortality on top of best-practice pharmacotherapy in heart failure (GISSI-HF) [79] seen with a 880 mg/day DHA + EPA dose. In a Japanese hypercholesterolemic patient group supplemented with 1800 mg of EPA (and with a higher population background intake of EPA + DHA in the diet), the Japan EPA Lipid Intervention Study noted a 19% reduction in major coronary events in those with a history of CAD [80]. As EPA and DHA have a wide variety of effects on the cardiovascular system, including antiarrhythmic and anti-inflammatory effects [81], the optimal dose for CVD prevention may vary between different patient populations.

A large-scale meta-analysis of usual blood pressure and vascular mortality, combining data from more than one million adults, found that even small proportional differences in blood pressure (in the order of 2 mmHg systolic) had the potential to result in a 10% reduction in stroke mortality and 7% reduction in mortality from ischemic heart disease and other causes [27]. Reductions in this order are potentially achievable by reducing daily salt intake by approximately 4 g/day (approximately one-third to one-half of daily intake) [82]. Advice to reduce salt intake is often difficult to follow, particularly when processed foods form a significant portion of the diet as these foods are thought to provide 75–80% of daily salt intake in developed nations. It has been suggested that reductions of this level could be achieved by mandated reductions in salt in the food supply, but it remains to be determined whether this could be achieved and what the implications would be for other aspects of dietary intake (e.g., sugar and fat, which may be substituted for the salt).

In the Aerobics Center Longitudinal Study from the US, low physical fitness was an independent predictor of mortality in both men and women, and was a stronger predictor in women. It also appeared that the risk associated with low physical fitness was of similar magnitude to that of other traditional CVD mortality risks, such as cholesterol and blood pressure [83]. Most clinical guidelines for CVD prevention now advocate at least 30 minutes of physical activity on all or most days of the week.

The expense and logistical implications of large-scale, event-driven, randomized trials of diet and physical activity make such trials largely unaffordable in most settings. Interesting observations have however been drawn from studies at the population level. The economic crisis in Cuba between 1989 and 2000 arising from the longstanding US trade embargo coupled with the loss of the Soviet Union as a trading partner following its collapse in 1989, resulted in dramatic reductions in the local availability of fuel supplies and food. This led to significant reductions in per capita energy intake and increased energy expenditure associated with greater use of walking and cycling for transport. Population-wide weight loss was noted, with the prevalence of obesity halving. The rates of mortality associated with diabetes and CHD decreased by 51% and 35%, respectively [84]. While causality cannot be definitively attributed within an observational epidemiological study such as this, and the "intervention" is clearly not one we would consider implementing, this study does provide further support for the importance of diet and physical activity in CVD prevention.

Adherence to advice to undertake at least 30 minutes of physical activity on a daily basis, reduce dietary salt intake, eat a diet low in saturated and *trans*-fats, and limit intake of highly processed foods is likely to be beneficial for cardiovascular health for all individuals, regardless of their level of CVD risk. The experience with uptake of these behaviors, in light of the considerable amounts of time and effort expended in promotion of such public health messages, suggests that it is "much easier said than done." Public health policy initiatives addressing these issues need to consider a wide range of influences, including urban planning (e.g., environments that facilitate physical activity), occupational issues, regulation of the food supply, and tax-based incentives to modify behavior (e.g., those used for tobacco and alcohol) amongst others.

Alcohol

The much vaunted "French paradox," which was used to describe the lower than expected rate of CVD in France given their relatively high-saturated fat diet, was suggested to be due the consumption of red wine. There exists a J-shaped curve in the relationship between alcohol consumption and CVD, with those consuming low-to-moderate amounts of alcohol having fewer CVD events than abstainers, while chronic alcohol consumption and binge-drinking are associated with increased risk of cardiovascular events [85]. However, it should be noted that there is insufficient evidence to suggest that non-drinkers should commence modest alcohol consumption for cardiovascular disease prevention.

Clinical trials that have informed our management of preventing CAD and other vascular diseases

Over the last 60 years, no other area of clinical medicine has had the extent of clinical trial activity as has CVD. Sound and extensive epidemiological evidence relating key risk factors, such as high blood pressure and elevated blood cholesterol levels, to the occurrence of coronary events began to accumulate in the middle part of the 20th century. The evidence base for risk factor intervention and management has since developed as a result of a number of key landmark clinical trials. The initiation and advancement of clinical trial activity in this area resulted from three critical "enabling factors." First, western industrialized countries were facing a CVD epidemic following the end of the World War II. Second, new drugs, particularly diuretics, had been developed and were highly effective in lowering blood pressure levels. Finally, the science of undertaking clinical trials had progressed with the development of multicenter clinical trial methodology, governance, and the statistical approaches required to analyze the comparative effectiveness of different treatment regimens on major clinical outcomes such as death and disability from CVD. The stage was now set for launching a new era in developing a robust evidence base for tackling the major killer in the western world.

High blood pressure

The early trials in high blood pressure in the 1950s focused predominantly on malignant hypertension and it was not until the 1960s that the first trial in essential or moderate hypertension was undertaken [86]. The Veterans Administration (VA) Cooperative Study was innovative in that it was the first long-term, multicenter, controlled trial in any type of CVD; setting the standards that are required to this day [87]. The VA study demonstrated convincingly the effectiveness of drug treatment in preventing the complications associated with hypertension in terms of reducing morbidity and mortality from cardiovascular events. Until this study was published in the 1960s, it was not accepted by most physicians that by controlling blood pressure with drug treatment, even without knowing the exact cause, cardiovascular event prevention was possible.

Over the next 20 years, the focus on prevention was further highlighted with the conduct of a number of hypertension studies, including the Hypertension Detection and Follow-up program [88], Australian National Blood Pressure Study [89], Medical Research Clinical Trial in Mild Hypertension [90], and European Working Party on High Blood Pressure in the Elderly (EWPHE) Trial [91]. Each of these studies furthered our understanding of the importance of lowering systolic and diastolic blood pressure across a range of elevated levels and age groups.

By 1990, the role of blood pressure and its lowering through antihypertensive treatment had been examined in nine prospective studies involving over 420 000 subjects followed for intervals of 6–25 years. This work demonstrated log-linear increases in the primary incidence of stroke and CHD with increasing levels of blood pressure [92]. Importantly, it projected that the 5–6-mmHg reduction in blood pressure normally seen in antihypertensive treatment studies would be expected to be associated with a reduction in stroke of about 35–40% and in coronary events of about 20–25%. A meta-analytic investigation of 14 randomized controlled studies involving 37 000 patients and 190 000 patient-years of follow-up, confirmed expected reduction in fatal and nonfatal stroke (42%), but concluded that the observed reduction in coronary events fell short (14%; 95% CI 4–22%) of the potential gain expected from the epidemiological studies [93]. Several factors were proposed to explain this apparent lack of benefit, including the balance of the net effect of blood pressure reduction weighed against any potential adverse effects of particular agents on other cardiovascular risk factors.

However, by the 1990s, the question of whether or not physicians should attempt to lower blood pressure in people with elevated blood pressure was diminishing as the evidence from these randomized trials was becoming very clear. The question was instead being refined towards whether different therapies influenced different outcomes and whether better outcomes could be achieved with lower levels of attained blood pressure.

Apart from two early studies comparing the effects of beta-blockers and diuretics to prevent cardiovascular events in hypertensive men [94,95], the last decade has seen a proliferation of comparative outcome studies looking at different blood pressure-lowering strategies in different populations. Much of the focus has been on newer versus older drug regimens with the underlying hypothesis that newer regimens will provide advantages beyond blood pressure lowering, and thus bring greater benefit in terms of disease prevention in comparison to the older regimens. All of these studies have strengths and weaknesses, but the common theme is that they have each provided further evidence to inform guidelines for practicing physicians as to appropriate management strategies to prevent disease.

The focus will now shift to a critical examination of two of these more recent studies in terms of their design, conduct, and reporting, and how this has further influenced current management practices in relation to blood pressure control for the prevention of cardiovascular events.

ASCOT–BPLA (Anglo-Scandinavian Cardiac Outcomes Trial–Blood Pressure Lowering)

ASCOT–BPLA was a prospective, multicenter randomized controlled trial in which 19257 patients (47–79 years) were randomly allocated to receive a calcium channel blocker (amlodipine; 5–10 mg) plus an angiotensin-converting enzyme (ACE)-inhibitor (perindopril; 4–8 mg) versus a beta-blocker (atenolol; 50–100 mg) plus a diuretic (bendroflumethiazide; 1.25–2.5 mg) (Table 12.3 and Figure 12.2). Treatment was titrated to achieve blood pressure targets of less than 140/90 mmHg for patients without diabetes or less than 130/80 mmHg for patients with diabetes. The study design was a prospective, randomized open-label, blinded endpoint study (PROBE) [96].

At study closure, blood pressure levels were lowered by an average of 28/18 mmHg in patients those on the amlodipine-based regimen and 26/16 mmHg in those on the atenolol-based regimen. The primary endpoints upon which the study was powered were non-fatal MI (including silent MI) and fatal CHD, and the intended duration of the study was to be the longer of either an average period of 5 years or until 1150 primary endpoint events had accrued. However, the study was stopped prematurely at 5.5 years/903 primary endpoints on the grounds that those on the beta-blocker–based regimen had significantly higher mortality and worse outcomes on a number of secondary endpoints. Although there were fewer primary endpoint events in the amlodipine-based treatment group (429 vs. 474 in the atenolol-based treatment group), this difference failed to reach statistical significance ($p = 0.1$). Significantly fewer of the individuals in the amlodipine-based regimen experienced strokes (327 vs. 422 in the atenolol-based treatment group; HR, 0.77;

Table 12.3 ASCOT–BPLA (Anglo-Scandinavian Cardiac Outcomes Trial- Blood Pressure Lowering Arm).

Disease focus	Hypertension
Main aim	To assess and compare the impact of amlodopine-based vs. atenolol-based antihypertensive regimens on non-fatal myocardial infarction and fatal coronary heart disease in hypertensive patients
Study design	Prospective, randomized, open, blinded endpoint trial with 2 x 2 factorial design
Study population	19257 patients with hypertension, aged 40–79 years (mean 63 years), 77% were male, with either untreated hypertension with BP ≥160/100 mmHg or treated hypertension with BP ≥140/90, with at least three of 11 specified cardiovascular disease risk factors
Intervention	Amlodopine (+ perindopril, if required) vs. atenolol (+ bendroflumethiazide, if required) titrated to achieve BP <140/90 mmHg
Results	Compared to patients on the atenolol-based regimen, fewer on the amlodopine regimen had a primary endpoint, although this was not significant (429 vs. 422; HR, 0.90; 95% CI, 0.79–1.02; p = 0.1052). However, there were significantly fewer strokes, total cardiovascular events and procedures, and all-cause mortality noted in the amlodopine-based treatment group

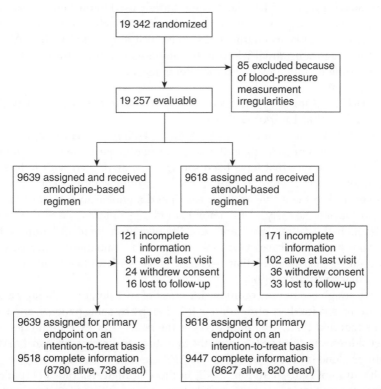

Figure 12.2 ASCOT–BPLA consort chart. MI, myocardial infarction. (Modified from Dahlöf B *et al.* [95], with permission.)

95% CI, 0.66–0.89; p < 0.0005), total cardiovascular events plus procedures (HR, 0.84; 95% CI, 0.78–0.90; p < 0.0001), all-cause mortality (HR, 0.89; 95% CI, 0.81–0.99; p = 0.025), and new-onset diabetes (HR, 0.70; 95% CI, 0.63–0.78; p < 0.0001).

By the end of the trial very few participants were taking single-agent antihypertensive agent therapy (with only 15% and 9% taking amlodipine and atenolol monotherapy, respectively). Only 53% of patients attained target blood pressure levels (32% of those with diabetes, 60% of those without diabetes). Given the relatively modest differences in blood pressure lowering between the two treatment arms, the authors suggested that the effects of the amlodipine-based regimen on major cardiovascular events and diabetes might not be entirely attributable to better control of blood pressure.

What were the implications for clinical practice? In line with most event-driven CVD prevention trials, ASCOT had enrolled relatively high-risk patients to ensure that the duration and cost of the trial was maintained at a feasible level. However, as the ASCOT participants were recruited from general practices across Scandinavia and the UK, they were likely to be representative of the high-risk population seen clinically in these regions. ASCOT confirmed the suggestion from other studies that beta-blockers may not be the most appropriate first-line therapeutic option in uncomplicated hypertension, and might be best targeted at patients with certain comorbidities (e.g., heart failure, previous MI). The dose of diuretic used in the beta-blocker arm of the study (≤2.5 mg) was much lower than that which had previously been shown to be effective in a number of studies, including ALLHAT; thus ASCOT was not able to substantially inform the discussion around utility of diuretics as a first-line therapeutic option for hypertension.

ONTARGET (Ongoing Telmisartan Alone and in Combination with Ramipril Global Endpoint Trial)

Angiotensin II, the major effector hormone within the renin–angiotensin–aldosterone system (RAAS), is the target of two major classes of antihypertensive therapeutics that have been shown to be associated with reductions in cardiovascular events [97]; ACE-inhibitors (which inhibit conversion of angiotensin I to the active angiotensin II) and angiotensin receptor blockers (ARBs). During the early 1990s, a number of large, randomized trials of ACE-inhibitors had noted a significant mortality benefit in the heart failure setting [98], and the HOPE (Heart Outcomes Prevention Evaluation) study was one of a number that noted similar benefit in those without heart failure or left ventricular dysfunction [97].

A dry cough is a not uncommon side effect of ACE-inhibitor therapy and is given as reason for discontinuation of this therapy by some patients, and it has been suggested that ARBs might confer the benefits of ACE-inhibitors with fewer side effects. ONTARGET was the first study to directly compare an ACE-inhibitor alone (ramipril 10 mg) to an ARB alone (telmisartan 80 mg) or the combination of ACE-inhibitor + ARB, in those at high risk of CVD (patients who had vascular disease or high-risk diabetes, but without heart failure).

Table 12.4 ONTARGET (Ongoing Telmisartan Alone and in Combination with Ramipril Global Endpoint Trial).

Disease focus	Hypertension
Main aim	To determine if the combination of the ARB temisartan and ACE-inhibitor ramipril is more effective in reducing mortality and morbidity from cardiovascular disease than either agent alone (primary outcome a composite of cardiovascular death, MI, stroke or hospitalization for heart failure)
Study design	Randomized, double-blinded, parallel group trial design
Study population	25620 patients with coronary, peripheral vascular or cerebrovascular disease, or diabetes with end-organ damage. Mean age 66 years, 73% were male
Intervention	Telmisartan (80mg/day), ramipril (5–10mg/day), or both
Results	Primary outcome occurred in 1412 (16.5%) in the ramipril group vs. 1423 (16.7%) in the telmisartan group vs. 1386 (16.3%) in the combination therapy group, with no significant differences between the treatment arms

ONTARGET was a double-blinded, randomized trial which enrolled a total of 25620 participants each assigned to one of the three study arms with a median follow-up of 56 months (Table 12.4). The primary outcome measure was a composite of death from cardiovascular causes, MI, stroke or hospitalization for heart failure. The primary objectives were to determine if the combination of telmisartan + ramipril was more effective than ramipril alone, and also to determine whether telmisartan alone was at least as effective (i.e. not inferior) to ramipril alone. There was no difference in primary outcomes between the ramipril alone and telmisartan alone arms of the study, and no additional benefit provided by the combination therapy group. Compared with ramipril alone, telmisartan alone was associated with lower rates of cough and angioedema, but higher rates of hypotensive symptoms. The combination of ACE-inhibitor + ARB was associated with more adverse events; with an increased risk of hypotensive symptoms (4.8% vs 1.7%; $p < 0.001$) and renal dysfunction (13.5% vs 10.2%; $p < 0.001$) compared to ramipril alone.

The results of ONTARGET provided evidence for clinicians that either ACE-inhibitors or ARBs can be used to reduce risk of CVD mortality and morbidity in patients at high risk of CVD (but without heart failure), and that dual RAAS blockade is unlikely to add benefit (despite providing additional lowering of blood pressure). Average blood pressure upon randomization into ONTARGET was less than 140/80mmHg, so the patients, whilst high risk, were considered to have BP in the "normal" range and most were on other cardioprotective agents such as statins or aspirin. The results of this study have prompted much debate, and there remain questions as to whether or not the specific agents used in ONTARGET are representative of their "class", with the suggestion that the pharmacokinetics of telmisartan might afford it advantages over other ARBs in blood pressure control [99].

High cholesterol

During the middle of the last century, epidemiological studies such as Framingham and the Seven Countries Study identified elevated circulating cholesterol levels as a risk factor for CVD, and in the mid-1980s MRFIT estimated that close to half of CHD deaths could be attributed to cholesterol levels above 4.65 mmol/L. During the 1970s and 1980s the Nobel laureates Goldstein and Brown [100] made the key discoveries of the pathways governing cholesterol homeostasis through feedback regulation of cellular cholesterol synthesis by the enzyme HMG-CoA reductase and uptake of LDL cholesterol into cells via the LDL receptor. This lead to the development of a class of cholesterol-lowering drugs; HMG-CoA reductase inhibitors or "statins," which were both powerful and relatively well tolerated. Until that time, whether lowering of elevated cholesterol conferred any benefit in those at greatest risk of a cardiovascular event had yet to be conclusively established.

The advent of the statin era of cholesterol-lowering therapy was heralded by the outcomes of 4S (Scandinavian Simvastatin Survival Study) [101]. 4S was designed to examine whether cholesterol lowering with statin therapy could prolong life in patients with existing CVD. This randomized, placebo-controlled trial of simvastatin (20–40 mg) in 4444 patients with CHD found a 30% reduction in all-cause mortality (RR, 0.70; 95% CI, 0.58–0.85; p = 0.0003) and a 34% reduction in risk of a major cardiovascular event (RR, 0.66; 95% CI, 0.59–0.75; p < 0.00001) in the simvastatin-treated group over the 5-year study period. However, there remained limited evidence of the effectiveness of statins in other high risk patients, in particular the elderly, those with diabetes but not overt CVD, and those who were considered high risk but had average or even below-average levels of LDL cholesterol. Such issues were addressed by the Heart Protection Study (HPS) which reported its outcomes in 2002 [102].

HPS (Heart Protection Study)

HPS was a prospective, randomized, placebo-controlled trial of 40 mg of simvastatin conducted across 69 hospitals in the UK (Table 12.5) [102]. The study population comprised 20 536 adults aged 40–80 years and considered to be at increased risk of death from coronary disease due to: history of coronary disease, occlusive disease of non-coronary arteries, diabetes, or treated hypertension. HPS was designed to examine whether statins conferred benefit even in those for whom cholesterol-lowering therapy might not have traditionally been indicated.

Over the 5-year study, the average compliance in the statin group was 85%, and in the placebo group the average "non-study" use of statins was 17%. The intention-to-treat analyses compared all the statin-allocated participants against all placebo-allocated participants, regardless of their compliance with

Table 12.5 HPS (Medical Research Council and British Heart Foundation Heart Protection Study)

Disease focus	Coronary heart disease
Main aim	To assess the effect of cholesterol-lowering therapy and antioxidant vitamin supplementation on cardiovascular disease mortality and major morbidity
Study design	Randomized, placebo-controlled trial with a 2 × 2 factorial design
Study population	20536 patients at increased risk of coronary heart disease due to previous myocardial infarction (MI), occlusive coronary or non-coronary artery disease, diabetes or treated hypertension, with total cholesterol ≥3.5mmol/L. Aged 40–80 years, 75% were male.
Intervention	Simvastatin (40mg/day) vs. placebo
Results	Simvastatin treatment significantly reduced all-cause mortality (12.9% vs. 14.7% in the placebo group; p = 0.0003), and was also associated with significantly lower rates of coronary death, first MI, stroke, and coronary and non-coronary revascularization

the study treatment. Thus, these analyses effectively assessed the impact of about two-thirds of the active treatment group taking a statin. Despite this, HPS noted a 13% reduction in all-cause mortality in those allocated to the simvastatin arm of the study (95% CI, 0.81–0.94; p = 0.0003). There were also significant reductions in rates of a number of the secondary study endpoints, including non-fatal MI, stroke, and revascularization (Figure 12.3).

In contrast to a combined analysis of three major pravastatin trials, which found no significant CHD benefit of statins in those with initial LDL-cholesterol levels below 3.2mmol/L (125mg/dL) [103], HPS showed clear differences in rates of major vascular events in those with pretreatment LDL of less than 3.00mmol/L (116mg/dL) (17.6% in the simvastatin allocated arm vs 22.2% in the placebo-allocated arm; P < 0.0001). This cardioprotective benefit was still evident in those with pretreatment LDL levels below 2.6mmol/L (100mg/dL). The results of HPS suggested that reducing LDL-cholesterol in high-risk patients by about 1mmol/L could reduce risk of a major vascular event by about one-quarter, regardless of whether the pretreatment LDL was 4mmol/L or 3mmol/L. This had tremendous implications for clinical practice as a number of guidelines of the time advocated LDL-cholesterol targets of 3.0mmol/L [104].

Statins: cardioprotection beyond cholesterol?

It has been suggested that 20% of cardiovascular events occur in those without conventional risk factors [105]. The inflammatory biomarker CRP has been heralded as a marker with some promise as a predictor of CVD risk. Building upon the laboratory studies suggesting that statins might have

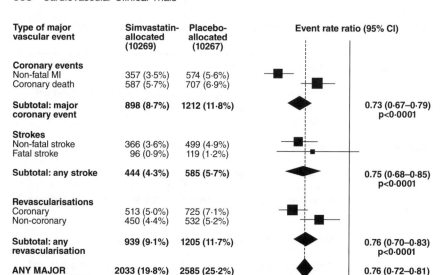

Type of major vascular event	Simvastatin-allocated (10269)	Placebo-allocated (10267)	Event rate ratio (95% CI)
Coronary events			
Non-fatal MI	357 (3·5%)	574 (5·6%)	
Coronary death	587 (5·7%)	707 (6·9%)	
Subtotal: major coronary event	**898 (8·7%)**	**1212 (11·8%)**	0.73 (0·67–0·79) p<0·0001
Strokes			
Non-fatal stroke	366 (3·6%)	499 (4·9%)	
Fatal stroke	96 (0·9%)	119 (1·2%)	
Subtotal: any stroke	**444 (4·3%)**	**585 (5·7%)**	0.75 (0·68–0·85) p<0·0001
Revascularisations			
Coronary	513 (5·0%)	725 (7·1%)	
Non-coronary	450 (4·4%)	532 (5·2%)	
Subtotal: any revascularisation	**939 (9·1%)**	**1205 (11·7%)**	0.76 (0·70–0·83) p<0·0001
ANY MAJOR VASCULAR EVENT	**2033 (19·8%)**	**2585 (25·2%)**	0.76 (0·72–0·81) p<0·0001

0·4   0·6   0·8   1·0   1·2   1·4

Simvastatin better   Placebo better

Figure 12.3 Effects of simvastatin allocation on first major coronary event, stroke, and revascularization (defined prospectively as "major vascular events"). (Modified from *Lancet* [101], with permission.)

anti-inflammatory effects [106], the PRINCE study noted that treatment with 40 mg/day of pravastatin over a 6-month period resulted in ~15% reductions in CRP, largely independent of reductions in LDL-cholesterol [107]. To study whether or not statin therapy is an effective primary prevention strategy in those with high CRP but levels of LDL cholesterol below the current treatment targets was the rationale for the JUPITER study, which reported outcomes in 2008 [108].

JUPITER (Justification for the Use of Statins in Primary Prevention: an Intervention Trial Evaluating Rosuvastatin)

The JUPITER primary CVD prevention study was a randomized, double-blind, placebo-controlled, multicenter trial (Table 12.6). JUPITER was designed to examine whether treatment with rosuvastatin in those with LDL-cholesterol below 130 mg/dL (3.4 mmol/L) but elevated CRP (>2 mg/L) was able to reduce the primary endpoint of a first major cardiovascular event (defined as either cardiovascular death, MI, stroke, hospitalization for unstable angina or arterial revascularization) over a 5-year period. An event-driven study, it planned to continue until 520 confirmed endpoints had been documented. In total 17802 participants were enrolled in the study, and upon the early termination of the study a total of 393 primary endpoints had accrued in a median of 1.9 years follow-up. The major outcome of the study was a 44% reduction

Table 12.6 JUPITER (Justification for the Use of Statins in Prevention: an Intervention Trial Evaluating Rosuvastatin)

Disease focus	Cardiovascular disease
Main aim	To determine whether rosuvastatin treatment in those with elevated high-sensitivity C-reactive protein, but without hyperlipidemia, will reduce the combined endpoint of MI, stroke, arterial revascularization, hospitalization for unstable angina or death from cardiovascular causes
Study design	Randomized, double-blinded, placebo-controlled trial
Study population	17 802 apparently healthy men and women with LDL <3.4 mmol/L and hs-CRP >2.0 mg/dL. Median age 60 years, 62% were male
Intervention	Rosuvastatin (20 mg/day) vs. placebo
Results	Rosuvastatin treatment significantly reduced primary endpoint occurrence (HR, 0.56; 95% CI 0.46–0.69; p < 0.00001)

in all vascular events (95% CI, 0.46–0.69; p < 0.00001), with a 20% reduction in all-cause mortality also seen (95% CI, 0.67–0.97; p = 0.02). As expected, treatment with rosuvastatin resulted in a 50% reduction in LDL and 37% reduction in CRP.

The results of the JUPITER study have promoted much debate. There are a number of important caveats to consider in evaluation of the JUPITER findings and their implication for clinical practice:

• There were significantly higher rates of diabetes and higher HbA1c levels in the rosuvastatin-treated group. Whether in the long-term the effects on diabetes and HbA1c might have changed the benefit–risk balance of the intervention cannot be fully evaluated due to truncation of the planned JUPITER study follow-up.

• The trial was stopped very early (median <2 years of follow-up) by the independent data safety and monitoring board. A meta-analysis of stopping randomized trials early has recently suggested that trials that stop early as a result of beneficial treatment effects may systematically overestimate the treatment effect that has prompted the early termination [109].

• There was no "low" or "normal" CRP group, so JUPITER cannot conclusively establish whether it was the effect of statins on CRP driving the cardiovascular risk reduction, or whether statins in fact benefit everyone with an LDL below 3.4 mmol/L. The pleiotropic effects of statins extend beyond reductions in CRP, with effects on other inflammatory markers (e.g., VCAM) and antioxidant activity.

• As can be seen from the cost-effectiveness analysis shown in Table 12.1, prescribing statins to those with low LDL levels has previously not been considered to be cost-effective. An analysis of the impact of JUPITER on the

US population suggests that an additional 11 million middle-aged to elderly adults would qualify for statin therapy if JUPITER criteria were applied [110].
• Recent studies suggest that while CRP levels may show associations with risk of CVD and all-cause mortality, these associations are not causal and the size of the associations is modest [52,111].

What are the clinical implications? In light of the JUPITER findings, the US FDA extended the approval of rosuvastatin to those with normal LDL-cholesterol levels but high hs-CRP in combination with one other CVD risk factor (e.g., smoking, low HDL-cholesterol, high blood pressure). However, there remain significant questions surrounding the cost-effectiveness of prescribing according to JUPITER criteria, and it would be reasonable to suggest that in a number of cases efforts to address other risk factors (such as smoking cessation, blood pressure lowering, physical activity, and diet) might confer a cardioprotective benefit of similar magnitude to that provided by rosuvastatin.

In recent years, professional societies that develop evidence-based clinical guidelines have ensured these undergo regular updates to include new large-scale, well-controlled clinical trials and meta-analyses. Given the aging populations in many nations and the predicted epidemics of diabetes and obesity, reduction of CVD burden will remain a major economic and social issue, with a priority to develop globally relevant and cost-effective strategies for CVD prevention. We look forward with interest to robust evaluation of new biomarkers, including genomic markers of risk, to further understand the relationships between genes, biomarkers, and the environment in the pathophysiology of CVD.

Update

"Hot-topics" in CVD prevention include the role of aspirin in primary prevention of CVD, the comparative effectiveness of the polypill in CVD prevention, and the evolution of new blood pressure-lowering therapies such as direct renin inhibitors. The low-cost and widely-accessible drug aspirin, is known to reduce incidence of non-fatal MI, but does increase risk of bleeding, and there has been some controversy surrounding the relative risk–benefit ratio in primary CVD prevention. In light of the aging populations being seen across the globe, there remains a lack of quality trial evidence for aspirin in the elderly, which will hopefully be addressed by the outcomes of the ASPREE (Aspirin in Reducing Events in the Elderly) placebo-controlled trial in the healthy elderly [112].

The polypill (a single tablet combination of aspirin, ACE-inhibitor, thiazide diuretic, and statin, for primary prevention of CVD) has shown promise in reducing CVD risk factors in short-to-medium term studies. Ongoing trials in Australia and India (amongst others) will inform our understanding of the effectiveness of the polypill in reducing CVD events.

The role of direct renin inhibitors in reducing risk of CVD remains unresolved.

References

1. Lloyd-Jones D, Adams RJ, Brown TM, *et al*. Heart disease and stroke statistics–2010 update: A report from the American Heart Association. *Circulation* 2010;121: e46–e215.
2. Yusuf S, Reddy S, Ounpuu S, Anand S. Global burden of cardiovascular diseases: Part i: General considerations, the epidemiologic transition, risk factors, and impact of urbanization. *Circulation* 2001;104:2746–2753.
3. Mackay J, Mensah GA. Atlas of heart disease and stroke. WHO, Editor 2004, World Health Organisation, Geneva.
4. Allender S, Peto V, Scarborough P, Kaur A, Rayner M. *Coronary Heart Disease Statistics*. London: British Heart Foundation, 2008.
5. Kher N, Marsh JD. Pathobiology of atherosclerosis–a brief review. *Semin Thromb Hemost* 2004;30:665–672.
6. Chambless LE, Heiss G, Folsom AR, *et al*. Association of coronary heart disease incidence with carotid arterial wall thickness and major risk factors: The atherosclerosis risk in communities (aric) study, 1987-1993. *Am J Epidemiol* 1997;146:483–494.
7. Vlachopoulos C, Aznaouridis K, Stefanadis C. Prediction of cardiovascular events and all-cause mortality with arterial stiffness: A systematic review and meta-analysis. *J Am Coll Cardiol* 2010;55:1318–1327.
8. Graham I, Atar D, Borch-Johnsen K, *et al*. European guidelines on cardiovascular disease prevention in clinical practice: Full text. Fourth joint task force of the European Society of Cardiology and other societies on cardiovascular disease prevention in clinical practice (constituted by representatives of nine societies and by invited experts). *Eur J Cardiovasc Prev Rehabil* 2007;14 (Suppl 2):S1–113.
9. Dawber TR. *The Framingham Study*. Cambridge, Massachusetts: Harvard University Press, 1980.
10. Verschuren WM, Jacobs DR, Bloemberg BP, *et al*. Serum total cholesterol and long-term coronary heart disease mortality in different cultures. Twenty-five-year follow-up of the seven countries study. *JAMA* 1995;274:131–136.
11. Menotti A, Keys A, Kromhout D, Blackburn H, Aravanis C, Bloemberg B, Buzina R, Dontas A, Fidanza F, Giampaoli S, et al. Inter-cohort differences in coronary heart disease mortality in the 25-year follow-up of the seven countries study. *Eur J Epidemiol* 1993;9:527–536.
12. Tunstall Pedoe H. *WHO MONICA Project Monograph*. Geneva, World Health Organization, 2003.
13. MRFIT Research Group. Multiple risk factor intervention trial. Risk factor changes and mortality results. Multiple risk factor intervention trial research group. *JAMA* 1982; 248:1465–1477.
14. Stamler J, Wentworth D, Neaton JD. Is relationship between serum cholesterol and risk of premature death from coronary heart disease continuous and graded? Findings in 356,222 primary screenees of the multiple risk factor intervention trial (mrfit). *JAMA* 1986;256:2823–2828.
15. EUROASPIRE. A European Society of Cardiology survey of secondary prevention of coronary heart disease: Principal results. EUROASPIRE Study Group. European action on secondary prevention through intervention to reduce events. *Eur Heart J* 1997;18: 1569–1582.
16. Bhatt DL, Steg PG, Ohman EM, *et al*. International prevalence, recognition, and treatment of cardiovascular risk factors in outpatients with atherothrombosis. *JAMA* 2006;295:180–189.

17. Yusuf S, Hawken S, Ounpuu S, *et al.* Effect of potentially modifiable risk factors associated with myocardial infarction in 52 countries (the interheart study): Case-control study. *Lancet* 2004;364:937–952.

18. Kearney PM, Blackwell L, Collins R, *et al.* Efficacy of cholesterol-lowering therapy in 18,686 people with diabetes in 14 randomised trials of statins: A meta-analysis. *Lancet* 2008;371:117–125.

19. Gordon DJ, Probstfield JL, Garrison RJ, *et al.* High-density lipoprotein cholesterol and cardiovascular disease. Four prospective american studies. *Circulation* 1989;79:8–15.

20. Erqou S, Kaptoge S, Perry PL, *et al.* Lipoprotein(a) concentration and the risk of coronary heart disease, stroke, and nonvascular mortality. *JAMA* 2009;302:412–423.

21. Clarke R, Peden JF, Hopewell JC, *et al.* Genetic variants associated with lp(a) lipoprotein level and coronary disease. *N Engl J Med* 2009;361:2518–2528.

22. Di Angelantonio E, Sarwar N, Perry P, *et al.* Major lipids, apolipoproteins, and risk of vascular disease. *JAMA* 2009;302:1993–2000.

23. Ingelsson E, Schaefer EJ, Contois JH, *et al.* Clinical utility of different lipid measures for prediction of coronary heart disease in men and women. *JAMA* 2007;298:776–785.

24. Expert Panel on Detection, Evaluation, and Treatment of High Blood Cholesterol in Adults, executive summary of the third report of the National Cholesterol Education Program (NCEP) expert panel on detection, evaluation, and treatment of high blood cholesterol in adults (adult treatment panel III). *JAMA* 2001;285:2486–2497.

25. Lawes CM, Vander Hoorn S, Rodgers A. Global burden of blood-pressure-related disease, 2001. *Lancet* 2008;371:1513–1518.

26. Chobanian AV, Bakris GL, Black HR, *et al.* The seventh report of the joint national committee on prevention, detection, evaluation, and treatment of high blood pressure: The JNC7 report. *JAMA* 2003;289:2560–2572.

27. Lewington S, Clarke R, Qizilbash N, Peto R, Collins R. Age-specific relevance of usual blood pressure to vascular mortality: A meta-analysis of individual data for one million adults in 61 prospective studies. *Lancet* 2002;360:1903–1913.

28. Law MR, Morris JK, Wald NJ. Use of blood pressure lowering drugs in the prevention of cardiovascular disease: Meta-analysis of 147 randomised trials in the context of expectations from prospective epidemiological studies. *BMJ* 2009;338:b1665.

29. Owen AJ, Retegan C, Rockell M, Jennings G, Reid CM. Inertia or inaction? Blood pressure management and cardiovascular risk in diabetes. *Clin Exp Pharmacol Physiol* 2009; 36:643–647.

30. Teo KK, Ounpuu S, Hawken S, *et al.* Tobacco use and risk of myocardial infarction in 52 countries in the interheart study: A case-control study. *Lancet* 2006;368:647–658.

31. Critchley JA, Capewell S. Mortality risk reduction associated with smoking cessation in patients with coronary heart disease: A systematic review. *JAMA* 2003;290:86–97.

32. Kahn R, Robertson RM, Smith R, Eddy D. The impact of prevention on reducing the burden of cardiovascular disease. *Diabetes Care* 2008;31:1686–1696.

33. Wild S, Roglic G, Green A, Sicree R, King H. Global prevalence of diabetes: Estimates for the year 2000 and projections for 2030. *Diabetes Care* 2004;27:1047–1053.

34. Huxley R, Barzi F, Woodward M. Excess risk of fatal coronary heart disease associated with diabetes in men and women: Meta-analysis of 37 prospective cohort studies. *BMJ* 2006;332:73–78.

35. Ceriello A, Assaloni R, Da Ros R, *et al.* Effect of atorvastatin and irbesartan, alone and in combination, on postprandial endothelial dysfunction, oxidative stress, and inflammation in type 2 diabetic patients. *Circulation* 2005;111:2518–2524.

36. Cavalot F, Petrelli A, Traversa M, *et al.* Postprandial blood glucose is a stronger predictor of cardiovascular events than fasting blood glucose in type 2 diabetes mellitus,

particularly in women: Lessons from the san luigi gonzaga diabetes study. *J Clin Endocrinol Metab* 2006;91:813–819.

37. Alberti KG, Eckel RH, Grundy SM, *et al*. Harmonizing the metabolic syndrome: A joint interim statement of the International Diabetes Federation task force on epidemiology and prevention; National Heart, Lung, and Blood Institute; American Heart Association; World Heart Federation; International Atherosclerosis Society; and International Association for the Study of Obesity. *Circulation* 2009;120:1640–1645.

38. Church TS, Thompson AM, Katzmarzyk PT, *et al*. Metabolic syndrome and diabetes, alone and in combination, as predictors of cardiovascular disease mortality among men. *Diabetes Care* 2009;32:1289–1294.

39. Mente A, Yusuf S, Islam S, *et al*. Metabolic syndrome and risk of acute myocardial infarction a case-control study of 26,903 subjects from 52 countries. *J Am Coll Cardiol* 2010;55:2390–2398.

40. WHO. Global database on body mass index. [cited 2010 May]; available from: www.who.int

41. Despres JP, Lemieux I, Bergeron J, *et al*. Abdominal obesity and the metabolic syndrome: Contribution to global cardiometabolic risk. *Arterioscler Thromb Vasc Biol* 2008;28: 1039–1049.

42. Poirier P, Giles TD, Bray GA, *et al*. Obesity and cardiovascular disease: Pathophysiology, evaluation, and effect of weight loss: An update of the 1997 American Heart Association scientific statement on obesity and heart disease from the Obesity Committee of the Council on Nutrition, Physical Activity, and Metabolism. *Circulation* 2006;113:898–918.

43. Deans KA, Bezlyak V, Ford I, *et al*. Differences in atherosclerosis according to area level socioeconomic deprivation: Cross sectional, population based study. *BMJ* 2009;339:b4170.

44. Lloyd-Jones DM, Larson MG, Beiser A, Levy D. Lifetime risk of developing coronary heart disease. *Lancet* 1999;353:89–92.

45. Friedlander Y, Kark JD, Stein Y. Family history of myocardial infarction as an independent risk factor for coronary heart disease. *Br Heart J* 1985;53:382–387

46. Cattin L, Fisicaro M, Tonizzo M, *et al*. Polymorphism of the apolipoprotein e gene and early carotid atherosclerosis defined by ultrasonography in asymptomatic adults. *Arterioscler Thromb Vasc Biol.* 1997;17:91–94

47. Musunuru K, Kathiresan S. Genetics of coronary artery disease. *Annu Rev Genomics Hum Genet.* 2010;11:91–108

48. Preuss M, Konig IR, Thompson JR, *et al*. Design of the coronary artery disease genome-wide replication and meta-analysis (CARDIOGRAM) study: A genome-wide association meta-analysis involving more than 22 000 cases and 60 000 controls. *Circ Cardiovasc Genet* 2010;3:475–483.

49. Boekholdt SM, Hack CE, Sandhu MS, *et al*. C-reactive protein levels and coronary artery disease incidence and mortality in apparently healthy men and women: The epic-norfolk prospective population study 1993-2003. *Atherosclerosis* 2006;187:415–422.

50. Ridker PM, Rifai N, Rose L, Buring JE, Cook NR. Comparison of C-reactive protein and low-density lipoprotein cholesterol levels in the prediction of first cardiovascular events. *N Engl J Med* 2002;347:1557–1565.

51. Hemingway H, Philipson P, Chen R, *et al*. Evaluating the quality of research into a single prognostic biomarker: A systematic review and meta-analysis of 83 studies of C-reactive protein in stable coronary artery disease. *PLoS Med* 2010;7:e1000286.

52. Kaptoge S, Di Angelantonio E, Lowe G, *et al*. C-reactive protein concentration and risk of coronary heart disease, stroke, and mortality: An individual participant meta-analysis. *Lancet* 2010;375:132–140.

53. Thompson A, Gao P, Orfei L, et al. Lipoprotein-associated phospholipase a(2) and risk of coronary disease, stroke, and mortality: Collaborative analysis of 32 prospective studies. *Lancet* 2010;375:1536–1544.

54. Porapakkham P, Porapakkham P, Zimmet H, Billah B, Krum H. B-type natriuretic peptide-guided heart failure therapy: A meta-analysis. *Arch Intern Med* 2010;170: 507–514.

55. Di Angelantonio E, Chowdhury R, Sarwar N, et al. B-type natriuretic peptides and cardiovascular risk: Systematic review and meta-analysis of 40 prospective studies. *Circulation* 2009;120:2177–2187.

56. Wald DS, Law M, Morris JK. Homocysteine and cardiovascular disease: Evidence on causality from a meta-analysis. *BMJ* 2002;325:1202.

57. Anderson KM, Odell PM, Wilson PW, Kannel WB. Cardiovascular disease risk profiles. *Am Heart J* 1991;121:293–298.

58. D'Agostino RB, Sr, Vasan RS, Pencina MJ, et al. General cardiovascular risk profile for use in primary care: The framingham heart study. *Circulation* 2008;117:743–753.

59. Hense HW, Schulte H, Lowel H, Assmann G, Keil U. Framingham risk function overestimates risk of coronary heart disease in men and women from germany–results from the MONICA Augsburg and the PROCAM cohorts. *Eur Heart J* 2003;24:937–945.

60. Wang Z, Hoy WE. Is the Framingham coronary heart disease absolute risk function applicable to Aboriginal people? *Med J Aust* 2005;182:66–69.

61. Kshirsagar AV, Carpenter M, Bang H, Wyatt SB, Colindres RE. Blood pressure usually considered normal is associated with an elevated risk of cardiovascular disease. *Am J Med* 2006;119:133–141.

62. Coleman RL, Stevens RJ, Retnakaran R, Holman RR. Framingham, SCORE, and DECODE risk equations do not provide reliable cardiovascular risk estimates in type 2 diabetes. *Diabetes Care* 2007;30:1292–1293.

63. Wilson PW, Bozeman SR, Burton TM, Hoaglin DC, Ben-Joseph R, Pashos CL. Prediction of first events of coronary heart disease and stroke with consideration of adiposity. *Circulation* 2008;118:124–130.

64. de Zeeuw D, Bakker SJ. Does the metabolic syndrome add to the diagnosis and treatment of cardiovascular disease? *Nat Clin Pract Cardiovasc Med* 2008;5 (Suppl 1): S10–14.

65. Redberg RF, Benjamin EJ, Bittner V, et al. AHA/ACCF 2009 performance measures for primary prevention of cardiovascular disease in adults. *Circulation* 2009;120: 1296–1336.

66. Sposito AC, Ramires JA, Jukema JW, et al. Physicians' attitudes and adherence to use of risk scores for primary prevention of cardiovascular disease: Cross-sectional survey in three world regions. *Curr Med Res Opin* 2009;25:1171–1178.

67. Chapman S, Freeman B. The cancer emperor's new clothes: Australia's historic legislation for plain tobacco packaging. *BMJ* 2010;340:c2436.

68. Wakefield MA, Durkin S, Spittal MJ, et al. Impact of tobacco control policies and mass media campaigns on monthly adult smoking prevalence. *Am J Public Health* 2008;98: 1443–1450.

69. Hopkins DP, Razi S, Leeks KD, Priya Kalra G, Chattopadhyay SK, Soler RE. Smokefree policies to reduce tobacco use. A systematic review. *Am J Prev Med* 2010;38:S275–289.

70. Meyers DG, Neuberger JS, He J. Cardiovascular effect of bans on smoking in public places: A systematic review and meta-analysis. *J Am Coll Cardiol* 2009;54:1249–1255.

71. Freeman B, Chapman S. British American Tobacco on Facebook: Undermining article 13 of the global World Health Organization framework convention on tobacco control. *Tob Control* 2010;19:e1–9.

72. Sacks FM, Svetkey LP, Vollmer WM, *et al.* Effects on blood pressure of reduced dietary sodium and the dietary approaches to stop hypertension (DASH) diet. DASH-sodium collaborative research group. *N Engl J Med* 2001;344:3–10.

73. Appel LJ, Sacks FM, Carey VJ, *et al.* Effects of protein, monounsaturated fat, and carbohydrate intake on blood pressure and serum lipids: Results of the OMNIHEART randomized trial. *JAMA* 2005;294:2455–2464.

74. Mozaffarian D, Katan MB, Ascherio A, Stampfer MJ, Willett WC. Trans fatty acids and cardiovascular disease. *N Engl J Med* 2006;354:1601–1613.

75. Angell SY, Silver LD, Goldstein GP, *et al.* Cholesterol control beyond the clinic: New York City's trans fat restriction. *Ann Intern Med* 2009;151:129–134.

76. Marchioli R, Levantesi G, Macchia A, *et al.* Antiarrhythmic mechanisms of n-3 PUFA and the results of the GISSI-Prevenzione trial. *J Membr Biol* 2005;206:117–128.

77. Kris-Etherton PM, Harris WS, Appel LJ. Fish consumption, fish oil, omega-3 fatty acids, and cardiovascular disease. *Circulation* 2002;106:2747–2757.

78. Marchioli R, Schweiger C, Tavazzi L, Valagussa F. Efficacy of n-3 polyunsaturated fatty acids after myocardial infarction: Results of GISSI-Prevenzione trial. Gruppo italiano per lo studio della sopravvivenza nell'infarto miocardico. *Lipids* 2001;36 (Suppl):S119–126.

79. Tavazzi L, Maggioni AP, Marchioli R, *et al.* Effect of n-3 polyunsaturated fatty acids in patients with chronic heart failure (the GISSI-HF trial): A randomised, double-blind, placebo-controlled trial. *Lancet* 2008;372:1223–1230.

80. Yokoyama M, Origasa H, Matsuzaki M, *et al.* Effects of eicosapentaenoic acid on major coronary events in hypercholesterolaemic patients (JELIS): A randomised open-label, blinded endpoint analysis. *Lancet* 2007;369:1090–1098.

81. Saravanan P, Davidson NC, Schmidt EB, Calder PC. Cardiovascular effects of marine omega-3 fatty acids. *Lancet* 2010;376:540–550.

82. He FJ, MacGregor GA. Effect of longer-term modest salt reduction on blood pressure. *Cochrane Database Syst Rev* 2004:CD004937.

83. Blair SN, Morris JN. Healthy hearts–and the universal benefits of being physically active: Physical activity and health. *Ann Epidemiol* 2009;19:253–256.

84. Franco M, Ordunez P, Caballero B, *et al.* Impact of energy intake, physical activity, and population-wide weight loss on cardiovascular disease and diabetes mortality in Cuba, 1980–2005. *Am J Epidemiol* 2007;166:1374–1380.

85. Djousse L, Lee IM, Buring JE, Gaziano JM. Alcohol consumption and risk of cardiovascular disease and death in women: Potential mediating mechanisms. *Circulation* 2009;120:237–244.

86. Mohler ER, Freis ED. Five-year survival of patients with malignant hypertension treated with antihypertensive agents. *Am Heart J* 1960;60:329–335.

87. Veterans Administration Cooperation Study on Antihypertensive Agents. Effects of treatment of morbidity in hypertension. Results in patients with diastolic blood pressure averaging 90 through 114mmhg. *JAMA* 1970;213:1143.

88. Hypertension Detection Follow-up Program Cooperative Group. Five-year findings of the hypertension detection and follow-up program: I. Reduction in mortality of persons with high blood pressure, including mild hypertension. *JAMA* 1979;242:2562–2571.

89. Australian National Blood Pressure Study Management Committee. The Australian therapeutic trial in mild hypertension. *Lancet* 1980;i:1261–1267.

90. Medical Research Council Working Party. Mrc trial of treatment of mild hypertension: Principal results. *BMJ* 1985;291:97–104.

91. Amery A, Brixko P, Clement D, *et al.* Mortality and morbidity results from the european working party on high blood pressure in the elderly trial. *Lancet.* 1985;1:1349–1354.

92. MacMahon S, Peto R, Cutler J. Blood pressure, stroke, and coronary heart disease. Part 1. Prolonged differences in blood pressure: Prospective observational studies corrected for the regression dilution bias. *Lancet* 1990;335:765–774.

93. Collins R, Peto R, MacMahon S. Blood pressure, stroke and coronary heart disease. Part 2: Short-term reductions in blood pressure: Overview of randomised drug trials in their epidemiological context. *Lancet* 1990;335:827–838.

94. Wilhelmsen L, Berglund G, Elmfeldt D, *et al.* Beta-blockers versus diuretics in hypertensive men: Main results from the happhy trial. *J Hypertension* 1987;5:561–572.

95. Wikstrand J, Warnold I, Olsson GA, *et al.* Primary prevention with metoprolol in patients with hypertension: Mortality results from the MAPHY study. *JAMA* 1988; 259:1976–1982.

96. Dahlöf B, Sever PS, Poulter NR, *et al.* Prevention of cardiovascular events with an antihypertensive regimen of amlodipine adding perindopril as required versus atenolol adding bendroflumethiazide as required, in the Anglo-Scandinavian Cardiac Outcomes Trial-Blood Pressure Lowering Arm (ASCOT-BPLA): A multicentre randomised controlled trial. *Lancet* 2005;366:895–906.

97. Turnbull F. Effects of different blood-pressure-lowering regimens on major cardiovascular events: Results of prospectively-designed overviews of randomised trials. *Lancet* 2003;362:1527–1535.

98. Garg R, Yusuf S. Overview of randomized trials of angiotensin-converting enzyme inhibitors on mortality and morbidity in patients with heart failure. Collaborative group on ACE inhibitor trials. *JAMA* 1995;273:1450–1456.

99. Burnier M. Telmisartan: A different angiotensin ii receptor blocker protecting a different population? *J Int Med Res* 2009;37:1662–1679.

100. Brown MS, Goldstein JL. A receptor-mediated pathway for cholesterol homeostasis. *Science* 1986;232:34–47.

101. Randomised trial of cholesterol lowering in 4444 patients with coronary heart disease: The Scandinavian Simvastatin Survival Study (4S). *Lancet* 1994;344:1383–1389.

102. MRC/BHF heart protection study of antioxidant vitamin supplementation in 20,536 high-risk individuals: A randomised placebo-controlled trial. *Lancet* 2002;360:23–33.

103. Sacks FM, Tonkin AM, Shepherd J, *et al.* Effect of pravastatin on coronary disease events in subgroups defined by coronary risk factors: The Prospective Pravastatin Pooling project. *Circulation* 2000;102:1893–1900.

104. Wood D, De Backer G, Faergeman O, Graham I, Mancia G, Pyorala K. Prevention of coronary heart disease in clinical practice: Recommendations of the second joint task force of european and other societies on coronary prevention. *Atherosclerosis* 1998; 140:199–270.

105. Khot UN, Khot MB, Bajzer CT, *et al.* Prevalence of conventional risk factors in patients with coronary heart disease. *JAMA* 2003;290:898–904.

106. Weber C, Erl W, Weber KS, Weber PC. HMG-CoA reductase inhibitors decrease CD11b expression and CD11b-dependent adhesion of monocytes to endothelium and reduce increased adhesiveness of monocytes isolated from patients with hypercholesterolemia. *J Am Coll Cardiol* 1997;30:1212–1217.

107. Albert MA, Danielson E, Rifai N, Ridker PM. Effect of statin therapy on c-reactive protein levels: The pravastatin inflammation/CRP evaluation (PRINCE): A randomized trial and cohort study. *JAMA* 2001;286:64–70.

108. Ridker PM, Danielson E, Fonseca FA, *et al.* Rosuvastatin to prevent vascular events in men and women with elevated c-reactive protein. *N Engl J Med* 2008;359:2195–2207.

109. Bassler D, Briel M, Montori VM, *et al.* Stopping randomized trials early for benefit and estimation of treatment effects: Systematic review and meta-regression analysis. *JAMA* 2010;303:1180–1187.

110. Spatz ES, Canavan ME, Desai MM. From here to Jupiter: Identifying new patients for statin therapy using data from the 1999-2004 National Health and Nutrition Examination Survey. *Circ Cardiovasc Qual Outcomes* 2009;2:41–48.

111. Zacho J, Tybjaerg-Hansen A, Nordestgaard BG. C-reactive protein and all-cause mortality–the Copenhagen City Heart Study. *Eur Heart J* 2010;31:1624–1632.

112. Nelson M, Reid C, Beilin L, *et al*. Rationale for a trial of low-dose aspirin for the primary prevention of major adverse cardiovascular events and vascular dementia in the elderly: Aspirin in Reducing Events in the Elderly (ASPREE). *Drugs Aging* 2003;20: 897–903.

Index

Page numbers in *italics* denote figures, those in **bold** denote tables.
The majority of clinical trials are referred to by their acronyms. Readers should
consult the list of abbreviations for a full explanation.

Cardiovascular Clinical Trials: Putting the Evidence into Practice, First Edition.
Edited by Marcus D. Flather, Deepak L. Bhatt, and Tobias Geisler.
© 2013 Blackwell Publishing Ltd. Published 2013 by Blackwell Publishing Ltd.

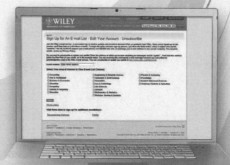
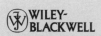